Craniosynostoses
Molecular Genetics, Principles of Diagnosis, and Treatment

Monographs in Human Genetics

Vol. 19

Series Editor

Michael Schmid Würzburg

Craniosynostoses

Molecular Genetics, Principles of Diagnosis, and Treatment

Volume Editors

Maximilian Muenke Bethesda, Md
Wolfram Kress Würzburg
Hartmut Collmann Würzburg
Benjamin D. Solomon Bethesda, Md

113 figures, 32 in color, and 17 tables, 2011

KARGER

Basel · Freiburg · Paris · London · New York · Bangalore · Bangkok · Shanghai · Singapore · Tokyo · Sydney

Maximilian Muenke
Medical Genetics Branch
National Human Genome Research Institute
National Institutes of Health
35 Convent Drive, MSC 3717
Building 35, Room 1B-203
Bethesda, MD 20892-3717 (USA)

Wolfram Kress
Institut für Humangenetik
Universität Würzburg
Biozentrum
Am Hubland
97074 Würzburg (Germany)

Hartmut Collmann
Neurochirurgische Klinik und Poliklinik der
Universität Würzburg
Abteilung Pädiatrische Neurochirurgie
Josef-Schneider-Straße 11
97080 Würzburg (Germany)

Benjamin D. Solomon
Medical Genetics Branch
National Human Genome Research Institute
National Institutes of Health
35 Convent Drive, Building 35
Bethesda, MD 20892-3717 (USA)

Library of Congress Cataloging-in-Publication Data

Craniosynostoses : molecular genetics, principles of diagnosis, and treatment / Volume Editors, Maximilian Muenke, Bethesda, Md, Wolfram Kress, Würzburg, Hartmut Collmann, Würzburg, Benjamin Solomon, Bethesda, Md.
p. ; cm. -- (Monographs in human genetics, ISSN 0077-0876 ; vol. 19)
Includes bibliographical references and indexes.
ISBN 978-3-8055-9594-0 (hard cover : alk. paper) -- ISBN 978-3-8055-9595-7 (e-ISBN)
1. Craniosynostoses. I. Muenke, Maximilian, editor. II. Kress, Wolfram, editor. III. Collmann, Hartmut, editor. IV. Solomon, Benjamin, editor. V. Series: Monographs in human genetics ; v. 19. 0077-0876
[DNLM: 1. Craniosynostoses--genetics. 2. Craniosynostoses--diagnosis. 3. Craniosynostoses--therapy. W1 MO567P v.19 2011 / WE 705]
RJ482.C73C69 2011
616'.042--dc22

2010051327

Bibliographic Indices. This publication is listed in bibliographic services, including Current Contents®.

www.karger.com
Printed in Switzerland on acid-free and non-aging paper (ISO 9706) by Reinhardt Druck, Basel
ISSN 0077–0876
ISBN 978–3–8055–9594–0
e-ISBN 978–3–8055–9595–7

Contents

VII **Editorial**
Schmid, M. (Würzburg)

VIII **Preface**
Muenke, M. (Bethesda, Md.); Kress, W.; Collmann, H. (Würzburg); Solomon, B.D. (Bethesda, Md.)

IX **Foreword**
Cohen Jr., M.M. (Halifax, N.S.)

Chapter 1
1 **Craniosynostosis: A Historical Overview**
Solomon, B.D. (Bethesda, Md.); Collmann, H.; Kress, W. (Würzburg); Muenke, M. (Bethesda, Md.)

Chapter 2
8 **Discovery of *MSX2* Mutation in Craniosynostosis: A Retrospective View**
Müller, U. (Gießen)

Chapter 3
13 **Regulation of Calvarial Bone Growth by Molecules Involved in the Craniosynostoses**
Benson, M.D.; Opperman, L.A. (Dallas, Tex.)

Chapter 4
28 **Signal Transduction Pathways and Their Impairment in Syndromic Craniosynostosis**
Connerney, J.J. (Boston, Mass.); Spicer, D.B. (Scarborough, Me.)

Chapter 5
45 **The Molecular Bases for FGF Receptor Activation in Craniosynostosis and Dwarfism Syndromes**
Beenken, A.; Mohammadi, M. (New York, N.Y.)

Chapter 6
58 **Recurrent Germline Mutations in the *FGFR2/3* Genes, High Mutation Frequency, Paternal Skewing and Age-Dependence**
Arnheim, N.; Calabrese, P. (Los Angeles, Calif.)

Chapter 7
67 **Apert, Crouzon, and Pfeiffer Syndromes**
Cohen Jr., M.M. (Halifax, N.S.)

Chapter 8
89 **Muenke Syndrome**
Solomon, B.D.; Muenke, M. (Bethesda, Md.)

Chapter 9
98 **Saethre-Chotzen Syndrome: Clinical and Molecular Genetic Aspects**
Kress, W.; Collmann, H. (Würzburg)

Chapter 10
107 **Craniofrontonasal Syndrome: Molecular Genetics, *EFNB1* Mutations and the Concept of Cellular Interference**
Wieland, I. (Magdeburg)

Chapter 11
119 **Uncommon Craniosynostosis Syndromes: A Review of Thirteen Conditions**
Raam, M.S. (Bethesda, Md./Chevy Chase, Md.); Muenke, M. (Bethesda, Md.)

Chapter 12
143 **Metopic Craniosynostosis Syndrome Due to Mutations in *GLI3***
McDonald-McGinn, D.M.; Feret, H.; Nah, H.-D.; Zackai, E.H. (Philadelphia, Pa.)

Chapter 13
152 **Craniosynostosis and Chromosomal Alterations**
Passos-Bueno, M.R.; Fanganiello, R.D.; Jehee, F.S. (São Paulo)

Chapter 14
165 **Nonsyndromic Craniosynostoses**
Collmann, H. (Würzburg); Solomon, B.D. (Bethesda, Md.); Schweitzer, T.; Kress, W. (Würzburg); Muenke, M. (Bethesda, Md.)

Chapter 15
177 **Molecular Genetic Testing of Patients with Craniosynostosis**
Hehr, U. (Regensburg)

Chapter 16
184 **Prenatal Sonographic Diagnosis of Craniosynostosis**
Schramm, T. (Munich)

Chapter 17
199 **Clinical Approach to Craniosynostosis**
Gripp, K.W. (Wilmington, Del.)

Chapter 18
216 **Imaging Studies and Neurosurgical Treatment**
Collmann, H.; Schweitzer, T.; Böhm, H. (Würzburg)

Chapter 19
232 **Maxillofacial Examination and Treatment**
Böhm, H.; Schweitzer, T.; Kübler, A. (Würzburg)

244 **Author Index**

245 **Subject Index**

Editorial

It is a great pleasure to introduce volume 19 of the book series *Monographs in Human Genetics* entitled 'Craniosynostoses: Molecular Genetics, Principles of Diagnosis and Treatment'. The initial idea for this book was born during a workshop on craniosynostoses held at the Academy of Human Genetics in Würzburg (Germany). Hartmut Collmann and Wolfram Kress brought together many seemingly diverse aspects of craniosynostoses, including clinical approaches, genetics, molecular mechanisms and, most importantly, treatments. As that course progressed, they realized how inspiring this subject was to their colleagues and medical students.

Craniosynostoses provide one of the best examples of today's molecular medicine, connecting simple anatomy and pathology with the structures of molecules that form the relevant signaling pathways. This book truly achieves the aim of *Monographs in Human Genetics* in dealing with the molecular causes of important hereditary diseases, their diagnosis, and their eventual prevention and clinical treatments. The volume has been organized in an exquisite way by Maximilian Muenke, Wolfram Kress, Hartmut Collmann and Benjamin Solomon. I express my gratitude to them for all the time they invested and the efforts they made in processing and refining all 19 chapters of this exciting book. The internationally renowned authors have contributed excellent manuscripts with astonishing illustrations. Their commitment has made the publication of this volume possible. The constant support of Thomas Karger with this ongoing and timely book series is highly appreciated.

Michael Schmid
Würzburg, November 2010

Preface

Craniosynostosis is a challenging and complex condition that has been recognized since the dawn of human history. Our understanding of the clinical manifestations of the disease process has advanced considerably in the last century, with molecular etiologies of many forms of syndromic craniosynostosis emerging in the last two decades. This increased knowledge has in turn enabled researchers and clinicians to probe normal and abnormal sutural biology from the atomic to the population-based level.

Just as important, and in parallel with the recent wave of basic biological understandings of craniosynostosis, advances in clinical diagnosis and treatment have been achieved, which include improvements in prenatal and postnatal imaging and craniofacial surgical techniques. These advances have been important for many reasons, and have allowed functional corrections and achievement of acceptable cosmesis in a broad range of patients.

Thus, given the growth of our knowledge base about craniosynostosis, the editors of this volume feel that the timing of publication comes at a very opportune moment. With the completion of the Human Genome Project and with the more recent availability of high-throughput investigative methods, we are now able to couple knowledge from previous accomplishments to newly emerging genomic technologies. We anticipate that through the critical mass of knowledge achieved to date, we can harness new tools of genome analysis in order to better understand craniosynostosis, both as relates to syndromic and nonsyndromic forms, as well as to normal cranial development more generally. This understanding is critical on many levels, but, most importantly perhaps, may be able to inform modalities of medical and surgical management to help improve the lives of affected patients and families.

We felt an international team of authors would be able to represent this difficult disorder in all its complexity; these are authors of diverse backgrounds, including clinicians and researchers whose careers are intimately involved in understanding the causes, effects, and treatments of craniosynostosis. Hence, this is a book intended for colleagues from a wide variety of disciplines. We hope this volume may prove useful whether a researcher is devoted to basic science at the bench or standing next to an operating table, and at every point in between.

The editors would like to thank all the authors who graciously contributed to this volume and who took the time to share their expertise and explain their most important discoveries to a wide audience. We also would like to extend our deepest gratitude to all the patients and families whom we have met over the course of our careers for their time, their generosity, and their compassionate spirits.

Maximilian Muenke, Wolfram Kress,
Hartmut Collmann, and Benjamin D. Solomon
Bethesda and Würzburg, August 2010

Foreword

The Editors – Max Muenke, Ben Solomon, Hartmut Collmann, and Wolfram Kress – have produced an epic-making volume on craniosynostosis that is a tour de force. They have done a remarkable job of selecting and coordinating many highly respected authorities in the field to write 19 chapters covering a wide range of subjects. It is also remarkable that these four editors have, in addition, written or been coauthors of six excellent articles, so that each one of them is magister mundi of craniosynostosis.

The rate of discovery in the molecular advances in craniosynostosis is very exciting, but it is equally true for the remarkable advances in craniofacial biology, imaging studies, neurosurgical treatment, craniofacial surgical treatment, and therapeutics and it means clearly that the future is now! However, we all know that advances in these fields will continue to flower tomorrow!

Chapter 1 by Ben Solomon, Hartmut Collmann, Wolfram Kress, and Max Muenke provides a historical review of craniosynostosis. The authors take us on a tour of ancient times, later historical developments, the advent of modern classifications, and the evolution of the molecular causes of craniosynostosis, and management. In Chapter 2, Ulrich Müller discusses Boston-type craniosynostosis and its molecular mutation on *MSX2* (p.Pro148His).

Some basic biological and molecular studies are grouped next. In Chapter 3 Douglas Benson and Lynne Opperman focus on the molecular regulation of calvarial bone growth by Ephrins, FGFs, and TGFβ. In Chapter 4, Jeanette Connerney and Douglas Spicer raise the question of how different signaling transduction pathways integrate with one another to regulate the formation and morphogenesis of craniofacial structures, which is only starting to be understood. In Chapter 5, Andrew Beenken and Moosa Mohammadi address the molecular mechanisms of FGFR activation in craniosynostosis and in some of the skeletal dysplasias, and discuss ligand-independent gain-of-function mutations, and also ligand-dependent gain-of-function mutations for those few disorders in the linker region between IgII and IgIII. In Chapter 6, Norman Arnheim and Peter Calabrese discuss recurrent germline mutations in *FGFR2* and *FGFR3,* which are paternally derived and age-dependent. The process is driven by a selective advantage of spermatogonial cells, as demonstrated in Apert syndrome.

Several chapters deal with various syndromes. Each of these is remarkably extensive and very thorough, analyzing both clinical and molecular aspects of the disorders. I have dealt with Apert syndrome, Crouzon syndrome, and Pfeiffer syndrome in Chapter 7. Ben Solomon and Max Muenke have analyzed the condition named after Max, namely Muenke syndrome in Chapter 8. Wolfram Kress and Hartmut Collmann have Saethre-Chotzen syndrome as their subject in Chapter 9. Ilse Wieland writes about craniofrontonasal syndrome in Chapter 10.

In Chapter 11, Manu Raam and Max Muenke tackle a large group of uncommon syndromes with craniosynostosis (Antley-Bixler syndrome, Baller-Gerold syndrome, Beare-Stevenson cutis gyrata syndrome, Bohring-Opitz syndrome, C syndrome (or Opitz trigonocephaly syndrome), Carpenter syndrome, Crouzon syndrome with acanthosis nigricans, Jackson-Weiss syndrome, Jacobsen syndrome, Loeys-Dietz syndrome type I, osteoglophonic dysplasia, P450 oxidoreductase deficiency, and Shprintzen-Goldberg syndrome).

In Chapter 12, Donna McDonald-McGinn, Elaine Zackai and their colleagues present two patients with trigonocephaly, one with postaxial polydactyly, the other with polysyndactyly. Both were shown to have *GLI3* mutations.

Chapters 13–17 deal with general problems of various kinds. In Chapter 13, Maria Rita Passos-Bueno and her colleagues deal with the difficult problems of analyzing chromosomal alterations associated with craniosynostosis. In Chapter 14, Hartmut Collman and his colleagues review non-syndromic craniosynostoses. In Chapter 15, Ute Hehr discusses the molecular genetic testing of patients with craniosynostosis, and in Chapter 16, Thomas Schramm discusses prenatal ultrasonography, pointing out that there are no data on the validity of prenatal ultrasound screening for craniosynostosis, although to a certain degree, syndromic forms of craniosynostosis with craniofacial and limb involvement may allow ultrasonic differentiation between syndromes. Karen Gripp in Chapter 17 provides a wonderful clinical approach to craniosynostosis and distinguishes isolated synostosis from the more complicated search for the causes of the craniosynostosis associated with other anomalies together with their more complicated medical needs.

The final two chapters discuss surgical treatment in the craniosynostoses. In Chaper 18, Hartmut Collmann and his colleagues deal with imaging studies and neurosurgical treatment. They indicate that the diagnosis of craniosynostosis is primarily a matter of careful clinical examination with the use of imaging to verify the clinical diagnosis, to detect other possible sutures involved, to look for signs of intracranial hypertension, and to assess possible associated anomalies. The earlier craniectomy techniques used have now been partially replaced by plastic surgical techniques. Long term postoperative surveillance is mandatory. In Chapter 19, Hartmut Böhm and his colleagues discuss maxillofacial treatment. Procedures developed have included Le Fort III distraction, frontoorbitomaxillary advancement, monobloc frontofacial advancement, and orbital transposition.

Finally, let me say that all these highly respected authorities have written remarkably excellent chapters, which are so provocative that this volume will be read by many clinicians, many residents, many craniofacial biologists, many molecular geneticists, and many students. This will be *the* definitive volume on craniosynostosis for many years to come!

M. Michael Cohen Jr.
Halifax (Canada), July 2010

Muenke M, Kress W, Collmann H, Solomon BD (eds): Craniosynostoses: Molecular Genetics, Principles of Diagnosis, and Treatment.
Monogr Hum Genet. Basel, Karger, 2011, vol 19, pp 1–7

Craniosynostosis: A Historical Overview

B.D. Solomon[a] · H. Collmann[b] · W. Kress[c] · M. Muenke[a]

[a]Medical Genetics Branch, National Human Genome Research Institute, National Insitutes of Health, Bethesda, Md., USA;
[b]Department of Neurosurgery, [c]Institute of Human Genetics, Julius-Maximilians University, Würzburg, Germany

Abstract

Craniosynostosis has been recognized since ancient times, and the condition has a colorful and diverse history. In this introductory chapter, we include a description of historical aspects of craniosynostosis, which touches upon ancient depictions of the condition, the advent of modern classification schemes, more recent gene discoveries involving the molecular causes of many types of craniosynostosis, and evolving aspects of the management of affected patients.

General History

Descriptions and definitions of craniosynostosis have a long and complicated history that stretches over many millenia. Depictions of affected individuals have appeared in numerous cultures spanning every part of the globe where investigations have been undertaken. The earliest evidence comes from an at least 500,000 year-old Middle Pleistocene human skull found in modern Spain, which was noted to have unilateral lambdoid synostosis (a relatively rare type of sutural fusion) and consequent predicted deformities in the shape of the skull. The skull also showed evidence for elevated intracranial pressure (ICP). Most interestingly, the age of the individual at death was estimated to be at least five to eight years of age (and likely at least several years older than that). The authors argue that the individual's age is evidence that the society to which this individual belonged cared for handicapped and otherwise impaired members, which has certainly not always been the rule, even in modern cultures [1].

There is good evidence to believe that since prehistoric times, humankind has associated deviated head shape with magic ideas and mythic imaginations, as well as with both positive and negative aesthetic appearances. Unintentional deformation of the head by external forces, for instance from tight fixing of an infant's head to a cradle board, may have resulted in the practice of intentional deformation by wrapping the head or applying pads or boards to the infantile head. The aim likely was to create an extraordinary outer appearance in order to emphasize the terrifying appearance of a warrior or the noble image of an aristocrat, or by simply following local cultural criteria of beauty. In fact, intentional deformation of the head has been practiced in almost all cultures for many hundreds of years, and was customary even in Europe until the 18th century [2].

Less ancient but equally interesting (and more speculative) examples abound. It has been hypothesized that the Egyptian pharaoh Akhenaten, who ruled around 1350 BCE, may have had craniosynostosis as a manifestation of a disorder similar to Antley-Bixler syndrome, as he and his family were also depicted as having features consistent with abnormal steroidogenesis [3]. Certain Chinese deities such as the god of longevity, Nan-ji-xian-weng, are sometimes shown with severe frontal bossing consistent with craniosynostosis [4, 5]. In the Iliad, Homer, who is thought to have lived around the 8th century BCE, though the exact date is controversial, described Thersites, a soldier in the Greek army during the Trojan war, as having a 'pointed head,' which may have been a reference to oxycephaly, a condition resulting from craniosynostosis of the lambdoid, sagittal, and coronal sutures. Thersites' odd behavior is sometimes attributed to neurocognitive impairment secondary to severe craniosynostosis. Busts of the renowned Athenian politician Pericles, who led Athens during the city's Golden Age in the 5th century BCE, show features consistent with sagittal synostosis, and he was described as 'handsome. . .but with the head enormously long.' Indeed, the great general was typically depicted wearing a helmet, presumably to hide the shape of his skull. Pericles was a brilliant polymath in many respects, and many individuals with isolated types of craniosynostosis have unaffected cognitive development even without the availability of surgical treatment [6].

Early systematic descriptions of craniosynostosis appear in the writings of Hippocrates, who around the 4th century BCE described cranial sutures as they relate to a broad spectrum of head shapes. Several centuries later, at the turn of the millennia, the Roman encylcopedist Cornelius Celsus described skulls with absent sutures [5]. Much later, in the 1500s, the Brussels-born physician and anatomist Andreas Vesalius, who spent his professional career in Italy, outlined a variety of skull deformities characteristic of craniosynostosis [7]. However, it was not until the late 1700s that Samuel Thomas Sömmering first clearly identified the sutures themselves as the sites of early cranial growth, and concluded that premature sutural fusion would consequently result in cranial deformity [8].

Modern concepts of craniosynostosis are based on the works of Otto and Virchow [5]. In 1851, the famed German scientist and physician Rudolf Virchow described a logical classification of deformities resulting from monosutural fusion. According to Virchow's law, expansion of the cranial vault is restricted in a direction perpendicular to the fused suture, while compensatory overgrowth occurs along the fused suture [9]. Virchow coined the related term 'craniostenosis', which implicates the potentially harmful effect that growth restriction due to craniosynostosis can have on brain function. Later, the Austrian radiologist Arthur Schüller confined the term to intracranial hypertension resulting from craniosynostosis [10]. Of note, in his 1851 study, Virchow did not clearly separate microcephaly due to primary osseous growth failure from deficient brain bulk growth (micrencephaly) resulting in secondary sutural fusion, which remains a critical distinction both in terms of diagnosis and treatment (see the discussion below on aspects of management) [9].

Syndromic Craniosynostosis and Genetic Discoveries

Like craniosynostosis more generally, syndromic craniosynostosis also has a complex and fascinating history. Many of these syndromes were first clinically defined in Europe in the first half of the 20th century. However, it was not until the end of the century that the precise molecular causes were unearthed, largely within a few years in the 1990s during a period in which emerging technology allowed for rapid discovery of the genetic causes of most Mendelian disorders. As several chapters in

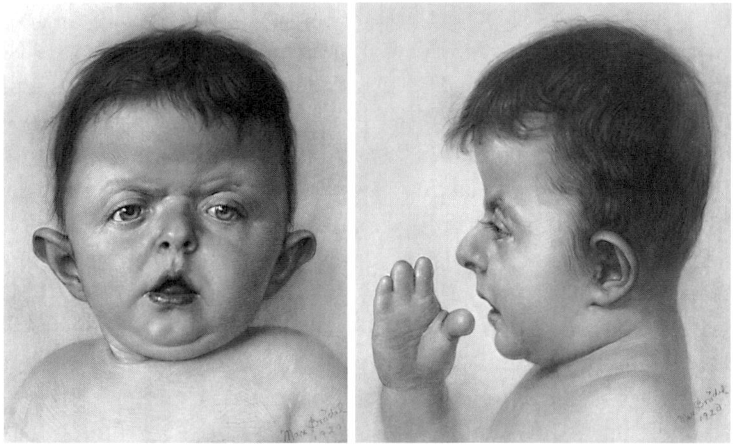

Fig. 1. Drawing of a child (approximately 18 months of age) with Apert syndrome, by Max Brödel, 1920. Brödel, who was trained in Germany, was brought to the Johns Hopkins School of Medicine in the United States in the 1890s in order to work with clinicians such as William Halsted, Howard Kelly, and Harvey Cushing, and is considered by some to be the father of modern medical illustration. Original art is #506 and #507 in the Walters Collection of the Max Brödel Archives in the Department of Art as Applied to Medicine, The Johns Hopkins University School of Medicine, Baltimore, Maryland, USA.

this book demonstrate, there remains active and healthy debate on both clinical and molecular definitions related to syndromic craniosynostosis (see Chapters 7 and 11 in this volume). While this historical introduction is not intended to exhaustively describe the history of every aspect and type of craniosynostosis, a discussion of the discovery of a number of craniosynostosis-related syndromes is nonetheless valuable and informative.

First, in 1906, Eugène Charles Apert, a French pediatrician, described a child affected with acrocephaly and syndactyly of the hands and feet [11]. (On a related but unfortunate side note, Apert was a vocal proponent of eugenics and euthanasia, and in fact was a founding member and later secretary general of the French Society of Eugenics [12]). Apert noted that 8 similar cases had already been reported, one of them by Wheaton in 1894 [13]. Apert termed the condition acrocephalosyndactyly [11] (see fig. 1 for an early illustration of a child with Apert syndrome). Almost exactly 100 years after Wheaton's description, in 1995, Wilkie et al. used a positional candidate gene approach to show that the genetic basis of the syndrome was due to specific mutations in *FGFR2* [14].

In 1912, Louis Edouard Octave Crouzon, a French neurologist who specialized in hereditary neurological diseases such as spinocerebellar ataxia, described a mother and her young son who both exhibited features of the syndrome that would take his name. After the initial description, Crouzon remained engaged with this entity and added several other studies to his first description [15]. As with many other craniosynostosis syndromes, linkage analysis established that *FGFR2* was the gene associated with this condition [16].

The history of Saethre-Chotzen syndrome is especially interesting, both in terms of the presentation of the patients and in terms of the eponymous physicians. Haakon Saethre, a Norwegian neurologist and psychiatrist, and Fritz Chotzen, a German psychiatrist, independently described patients with hereditary turricephaly associated with additional minor abnormalities [17, 18]. In 1930, Saethre saw a 32-year-old woman, who had been admitted to the psychiatric department of Oslo because of a catatonic crisis. He noticed characteristic craniofacial and limb features, as well as signs of intracranial hypertension. Her mother and sister were similarly affected, suggesting autosomal dominant inheritance. In the same study, he reported another adult woman who appeared to be similarly affected. In 1932, Chotzen reported a father and his 2 sons with similar findings. Chotzen also noted signs of elevated intracranial pressure in 2 members of this family. Chotzen categorized this family along with the acrocephalosyndactylies, emphasizing a commonality with Apert syndrome and Crouzon cranio-facial dysostosis. The molecular cause of Saethre-Chotzen syndrome was defined by both cytogenetic mapping and linkage analysis, in contrast to other syndromic forms of craniosynostosis. While the first cytogenetic clues emerged in the 1970s, mutations in *TWIST* were shown to be causative only in 1997 [19, 20].

Saethre-Chotzen syndrome particularly carries the stigma of German political history. Fritz Chotzen, the chairman of the Breslau hospital for nervous diseases, was Jewish. In 1933, he was expelled from his position by the Nazis, and died in 1937 at age 66. In Norway, Saethre was kept hostage and shot by German occupiers in February 1945, only a few short months before the end of WWII, in reprisal for an attack on a police officer by the Norwegian resistance movement.

It was not until 1964 that Rudolf Pfeiffer, a contemporary German geneticist, described 8 members of a family who were affected with acrocephaly and striking first digit anomalies. Pfeiffer saw the first member of this family, an affected child, during his pediatric residency in Münster, Germany, and this experience at least contributed to his decision to pursue a career in genetics. In 1991, Max Muenke, after whom Muenke syndrome is named, visited this family in their small Westphalian hometown (which is very close to his own childhood home) in order to obtain the necessary samples for linkage. Linkage analysis and sequencing of candidate genes led to the determination that Pfeiffer syndrome was due to mutations in *FGFR1* and *FGFR2* [21–24]. Interestingly, the mutation in the original Pfeiffer syndrome family, described years later, was in an unusual location in *FGFR2* [25].

Finally, Muenke syndrome offers an example of a craniosynostosis syndrome that was first defined molecularly, rather than clinically. Muenke syndrome, which is due to a specific mutation in *FGFR3*, was established when in a number of kindreds who were previously clinically diagnosed with Pfeiffer syndrome, the disease was shown to be linked to markers on chromosome 4 and to segregate with a common mutation in *FGFR3* [26, 27].

The case of Muenke syndrome highlights tensions within the field of genetics between historic clinical diagnoses and more recent molecular definitions. Only within the last few decades has the latter become possible for the vast majority of Mendelian disorders, and even now, there are many syndromic forms of craniosynostosis whose etiologies remain unknown (see Chapter 11 in this volume). Continued advances in genomic research will certainly accelerate the process of molecular definitions, but careful clinical dissections remain critical to understanding of the disease, and must continue in a fashion coupled to purely genetic knowledge. Indeed, the lesson of the discovery of Muenke syndrome is that thorough clinical and molecular investigations must proceed together in order to advance our understanding of rare diseases.

Overall, the *FGFR*-associated craniosynostoses are a prime example of current trends in 'molecular medicine', which allow clinicians and researchers a glimpse of the future of genetic medicine. Using molecular medicine, clinical problems might be addressed on the molecular and even the atomic level. The highly complex and likely redundant network of signal transduction pathways controlling growth, differentiation, demarcation and apoptosis of cells in the sutures is only partly understood. However, crystallographic data makes use of atomic information in order to explore how differences in hydrogen bridges affect receptor stabilization and ligand binding. This type of data has been used to clarify how specific phenotypes may result from specific atomic changes, as in the case of FGFR2 and Apert syndrome (see Chapter 5 in this volume for detailed discussion). Further, the observation that the same signal transduction cascades are important both in embryologic development and later on in life (for example, in cancer) has led to fascinating hypotheses, such as the idea that cancer therapies designed to impede a certain signaling cascade might also be used in the treatment of birth defects [28]. The future will undoubtedly bring many exciting developments in this field.

History of Treatment Aspects of Craniosynostosis

The first attempts to surgically treat craniosynostosis were performed on microcephalic children with deficient brain bulk growth [29, 30]. In these cases, the mortality was extremely high. Since the problem of micrencephaly was well known at that time, surgical enthusiasm soon met with harsh criticism. The most famous voice was that of Abraham Jacoby, a New York pediatrician, who at the American Annual Meeting in 1893 accused the surgeons with the following declaration: 'The hands take too frequently the place of brains... Is it sufficient glory to let daylight into a deformed cranium and on top of a hopelessly defective brain, and to proclaim a success because a victim consented not to die of the assault?... Such rash feats of indiscriminate surgery, if continued, moreover in the presence of 14 deaths in 33 cases, are stains on your hands and sins on your souls. No ocean of soap and water will clean those hands...' [2, 31, 32]. Thereafter, surgery on craniosynostosis was abandoned for nearly two decades.

Today, neurosurgery (in cooperation with maxillofacial or plastic surgery) is a mainstay of treatment, though the optimal technique continues to evolve and remain controversial at times. An important related consideration has been the ability to assess for the presence of elevated intracranial pressure (ICP) and to precisely define the involved sutures (see Chapter 18 for a more in-depth analysis of these issues). Naturally, these techniques are intimately connected with treatment approaches. In the patients they first described, both Saethre and Chotzen were able to assess intracranial hypertension via ophthalmologic examination and by detecting signs on plain radiographs. At this time, elevated ICP was evident only in its more advanced stages. Improvements in ophthalmologic instruments allow for the ability to detect earlier and less obvious degrees of elevated ICP, as does the ability to perform intracranial pressure monitoring. In addition, the widespread availability of more sophisticated neuroimaging techniques, including plain radiographs, ultrasonography, computerized tomography, and magnetic resonance imaging, allows for better detection. As discussed by Collmann et al. (Chapter 18 this volume), all or any of these techniques may be useful in a given scenario, and it is up to the clinicians' expertise to select the appropriate modality. Finally, the value of dedicated teams of professionals and dedicated services to care for affected patients cannot be overstated. These services include intensive care units familiar with caring for patients in the postoperative period, diverse craniofacial and neurosurgical teams who are capable and willing to manage a wide variety of needs, ranging from genetic counseling to precise neurosurgical techniques, and laboratory-based researchers dedicated to dissecting the precise pathogenetic mechanisms in order to design molecularly-derived treatments.

Concluding Remarks

From human ancestors and relatives living long before recorded history to cutting-edge researchers using the most precise instruments available in the modern laboratory setting, countless aspects of craniosynostosis provide a view on many facets of the human condition. In the last few decades, new treatment and diagnostic modalities allow a dramatically improved understanding of the condition. Further, the prognosis for affected individuals continues to improve. Still, the story of the earliest known affected patient, a child with lambdoid craniosynostosis and accompanying severe facial deformities who lived half-a-million years ago, underscores the most important lesson that can be taken from this dramatic and fascinating disease: we must strive to care for the less fortunate to the extent of our collective abilities.

Acknowledgements

This work was supported in part by the Division of Intramural Research, National Human Genome Research Institute, National Institutes of Health, Department of Health and Human Services, United States of America.

References

1 Gracia A, Arsuaga JL, Martínez I, Lorenzo C, Carretero JM, Bermúdez de Castro JM, Carbonell E: Craniosynostosis in the Middle Pleistocene human Cranium 14 from the Sima de los Huesos, Atapuerca, Spain. Proc Natl Acad Sci USA 2009;106:6573–6578.

2 Goodrich JT, Tutino M: An annotated history of craniofacial surgery and intentional cranial deformation. Neurosurg Clin N Am 2001;12:45–68.

3 Braverman IM, Redford DB, Mackowiak PA: Akhenaten and the strange physiques of Egypt's 18th dynasty. Ann Intern Med 2009;150:556–560.

4 Wang HS, Kuo MF: Nan-ji-xian-weng: the god of longevity. Childs Nerv Syst 2010;26:1–2.

5 Cohen MM Jr: History, terminology, and classifications of craniosynostosis, in Cohen MM Jr, MacLean RE (eds): Craniosynostosis: Diagnosis, Evaluation, and Management, ch 9, pp 103–111 (Oxford University Press, New York, Oxford 2000).

6 Di Rocco C: Craniosynostosis in old Greece: political power and physical deformity. Childs Nerv Syst 2005;21:859.

7 Vesalius A: De humanis corporis fabrica (Oporinus, Basel 1543).

8 Sömmering ST: Vom Baue des menschlichen Körpers. Erster Teil: Knochenlehre (Warentrapp & Brenner, Frankfurt/M 1791).

9 Virchow R: Über den Cretinismus, namentlich in Franken, und über pathologische Schädelformen. Verhandl Phys Med Ges Würzburg 1851;2:230–270.

10 Schüller A: Craniostenosis. Radiology 1929;13:377–382.

11 Apert E: De l'acrocéphalosyndactylie. Bull Soc Méd Paris 1906;23:1310–1330.

12 Strous RD, Edelman MC: Eponyms and the Nazi era: time to remember and time for change. Isr Med Assoc J 2007;9:207–214.

13 Wheaton SW: Two specimens of congenital cranial deformity in infants associated with fusion of the fingers and toes. Trans Path Soc London 1894;45:238–241.

14 Wilkie AO, Slaney SF, Oldridge M, Poole MD, Ashworth GJ, et al: Apert syndrome results from localized mutations of *FGFR2* and is allelic with Crouzon syndrome. Nat Genet 1995;9:165–172.

15 Crouzon O: Dysostose cranio-faciale héréditaire. Bull Soc Méd Paris 1912;33:545–555.

16 Jabs EW, Li X, Scott AF, Meyers G, Chen W, et al: Jackson-Weiss and Crouzon syndromes are allelic with mutations in fibroblast growth factor receptor 2. Nat Genet 1994;8:275–279. Erratum in: Nat Genet 1995;9:451.

17 Saethre H: Ein Beitrag zum Turmschädelproblem (Pathogenese, Erblichkeit und Symptomatologie). Dtsch Z Nervenheilk 1931;117:533–555.

18 Chotzen F: Eine eigenartige familiäre Entwicklungsstörung (Akrocephalosyndaktylie, Dysostosis craniofacialis und Hypertelorismus). Monatsschr Kinderheilk 1932;55:97–122.

19 el Ghouzzi V, Le Merrer M, Perrin-Schmitt F, Lajeunie E, Benit P, et al: Mutations of the *TWIST* gene in the Saethre-Chotzen syndrome. Nat Genet 1997;15:42–46.

20 Howard TD, Paznekas WA, Green ED, Chiang LC, Ma N, et al: Mutations in *TWIST*, a basic helix-loop-helix transcription factor, in Saethre-Chotzen syndrome. Nat Genet 1997;15:36–41.

21 Muenke M, Schell U, Hehr A, Robin NH, Losken HW, et al: A common mutation in the fibroblast growth factor receptor 1 gene in Pfeiffer syndrome. Nat Genet 1994;8:269–274.

22 Lajeunie E, Ma HW, Bonaventure J, Munnich A, Le Merrer M, Renier D: *FGFR2* mutations in Pfeiffer syndrome. Nat Genet 1995;9:108.

23 Rutland P, Pulleyn LJ, Reardon W, Baraitser M, Hayward R, et al: Identical mutations in the *FGFR2* gene cause both Pfeiffer and Crouzon syndrome phenotypes. Nat Genet 1995;9:173–176.

24 Schell U, Hehr A, Feldman GJ, Robin NH, Zackai EH, et al: Mutations in *FGFR1* and *FGFR2* cause familial and sporadic Pfeiffer syndrome. Hum Mol Genet 1995;4:323–328.
25 Kan SH, Elanko N, Johnson D, Cornejo-Roldan L, Cook J, et al: Genomic screening of fibroblast growth-factor receptor 2 reveals a wide spectrum of mutations in patients with syndromic craniosynostosis. Am J Hum Genet 2002;70:472–486.
26 Bellus GA, Gaudenz K, Zackai EH, Clarke LA, Szabo J, Francomano CA, Muenke M: Identical mutations in three different fibroblast growth factor receptor genes in autosomal dominant craniosynostosis syndromes. Nat Genet 1996;14:174–176.
27 Muenke M, Gripp KW, McDonald-McGinn DM, Gaudenz K, Whitaker LA, et al: A unique point mutation in the fibroblast growth factor receptor 3 gene *(FGFR3)* defines a new craniosynostosis syndrome. Am J Hum Genet 1997;60:555–564.
28 Wilkie AO: Cancer drugs to treat birth defects. Nat Genet 2007;39:1057–1059.
29 Lane LC: Pioneer craniectomy for relief of imbecillity due to premature sutural closure and microcephalus. JAMA 1892;18:49–50.
30 Lannelongue O: De la craniectomie dans la microcéphalie. L'Union Medicale 1890;50:42–45.
31 Jacobi A: Nil nocere. Med Report 1894;45:609–618.
32 Fisher RG: Surgery of the congenital anomalies, in Walker AE (ed): A history of neurological surgery, pp 334–361 (Hafner, New York 1967).

Maximilian Muenke
NIH, MSC 3717
Building 35, Room 1B-203
Bethesda, MD, 20892–3717 (USA)
Tel. +1 301 402 8167, Fax +1 301 496 7184, E-Mail mamuenke@mail.nih.gov

Muenke M, Kress W, Collmann H, Solomon BD (eds): Craniosynostoses: Molecular Genetics, Principles of Diagnosis, and Treatment.
Monogr Hum Genet. Basel, Karger, 2011, vol 19, pp 8–12

Discovery of *MSX2* Mutation in Craniosynostosis: A Retrospective View

U. Müller

Institut für Humangenetik, Justus-Liebig-Universität, Gießen, Germany

Abstract
This is a historical review of the discovery of the first mutation detected in autosomal dominant craniosynostosis. The mutation was found in one large family in whom craniosynostosis segregated as an autosomal dominant trait. Craniosynostosis in this family was highly variable and could present as frontal recession, turribrachycephaly, frontal bossing, or clover-leaf malformation. Craniosynostosis is the only or main sign in this syndrome, now referred to as craniosynostosis, Boston type, based on the location of its discovery. A gain-of-function mutation was identified in the gene *MSX2* in this disorder. The mutation results in replacement of an evolutionarily highly conserved proline within the homeodomain of the gene by a histidine (p.Pro148His). The causative role of the mutation in craniosynostosis was borne out in transgenic mice. To date affected members of the Boston family are the only ones in whom a mutation in *MSX2* has been shown to cause craniosynostosis.

Family Identification

A patient with a clinically undescribed form of craniosynostosis was presented at medical genetics rounds at Children's Hospital in Boston in 1991. The family history revealed many affected members in several generations, consistent with autosomal dominant inheritance of the trait in this family. Together with Matt Warman, then a fellow in medical genetics, and John B. Mulliken, professor of craniofacial surgery at Children's hospital, I decided to study the genetic basis of the disorder in this family. The three of us contacted the family, who was excited to participate in an investigation and invited us to what they called a 'DNA party' at their home. This gave us an opportunity to clinically examine all affected family members from 3 generations (fig. 1). The phenotype varied dramatically in affected persons (fig. 2). While the grandmother was affected only slightly, mainly displaying fronto-orbital recession and absence of midface hypoplasia, persons in subsequent generations were more severely affected. Their findings included frontal bossing, turribrachycephaly, and clover-leaf anomaly. Seven affected members of the family required surgical intervention. Three had turribrachycephaly, 2 clover-leaf skulls, 1 fronto-orbital recession, and 1 frontal bossing. Figure 3 shows the radiograph of a severely affected patient with turribrachycephaly, who later underwent surgery. Almost all affected individuals had myopia or hyperopia and 2 had tunnel vision and visual field loss. In addition, several patients suffered from severe headaches and 4 had seizures. A triphalangeal thumb was found in 1 individual

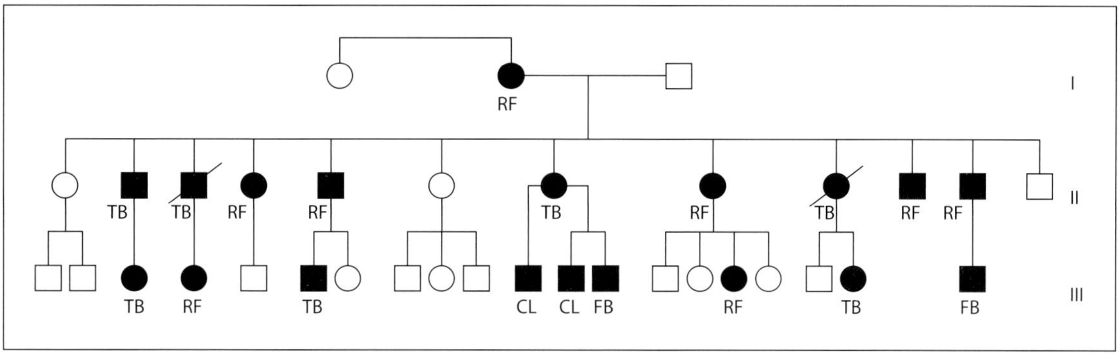

Fig. 1. Pedigree of the Boston family. CL, clover-leaf skull; FB, frontal bossing; RF, fronto-orbital recession; TB, turribrachycephaly.

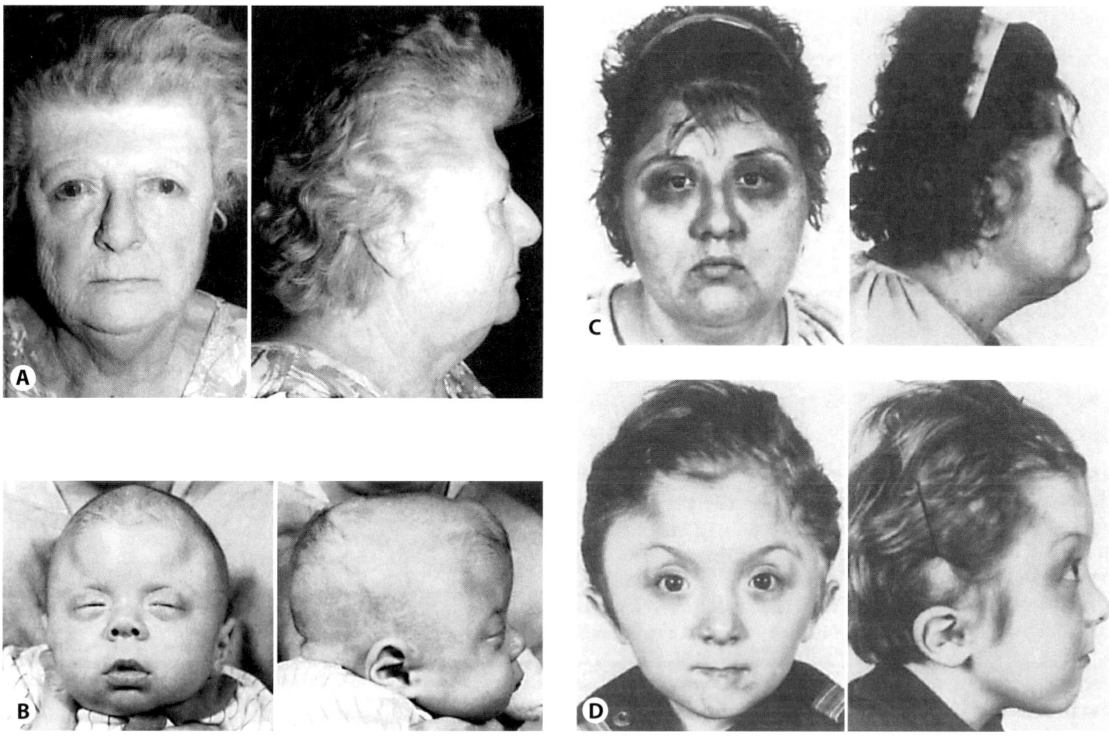

Fig. 2. Phenotypic spectrum in affected members of the Boston family. **A** Fronto-orbital recession and absence of midface hypoplasia. **B** Frontal bossing. Lateral photograph shows markedly retropositioned supraorbital rims without midface retrusion. **C** Turribrachycephaly as the result of pancraniosynostosis. Lateral photograph shows retrusion of the supraorbital rims in presence of normal midface position. **D** Clover-leaf skull. The malformation is still apparent despite coronal, lambdoidal and temporal craniectomies were performed during infancy (from [1, 2]).

Fig. 3. Frontal (left) and lateral (right) radiograph of a patient from the Boston family, demonstrating signs of turribrachycephaly. Note bony extensions between frontal and middle lobes (frontal view) and frontal and supraorbital retrusion, short cranial base, platybasia, and marked convolutional impressions on the endocranial surface (lateral view) (from [1]).

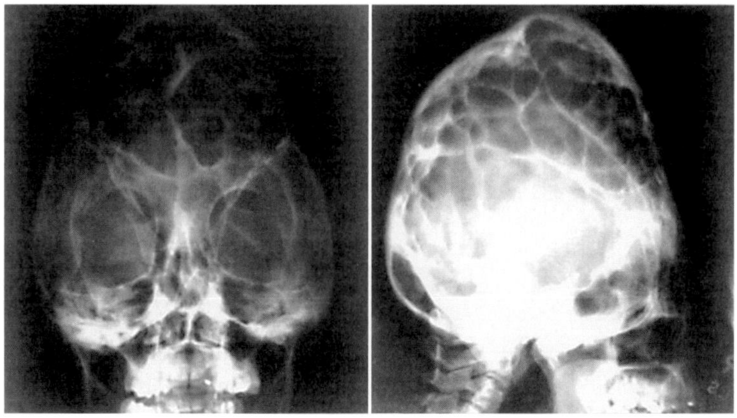

and radiographs revealed short first metatarsals in 3 out of 4 patients examined. Taken together, limb involvement was very mild if present at all in this mainly 'pure' form of craniosynostosis [1].

Discovery of the Causative Mutation

DNA was available from 23 members of the family. In order to chromosomally assign the disease locus by linkage analysis, I joined Jim Weber's lab in Marshfield Wisconsin for several weeks in 1992. Jim had established a panel of short tandem repeat polymorphic (STRP) markers that allowed investigation of the entire genome. At this time STRPs were amplified in the presence of a radiolabeled nucleotide (α-^{32}P-dCTP) and investigated by autoradiography after gel electrophoretic separation. Time to perform a whole genome scan was dramatically abbreviated by finding highly significant linkage to the first marker tested (Mfd 154 at locus D5S211). With a maximum logarithm of the odds (LOD) score (Zmax) of 4.82 at zero recombination ($\theta = 0.00$) the craniosynostosis locus was assigned to the distal long arm of chromosome 5 in this Boston family [2].

At the same time, Ethlyn Jabs at Johns Hopkins Medical School in Baltimore and Robert Maxson, at the Institute for Genetic Medicine of the Kenneth R. Norris Cancer Hospital, Los Angeles, had cloned the human homologue of the mouse *Msx2* gene and assigned it to the distal long arm of human chromosome 5. *MSX2*, composed of 2 exons separated by a large intron, is a member of the vertebrate *Msx* family of homeobox genes that were originally identified on the basis of their homology to the *Drosophila* gene *Msh* (muscle segment homeobox gene) (summarized in [3]). The chromosomal location of *MSX2* and its function in epithelial-mesenchymal interactions made it a good candidate gene for craniosynostosis, Boston type. In collaboration with the Baltimore/Los Angeles groups, we identified a C-A transversion at nucleotide 64 in exon 2 of *MSX2*. This mutation results in an amino acid change from proline (Pro, encoded by CCC) to histidine (His, encoded by CAC) at position 7 of the homeodomain of *MSX2* (p.Pro148His) and segregated with the disorder in the family.

Functional Analyses of the Mutation

Proline has been highly conserved during evolution and occurs at a position that has been invariant in Msx homeodomains of numerous phyla for approximately 600 million years [4]. These observations together with expression of *Msx2* in

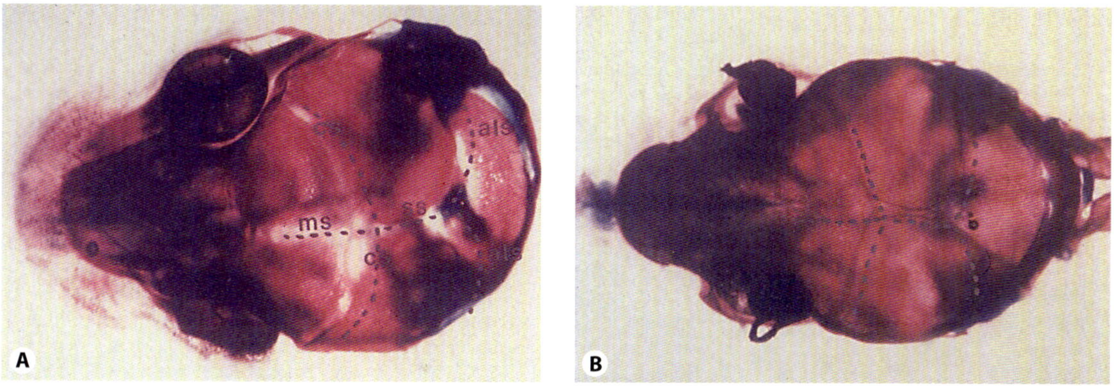

Fig. 4. **A** Skull of a 1-day-old normal mouse. **B** Skull of a 1-day-old transgenic animal expressing the mouse counterpart of the human p.Pro148His mutation in the *Msx2* gene. Skulls were stained with alcian blue to demonstrate cartilage (blue) and with alizarin red S to reveal mineralized bone (red). Note complete occlusion of coronal and sagittal sutures and partial closure of lambdoid suture in the transgenic animal (Photograph kindly provided by Dr. R.E. Maxson; see also [5]). als, lambdoid suture; cs, coronal suture; ms = metopic suture; ss = sagittal suture.

membranous bone of the calvaria and in adjacent mesenchymal cells in the mouse convincingly suggested that the *MSX2* mutation causes craniosynostosis, Boston type [4]. A role of the *MSX2* (p.Pro148His) mutation was borne out in transgenic mice. Both, overexpression of human *MSX2* in mice and introduction of the murine counterpart of the p.Pro148His mutation, result in craniosynostosis [5, 6]. Figure 4 depicts the skull of a normal mouse and of a transgenic animal with synostosis of the coronal and sagittal suture and partial occlusion of the lambdoid suture.

The mutation increases the affinity of Msx2 for its target sequence without interfering with site specificity of Msx2 binding. In comparison to wild-type Msx2, gel shift analysis revealed drastically enhanced binding of p.Pro148His Msx2 to a sequence containing the consensus Msx binding site, TAATTG [7]. This suggests that the dominant mutation acts by a gain-of-function mechanism by overstimulating Msx2 target sequences. Interestingly, some patients with partial trisomy of the long arm of chromosome 5 have craniosynostosis [8]. This may thus be caused by the increased dosage of MSX2 expected in these patients.

Conclusion

MSX2 was the first gene found to be associated with autosomal dominant craniosynostosis in the absence of gross limb deformities. Ironically, no additional families with craniosynostosis and an *MSX2* mutation have been identified to date. It appears that only the specific mutation at position 7 of the homeodomain of *MSX2* found in the Boston family results in increased binding, overstimulation of target sequences, and eventually in craniosynostosis. Other mutations might not have such an effect. Interestingly, haploinsufficiency of *MSX2* causes the opposite of craniosynostosis, i.e. parietal foramina (delayed ossification along the sagittal sutures) [9, 10].

Acknowledgement

The enthusiastic participation of the Boston family in the work reported is highly appreciated.

References

1 Warman ML, Mulliken JB, Hayward PG, Müller U: Newly recognized autosomal dominant disorder with craniosynostosis. Am J Med Genet 1993;46:444–449.
2 Müller U, Warman ML, Mulliken JB, Weber JL: Assignment of a gene locus involved in craniosynostosis to chromosome 5qter. Hum Mol Genet 1993;2:119–122.
3 Müller U: MSX2 and ALX4: craniosynostosis and defects in skull ossification; in Epstein CJ, Erickson RP, Wynshaw-Boris AJ (eds): Inborn Errors of Development – The Molecular Basis of Clinical Disorders of Morphogenesis. Oxford, Oxford University Press, 2nd ed., 2008, pp 730–773.
4 Jabs EW, Müller U, Li X, Ma L, Luo W, et al: A mutation in the homeodomain of the human *MSX2* gene in a family affected with autosomal dominant craniosynostosis. Cell 1993;75:443–450.
5 Liu YH, Kundu R, Wu L, Luo W, Ignelzi MA Jr, et al: Premature suture closure and ectopic cranial bone in mice expressing *Msx2* transgenes in the developing skull. Proc Natl Acad Sci USA 1995;92:6137–6141.
6 Liu YH, Tang Z, Kundu RK, Wu L, Luo W, et al: *Msx2* gene dosage influences the number of proliferative osteogenic cells in growth centers of the developing murine skull: a possible mechanism for MSX2-mediated craniosynostosis in humans. Dev Biol 1999;205:260–274.
7 Ma L, Golden S, Wu L, Maxson R: The molecular basis of Boston-type craniosynostosis: the Pro148→His mutation in the N-terminal arm of the MSX2 homeodomain stabilizes DNA binding without altering nucleotide sequence preferences. Hum Mol Genet 1996;5:1915–1920.
8 Kariminejad A, Kariminejad R, Tzschach A, Ullmann R, Ahmed A, et al: Craniosynostosis in a patient with 2q37.3 deletion 5q34 duplication: association of extra copy of *MSX2* with craniosynostosis. Am J Med Genet 2009;149A:1544–1549.
9 Wilkie AO, Tang Z, Elanko N, Walsh S, Twigg SR, et al: Functional haploinsufficiency of the human homeobox gene *MSX2* causes defects in skull ossification. Nat Genet 2000;24:387–390.
10 Wuyts W, Reardon W, Preis S, Homfray T, Rasore-Quartino A, et al: Identification of mutations in the *MSX2* homeobox gene in families affected with foramina parietalia permagna. Hum Mol Genet 2000;9:1251–1255.

Prof. Dr. Ulrich Müller
Institut für Humangenetik
Schlangenzahl 14
35392 Gießen (Germany)
Tel. +49 641 9941601, Fax +49 641 9941609, E-Mail ulrich.mueller@humangenetik.med.uni-giessen.de

Muenke M, Kress W, Collmann H, Solomon BD (eds): Craniosynostoses: Molecular Genetics, Principles of Diagnosis, and Treatment.
Monogr Hum Genet. Basel, Karger, 2011, vol 19, pp 13–27

Regulation of Calvarial Bone Growth by Molecules Involved in the Craniosynostoses

M.D. Benson · L.A. Opperman

Texas A&M Health Science Center, Baylor College of Dentistry, Dallas, Tex., USA

Abstract

The development and growth of the mammalian cranium is choreographed by a complex interplay of dynamic interactions between its constituent bone plates and the sutures that buffer them. These interactions are governed by several families of cytokines and growth factors that act to control osteoblast proliferation, migration and maturation. In this chapter, we discuss 3 of those families whose central roles in bone growth are highlighted by their association with dysregulated growth in craniosynostosis. It is hoped that study of the interplay between these – the ephrins, fibroblast growth factors, and transforming growth factors beta – will reveal molecular targets for future treatment in a clinical setting.

Classical anatomy divides the human skull into the neurocranium, so called because it surrounds the brain, and the viscerocranium, which contains the orbits and the entries to the respiratory and digestive tracts. The neurocranium is further divided into the skull base and the cranial vault. The largest part of the cranial base is termed the chondrocranium because of its endochondral ossification, while the cranial vault may also be called the dermatocranium due to its direct, intramembranous mode of ossification.

The mammalian cranial vault consists of an assembly of bones that fit against one another and are buffered by the fibrous sutural tissue that allows for lateral bone growth. The skull bones form during embryogenesis from condensations of neural crest and mesodermal tissues, and, once pattern formation is complete, they will continue to grow laterally and in thickness for much of postnatal life. This means that the story of cranial expansion is essentially one of how bone growth is regulated in three dimensions. The two main sites of action in this process are on the bone surfaces (the periosteum) and the sutures, where complex interactions between cells of the suture mesenchyme and osteoblastic stem cells on the bone fronts tightly regulate bone synthesis. This coordination between suture and expanding bone is what allows for optimal protection of the brain throughout its period of rapid growth in early childhood, during which the brain reaches 50% of its final volume in the first seven months and 95% by the eighth year. As with so many other sophisticated biological processes, insights into the nature of these interactions are to be found in the cases where they go awry. In this regard, the study of the cranial synostoses (premature fusion of the calvarial bones) has revealed the importance of three key families of growth factors and their signaling

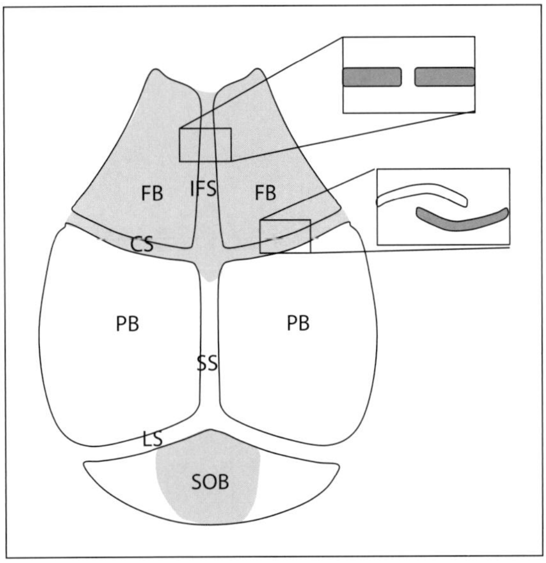

Fig. 1. Origins and anatomy of the cranial bones. Gray areas denote cranial neural crest derived tissue. White areas denote mesodermally-derived tissues. PB, parietal bone; FB, frontal bone; SOB, supraoccipital bone; CS, coronal suture; IFS, interfrontal suture; SS, sagittal suture; LS, lambdoid suture. Insets show coronal sections of interfrontal and coronal sutures. The IFS (and SS, by extension) are abutting sutures, while the CS is overlapping. The CS represents a neural crest/mesoderm boundary.

effectors in cranial growth by virtue of the dramatic consequences of their dysregulation.

The primary focus of this review then is on regulation of bone growth in the cranium by these three families: The ephrins, the fibroblast growth factors (FGFs), and the transforming growth factors β (TGFβ), mutations in the pathways of which have been linked to the majority of the heritable and acquired synostoses. As the discussion that follows is primarily a story of bone growth, we will begin with a brief review of the cranial bones and their origins, followed by a primer on the molecular basis of osteoblast (OB) differentiation, as this is the bone-forming cell. We will then address the regulation of OB commitment and differentiation by the three families of signals that are so dramatically associated with cranial deformities. As we will see, the signaling pathways for these factors are interwoven into a complex web that is only now beginning to be unraveled on a molecular basis.

Anatomy and Origins of the Cranial Vault

After cranial expansion is complete in humans, sometime in the third decade of life, the suture tissue is obliterated and the bones of the calvaria fuse to form a confluent mineralized dome. In mice, the majority of sutures remain patent throughout the two-year lifespan of the animal. Nevertheless, the developmental anatomy of the rodent skull otherwise closely parallels that of the human, and provides examples of both patent and fused sutures. Thus, it is to this system that we will refer in our discussion.

The calvaria is composed of five separate bones: the two frontal bones, behind which are the two parietal bones and the supraoccipital bone (fig. 1). Disputes about the embryonic origins of these have only recently been resolved by definitive genetic lineage tracing experiments in the mouse [1, 2]. Mice bearing the neural crest-specific Wnt1-cre and the Rosa26-STOP-LacZ indicator to label neural crest cell (NCC)-derived structures showed that the frontal bones and the medial section of the supraoccipital bone come from cells of the trigeminal neural crest, which migrate from the closing neural folds during E8 to E10. By contrast, the parietal bones and the lateral parts of the supraoccipital are derived from paraxial mesoderm. The edges where these bones meet define the calvarial sutures, which are composed of fibrous mesenchymal tissue that acts as a buffer between the bone fronts. Interestingly, the abutting sutures are those that form between bones of the same lineage (the interfrontal, sagittal, and lambdoid), while the coronal suture that forms between the bones of neural crest (frontal) and mesodermal (parietal) origins is an overlapping one. The coronal suture is thus a

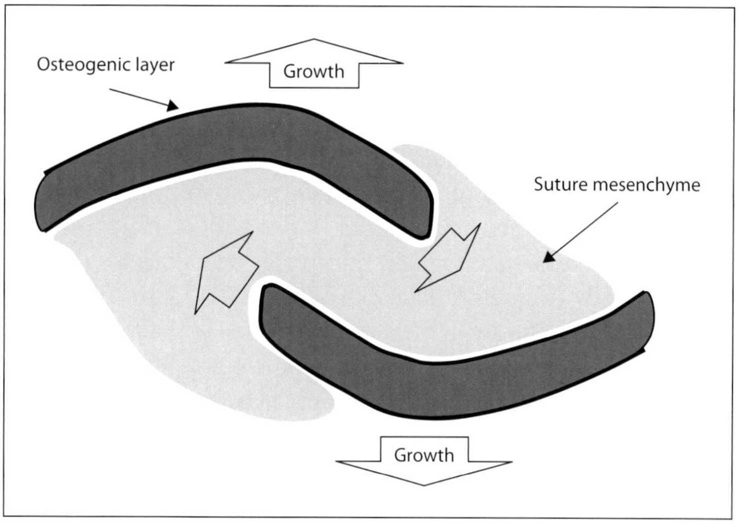

Fig. 2. Bone growth in calvariae. The 2 opposing bones are buffered by the suture mesenchyme (light gray). On their surfaces is the osteogenic layer (dark gray band) that holds committed osteoprogenitor cells and the stem cells from which they derive. Bone thickness is increased as these surface periosteal cells secrete a collagen matrix, become embedded within it, and differentiate to produce mineralized bone. Similarly, lateral bone growth proceeds from cells in the same layer that migrate to the leading edge of the bone and both proliferate to extend that edge and differentiate to produce bone. Signals in the suture must prevent leading edge cells from extending too far into the buffer zone that keeps the suture patent.

boundary between two lineages, and provides an opportunity to study the molecular regulation of suture morphogenesis.

Calvarial Sutures as Intramembranous Bone Growth Sites

The calvarial bones are initially separated by a wide distance in the embryo, but shortly before birth, the expanding bone fronts interact to form the presumptive sutures, the tissue of which is composed of mesenchymal cells in a primarily type III collagen matrix (fig. 2). At this point, the bones either abut or begin to change direction and slide over each other to form an overlap, with sutural tissue buffering the edges. Unlike in humans, the only suture that fuses naturally in the mouse is the posterior part of the interfrontal suture. However, the establishment of several mouse models of craniosynostosis has guided us in the identification of a number of factors that contribute to maintenance of suture patency. Transplantation studies done in the mid-1990s defined the contribution of the surrounding tissue environment to formation and maintenance of this critical structure. Opperman and colleagues implanted late fetal or early postnatal mouse coronal sutures into surgically prepared defects in adult mouse host skulls. The transplants were able to form and maintain morphologically normal coronal sutures. However, after three weeks, these sutures fused unless they were transplanted along with their associated fetal dura mater. These experiments showed that signals from the frontal and parietal bone fronts are sufficient to instruct the proper formation of the suture, but that signals from the pre- or neonatal dura are required to keep it patent. And, these dura-derived signals are absent in the adult, where the sutures become self-sustaining. Follow-up experiments showed that embryonic calvariae co-cultured ex vivo with, but physically separated from, the dura mater were able to avoid osseous suture obliteration the same as if they were in contact with the dura. Interestingly, overall bone growth, as measured by calcium content, was significantly reduced in calvariae grown separated from the dura as compared to those grown in contact with it. Collectively, these studies demonstrated that the embryonic dura mater produces a soluble activity that diffuses into the suture to keep it patent while also manufacturing an insoluble factor that spurs bone growth elsewhere [3, 4]. Sutural function also depends on mechanical forces, i.e. the intracranial pressure created by the growing brain and the continuously secreted cerebrospinal fluid. In childhood, abnormally increased pressure of any origin causes splitting of the sutures while grossly subnormal brain growth eventually may result in premature fusion of the sutures. This latter process is called secondary synostosis, a reaction to abnormal environmental conditions of an otherwise normal suture.

Normal bone growth proceeds in two directions, laterally (to expand the edges of the bones) and longitudinally (to increase bone thickness). Longitudinal growth is accomplished by mesenchymal osteoprogenitor cells in the layer of periosteum lining both inside and outside of the bone. Lateral growth is maintained by these same osteoprogenitors, which migrate from the periosteum into the bone front at the edge of the suture such that this front can be thought of as contiguous with the periosteum (fig. 2). Thus, the process of intramembranous bone growth can be thought of in three stages: proliferation of osteoprogenitors, their migration into the leading edge of the bone fronts, and their differentiation into mineralizing OBs.

Transcriptional Control of Osteoblast Commitment and Differentiation

Mesenchymal cells that have condensed into the pattern of the presumptive calvarial bones are induced into the OB lineage by the actions of growth factors including FGFs, platelet derived growth factor (PDGF), and members of the transforming growth factor β superfamily (including the TGFs and BMPs). Once committed to the OB lineage, the cells begin to secrete and embed themselves in a type I collagen extracellular matrix (ECM), which in turn mediates the final stage of OB differentiation through interactions with cell surface α2β1 integrin [5]. That this ECM interaction is required for OB differentiation is demonstrated by the fact that proline hydroxylation inhibitors such as 3,4-dehydroproline, which block triple helix formation and secretion, also block expression of the differentiated phenotype. Integrin activation stimulates focal adhesion kinase and subsequent activation of the mitogen activated protein kinase (MAPK) pathway. This leads to synthesis and secretion of the characteristic bone matrix proteins such as alkaline phosphatase (Alp), bone sialoprotein (Bsp), osteopontin (Opn), and osteocalcin (Ocn). It is this mature matrix that finally mineralizes into bone (reviewed in more detail in [6]).

The transcription factor Runx2 (a.k.a. Pebp2a1, AML-3, Osf2, or Cbfa1) is the lynch pin in the control of both osteoprogenitor commitment and terminal OB differentiation. Mesenchymal stem cells in the skeletal condensations require Runx2 to proceed along the OB lineage. Without it, these cells instead fall under the control of Sox9 and proceed to become chondrocytes [7]. Later on in committed preosteoblasts, Runx2 is required to activate the transcription of specific genes in the OB differentiation program [8–10]. In fact, Runx2 was first identified through its binding to specific sites in the *Ocn* promoter that are required for OB-specific expression [11]. The need for Runx2 is dosage-dependent; Runx2$^{+/-}$ mice have the equivalent of the human disease cleidocranial dysplasia

(CCD), characterized by hypoplastic clavicles and delayed fontanel closure owing to impaired OB differentiation, while Runx2$^{-/-}$ mice completely lack OBs.

Runx2 activity is regulated by phosphorylation of its proline-serine-threonine (PST) domain through the Erk1/2 branch of the MAPK pathway. Phosphorylated Runx2 enters the nucleus to activate transcription from the promoters of OB-specific genes [12]. Thus, growth factors that act through the Ras/MAPK/Erk pathway can regulate bone formation at both the commitment and differentiation control points through modulation of Runx2 activity. Runx2 is also directly regulated by the basic-helix-loop-helix protein Twist1. Twist1 is of particular interest in cranial biology because it is expressed in the mesenchyme of the coronal sutures where it binds to the DNA-binding domain of Runx2 to inhibit its activity and thus bone formation [13]. Heterozygous loss of Twist1 causes synostosis of the coronal suture in mice and Saethre-Chotzen syndrome in humans [14, 15]. Msx2, the mammalian homolog of the *Drosophila* homeodomain protein Mash, is an indirect regulator of Runx2 with particular relevance to cranial bone growth. It stimulates expression of Runx2 and thereby increases OB differentiation [16]. Msx2 loss of function mutations result in enlarged parietal foramina, while a gain of function mutation is responsible for Boston-type craniosynostosis [17, 18]. The close epistatic relationship of these 3 genes is illustrated in the cranial symptoms of their mouse mutants. The enlarged foramina in Runx2$^{+/-}$ mice can be rescued by loss of one Twist1 allele [13], while loss of one Msx2 allele rescues coronal synostosis in Twist1$^{+/-}$ mice [19].

Ephrins, Boundary Formation, and Directed Bone Growth

We now turn our attention to the growth and guidance factors that regulate the behavior of OBs and their progenitors in the sutural milieu. As mentioned above, the suture mesenchyme forms a buffer region between growing bone fronts. Signaling between the suture and bone is critical for restricting lateral growth, and disruption of these signals results in the unregulated ossification of the sutures seen in the craniosynostoses. Thus, the first priority in development of the suture buffer is establishment of the boundaries that segregate bone and suture cells into these tissues.

Ephrins are membrane-bound ligands that are used throughout development as guidance and migration cues and to signal tissue segregation and boundary maintenance [20, 21]. Three B and eight A ephrins have so far been identified. B-class ephrins are single-pass transmembrane domain proteins while the A-class members are glycosylphosphatidyl inositol (GPI)-linked to the extracellular membrane. Their receptors are the Eph family of receptor tyrosine kinases (RTKs), 14 of which have been identified. The Ephs are also classified into A and B based on preferential binding for the corresponding class of ligand. However, several members are promiscuous in that regard. Most notable is EphA4, which receives biologically important signals from all three B ephrins [22]. Twenty-six known loss of function mutations in the human EFNB1 gene have been linked to craniofrontonasal syndrome, which includes as a feature cranial synostosis [23]. This suggests an important role for the ephrin-B1 protein in cranial development, and indeed, mouse genetic studies have demonstrated a requirement for ephrins B1 and B2 in neural crest cell migration and subsequent craniofacial patterning [24]. A unique feature of Eph/ephrin signaling is the phenomenon of 'reverse signaling', in which ephrins act as receptors and the Ephs are their ligands [25]. The cytoplasmic domains of B ephrins contain tyrosine residues that can be phosphorylated by src-family kinases and serve as docking sites for SH2-domain signaling proteins such as Grb4 [26–28]. Their C-terminal tails also contain PDZ-binding sequences that bind PDZ-domain containing proteins. Neural crest cell migration

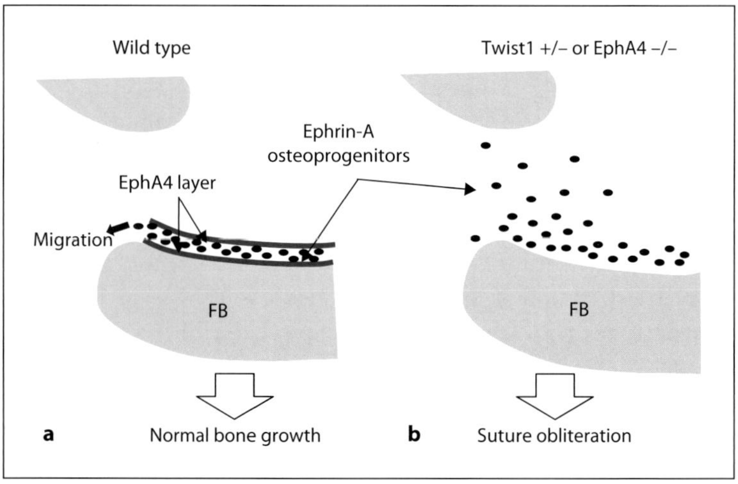

Fig. 3. Eph/ephrin signaling controls osteoprogenitor migration during development of the coronal suture. **a** EphA4 is expressed in twin layers along the surface of the NCC-derived frontal bone (FB) and forms a guidance 'corridor' along which ephrin A2 and A4 expressing osteoprogenitor cells migrate to the leading edge of the extending bone. This preserves the boundary during suture patterning that prevents proliferating frontal bone cells from mineralizing the suture. After E16.5, the suture is formed and is sustained without the action of EphA4. **b** In the Twist1 heterozygous or EphA4 knockout lines, osteoprogenitors are free to migrate into the coronal suture during the developmental period and differentiate, causing osseous obliteration of the suture.

depends on ephrin-B1 reverse signaling from its PDZ-binding tail, as deletion of this tail in mice results in aberrant NCC migration [24].

Two studies from the Maxson group recently described a critical role for EphA4 and its ligands in control of coronal suture formation [19, 29]. They detected EphA4 in two layers on the periosteal surface of the developing frontal bone between E13.5 and E16.5 and in the mesenchyme of the presumptive suture. The upper layer was found to be mesodermally-derived, while the lower was NCC in origin. The layer of NCC-derived frontal bone osteoprogenitor cells between these two layers expressed ephrins -A2 and -A4. These authors' data support a model whereby domains of EphA4 expression activate repulsive reverse signaling in these osteoprogenitors to maintain them in a discreet layer and to direct them along a 'corridor' to the bone front (fig. 3). Twist1$^{+/-}$ mice displayed reduced EphA4 expression, and thus loss of frontal bone NCC 'containment'. In these mutants, the cells migrated into the presumptive suture and differentiated inappropriately to cause suture fusion. The importance of this mechanism in cranial pathology was highlighted by the identification of *EFNA4* mutations in patients with non-syndromic coronal synostosis. Thus, it would appear that a major conserved role of Twist1 is to maintain EphA4/ephrin-A signaling at this particular mesoderm/neural crest boundary.

There is also cause to suspect that Eph/ephrin signaling is involved in regulating bone formation in the calvarial bones long after the developmental period. Zhao et al. recently documented a role for Eph/ephrin signaling in regulation of bone homeostasis [30]. These authors found expression of multiple Ephs and ephrins in primary mouse calvarial OBs. Their data demonstrated that ephrin-B2 expressed on osteoclast precursors inhibited differentiation into multinucleated osteoclasts when stimulated with EphB4 on OBs. At the same time, stimulation of EphB4 forward signaling on OBs by ephrin-B2 induced OB differentiation marker expression and mineralization. We observed ephrin-B2 expression in the periosteal layer and in the dura mater beginning at E14.5. EphB2, a known receptor for ephrin-B2, was also in the same layers and in the bone fronts of the frontal bone. Further, we found that EphB1 is expressed in these bones postnatally (unpublished observations). Treatment with recombinant ephrin-B2 increased bone mass of calvariae in ex vivo culture. This suggests that the unidentified, osteogenic, dura-associated 'insoluble factor' noted in Opperman's earlier work may be ephrin-B2. Our findings thus support a role for ephrins in maintenance of bone growth through Eph forward signaling.

As noted above, the Ephs are RTKs, and, like other RTKs, their activation causes transphosphorylation of specific conserved intracellular tyrosine residues that are necessary for forward signaling-mediated events. The bewildering array of intracellular effectors downstream of activated Ephs has been the subject of other recent reviews ([31] and above), and we will review them only in the depth required by the current discussion (fig. 4). The predominant theme of Eph/ephrin action is modulation of actin dynamics through the Rho family of small GTPases to control cell motility and morphology. RhoA, Rac, and Cdc42 are the prototypical members of this family. All three are activated to bind their downstream effectors when GTP-bound and deactivated when GDP-bound. RhoGTP binds to Rho kinase (ROCK), which ultimately leads to inhibition of actin filament severing and stabilization of actin structures. Globally, this induces structures such as stress fibers and inhibits membrane outgrowth, fluidity, and cell migration. Rac and Cdc42 oppose the action of RhoA in that they stimulate polymerization of new actin filaments to promote lamellipodia and filipodia extension, respectively. Ephs modulate these opposing activities by binding and controlling Rho and Rac guanine nucleotide exchange factors (GEFs), activating proteins (GAPs) and dissociation inhibitors (GDIs). In the case of EphA4, receptor activation of the ephexin RhoGEFs stimulates RhoA, while activation of the RacGAP alpha2-chimaerin inhibits filopodial extension, and activation of the Vav2 RacGEF appears to induce Rac-mediated endocytosis of the receptor [32–34]. How these various signals are integrated in space, magnitude, and time is still largely unknown, but the end result is a repulsive event such as seen in the migratory boundary to osteoprogenitors described above.

But how might Eph forward signaling influence the transcriptional events associated with OB differentiation? One way is through conventional binding of SH2-domain proteins to conserved receptor phosphotyrosines. Phospholipase C gamma (PLCγ), in particular, has been identified as a binding partner for EphA4 [35]. This enzyme is activated by receptor binding to cleave phosphotidylinositol 4,5-bisphosphate (PIP_2) into diacyglycerol (DAG) and inositol 1,4,5 trisphosphate (IP_3). IP_3 binds to its receptors on mitochondria to release intracellular calcium and activate calcium-dependent transcription factors such as the NFATs that regulate Osterix function [36].

Fibroblast Growth Factor Receptors in Cranial Osteoblast Proliferation and Differentiation

The fibroblast growth factors are a family of 18 soluble ligands that guide skeletal patterning through their activation of the 4 FGF receptor (FGFR) tyrosine kinases. The extracellular domains of the FGFRs contain 3 immunoglobulin (Ig)-like domains. Alternative splicing of the Ig III domain (the one closest to the transmembrane domain) into 'b' and 'c' variants influences

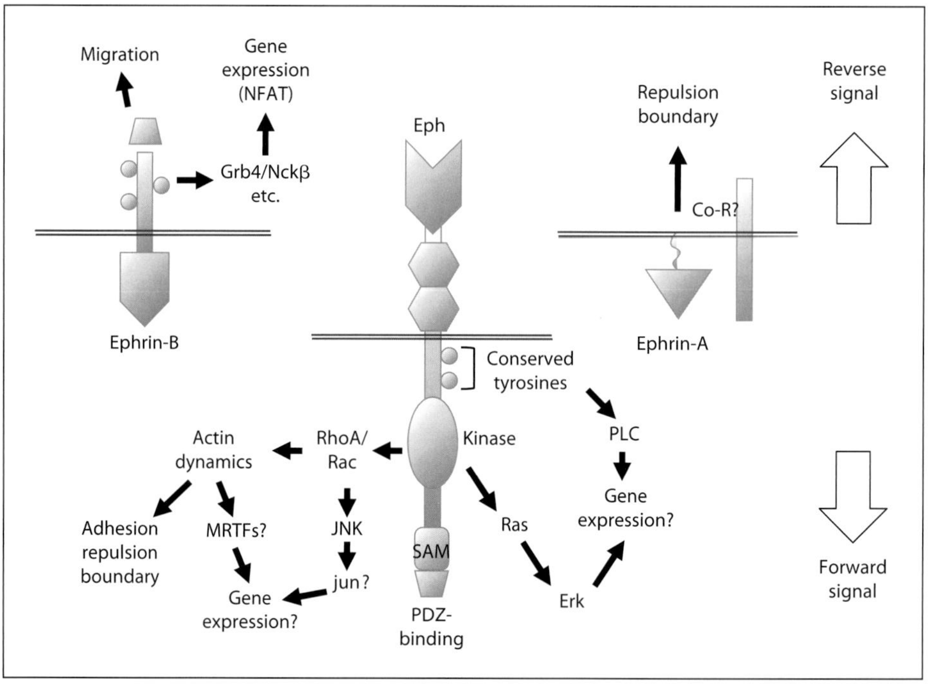

Fig. 4. Simplified diagram of Eph/ephrin signaling. The Eph receptor tyrosine kinases consist of a ligand binding domain and twin fibronectin-like domains on the extracellular domain, a juxtamembrane region containing 2 conserved tyrosine residues that form SH2 binding sites when phosphorylated, and protein tyrosine kinase, sterile alpha motif (SAM), and PDZ-binding sequence in the intracellular domain. Signaling through Ephs proceeds via modulation of receptor-bound Rho and Rac GAPs and GEFs to modulate actin cytoskeletal motility and thereby affect migration and cell morphology. These same pathways may also signal to the nucleus. Binding of SH2 proteins such as PLCγ may also provide for transcriptional regulation. Some reports have also documented Ras/MAPK activation by Ephs (see text). Ephrins may also signal as receptors when bound by Ephs acting as ligands (reverse signaling). The B ephrins have cytoplasmic tails with conserved tyrosines that bind adaptor proteins such as Grb4 when phosphorylated. A ephrins have no cytoplasmic domain and are presumed to couple with a signaling co-receptor to transduce reverse signals.

binding specificity for subsets of FGFs, with the IIIc variants preferentially expressed in mesenchymal cells [37, 38]. The FGFRs 1 and 2 are the most prominently expressed in the cranial sutures, and the number of mutations of these receptors in or near their IgIII domains associated with syndromic craniosynostoses points to their importance in cranial growth. Point mutations in *FGFR1* and *R2* are linked to Pfeiffer syndrome, while *FGFR2* mutations are associated with Apert and Crouzon syndromes. These disease-causing mutations (catalogued in [39] and discussed in further detail in Chapters 5 and 7) are gain-of-function, as they increase ligand binding, receptor dimerization, or tyrosine kinase activity.

Fgfr2 is expressed in a band of undifferentiated osteoprogenitor cells along the outside edge of the developing mouse calvarial bones, while Fgfr1 is expressed in an interior, concentric band made up of an osteoblast layer of cells that rest atop

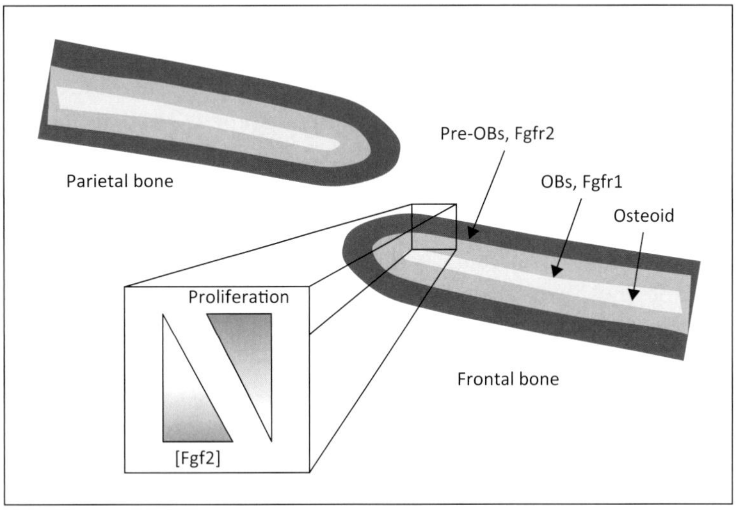

Fig. 5. Diagram of Fgf2 and Fgfr expression patterns in cranial bones. The developing bones contain an inner layer of osteoid that becomes mineralized bone upon OB differentiation. On top of this is a layer of newly formed OBs that primarily express the Fgfr1 and secrete soluble Fgf2, which diffuses to the outer layer of pre-OB cells. These respond to Fgf2 by proliferating due to their expression of the Fgfr2.

the domain of osteoid at the center, but are not yet mineralizing (fig. 5) [40, 41]. Iseki et al. [41] perturbed Fgfr signaling in this system by placing Fgf2-soaked beads (to mimic activating mutations of the receptors) onto E15 mouse coronal sutures. Within 24 hours of this application, they documented downregulation of *Fgfr2* mRNA and expansion of *Fgfr1* mRNA into the suture mesenchyme, where they also found increased osteopontin expression. Based on these results, these authors proposed a model in which Fgfs are secreted from the osteoblast layer in a gradient to control the balance of *Fgfr* expression. The less differentiated osteoprogenitors exposed to the lower concentration express Fgfr2, which stimulates their proliferation in response to the Fgf. The more interior cells express *Fgfr1* and downregulate *Fgfr2* in response to their locally perceived higher Fgf concentration. This model stipulates that Fgfr2 signaling promotes osteoprogenitor proliferation while Fgfr1 promotes OB differentiation.

Loss of function experiments in which the effects of knockout of these receptors were studied in cells of the OB lineage (albeit in long bones) support such a division of labor between the Fgfrs. Yu et al. created a knockout of *Fgfr2* early in the osteo-chondro lineage by crossing a conditional *Fgfr2* allele with a Twist2 cre [42]. These conditional knockout mice exhibited dwarfism and a severe reduction in bone mass throughout the skeleton. Skeletal development and OB commitment/differentiation (including Runx2 expression) in utero were unchanged, but postnatal osteoprogenitor proliferation was dramatically reduced. By contrast, osteoprogenitor proliferation was accelerated in the *Fgfr1*;col2-cre knockout mouse recently created by Jacob et al. [43]. In these mice, the cre was expressed in cells before the division of the chondrocyte and OB lineages, essentially removing Fgfr1 from all stages of OB development. The bones of these mice did not have reduced levels of Runx2 positive cells, indicating no failure in OB fate commitment, but they did display reduced type 1 collagen and osteocalcin, suggesting a deficiency in OB function or differentiation. The same study also examined a conditional knockout of *Fgfr1* in committed pre-osteoblasts by using a col1 cre. These mice had increased bone mass, implying that Fgfr1 functions to inhibit the final transition to the mineralizing OB. One caveat to this finding is that the osteoclast function was reduced in the *Fgfr1*;col1-cre mice. Their increased bone mass could therefore be attributed to decreased resorption, and it is unclear how this would affect bone deposition in the cranial sutures. Nevertheless, accompanying in vitro experiments with primary OB cultures verified increased proliferation in the col2-cre knockout cells with ultimately reduced mineralization, while col1-cre knockout cells showed unchanged alkaline phosphatase activity and increased mineral formation. Taken together, these data support a model in which Fgfr1 acts to increase the abundance of committed pre-osteoblastic cells but discourages final ossification of bone.

Overall then, activating mutations of Fgfr2 may act to increase production of osteoprogenitors in the suture, while activating mutations of Fgfr1 might drive them down the osteoblast lineage. Both lead to bone formation in the suture and premature fusion. But, if Fgfr1 acts to inhibit the final stage of mineralization, why would bone formation not be slowed, thus forestalling fusion? One answer may lie in the production of Fgfr3 by osteoblasts and adjacent cartilage. The Fgfr3c splice variant appears to stimulate OB differentiation in mice and bone marrow stromal cells [44, 45], and while it is downregulated by Fgf2 treatment [41], may tip the final balance toward ossification of the osteoblasts in the suture.

A mystery that remains to be solved is how intracellular signaling downstream of the individual Fgfrs varies such that activation of the different receptors can have such divergent actions on OBs. Fgfrs require the Fgfr Receptor Substrate 2 (FRS2) to signal Fgf actions in target cells (fig. 6). Upon phosphorylation and dimerization, the activated Fgfr phosphorylates FRS on several tyrosine residues, creating docking sites for SH2 domain proteins such as Grb2 and Sos. These, in turn, activate the Ras/MAPK/Erk and PI3K pathways [46, 47]. As Runx2 is a direct substrate for Erks, this raises the possibility that Fgfs may activate OB differentiation through phosphorylation of this transcription factor. Indeed, overexpression of the wild type Fgfr1 or the activated Fgfr1 point mutant in Pfeiffer syndrome (P250R), have been shown to activate Runx2 in OBs. Fgfr2, however, has not been associated with Runx2 activation, and such activation would seem to run counter to the proposed role of Fgfr2 in promoting osteoprogenitor proliferation over differentiation. Fgfrs also bind the SH2 domain of PLCγ independently of FRS2 [48]. Thus, Fgf signaling can activate calcium-mediated events through IP_3 release, and stimulate PKC, which in turn potentiates the MAPK signal.

How then might the cell discriminate between signaling from the two receptors? There are several possible explanations, none of which are mutually exclusive. One lies in the role of FRS2 as a signal integrator. Phosphorylation on FRS2 serine and threonine residues by MAPK reduces its tyrosine phosphorylation, thereby reducing its ability to act as an SH2 adaptor. Thus, FRS2 can function to limit signaling from its own Fgfr in a negative feedback loop, or to allow inhibition of Fgfr signal by other tyrosine kinase receptors such as EGF, which also activate the Ras/MAPK pathway [49]. In the suture milieu, the cell's decision on how to respond to a given level of Fgfr activation will depend greatly on the contribution signals from other elements surrounding it, including MAPK activation/inbition generated from integrins, other Fgfrs, Ephs, and Tgfβrs. This crosstalk is often indirect through shared intracellular intermediates, but can also be direct, as in one recent report of direct binding of EphA4 to Fgfr1 to form a complex that enhances MAPK and PI3K signaling [50]. Since Fgfr1 is predominantly expressed in the OB layer of the calvarial bones, it could be that ephrin stimulation of EphA4 (or other Ephs) acts to promote OB differentiation through potentiation of Fgfr1.

Differential regulation of signal duration from the same signaling pathway can also produce vastly different results in the same cell. A recent study by Xian and coworkers implicates a similar mechanism of Fgfr signal regulation in mammary epithelial cells. These authors found that

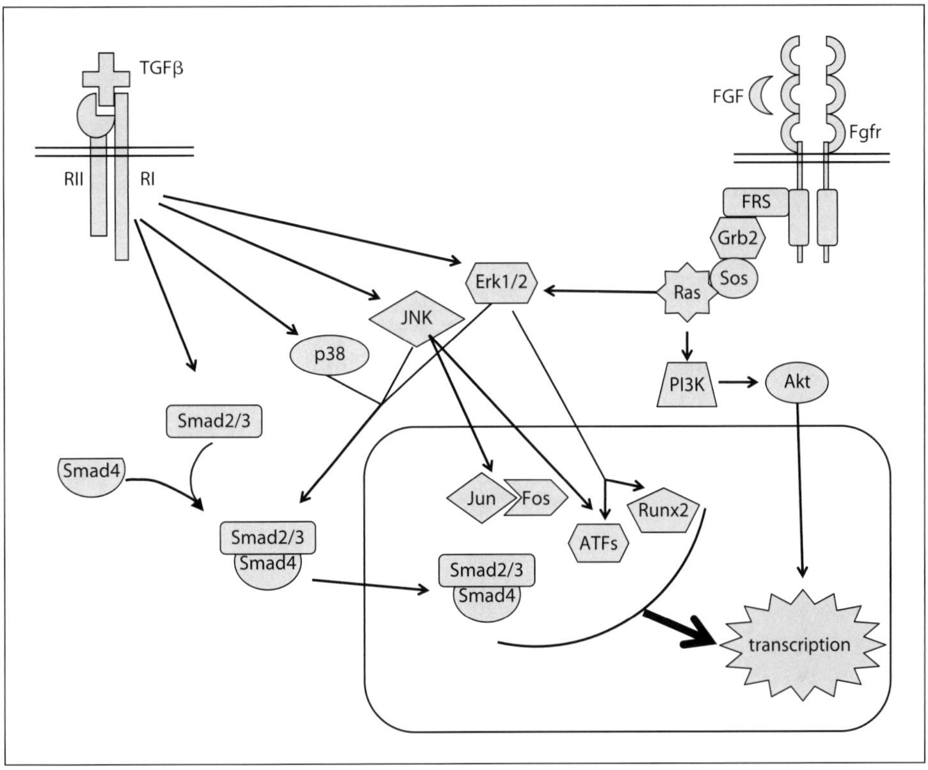

Fig. 6. Diagram in intracellular signaling pathways downstream of the Tgfβr and Fgfrs in osteoblasts. Canonical Tgfβr signaling via the R-Smads 2 and 3 occurs when liganded type II receptor complexes with the type I and phosphorylates it on specific serine and threonine residues. The R-Smads bind to Smad4 and enter the nucleus to activate transcription. The Tgfβr also signals through the MAPK pathways, which are shared with the Fgfrs. Thus, both receptors can regulate transcription factors that control osteoblast differentiation, as well as modulate each others' signals. Thus, levels and duration of activation of each signaling pathway likely combine to fine tune gene expression according to the cell's position in the extracellular matrix and its exposure to different levels/combinations of ligands.

activation of Fgfr2 induced rapid internalization of the receptor and proteosome degradation resulting in a transient Erk signal, while Fgfr1 activation yielded a much more sustained level of Erk activation. The result of this discrimination was that Fgfr1 promoted proliferation and survival while Fgfr2 promoted apoptosis. Both functions were Erk-dependent. Recalling that stimulation in the coronal suture with FGF2 beads led to a dramatic reduction of Fgfr2 and an increase in Fgfr1, it is entirely possible that the difference between Fgfr 1 and 2 actions may stem from this MAPK regulatory mechanism. In support of this scenario, Xian et al. noted that Fgfr1 activation in epithelial cells promoted b1 integrin expression and FAK activation, whereas Fgfr2 activation reduced them [51]. As integrin-induced MAPK activation leads to OB differentiation, these observations are consistent with a role for Fgfr1 in OB differentiation. Different binding affinities for individual Fgfs present in the suture may also influence the delicate balance of Fgfr activation, as strength of ligand binding might affect duration or strength of receptor activation.

Transforming Growth Factor Beta, Osteoblast Function, and Suture Maintenance

The members of the TGF beta superfamily are grouped into three subfamilies based on structure and receptor binding: the TGFβs, the activins, and the bone morphogenetic proteins (BMPs) [52]. We will focus here on the TGFβs and their manifest role in suture maintenance. TGFβ1, β2, and β3 – the forms expressed in mammals – are highly homologous secreted polypeptides that control a variety of developmental processes, including growth, differentiation, and apoptosis [53, 54]. They are secreted as pro-peptides that are proteolytically cleaved and dimerize into the mature, active forms. The expression patterns of each throughout the stages of suture morphogenesis bespeak dynamic and distinct roles in suture formation and stability. While all three are expressed in the bone fronts of patent sutures, TGFβ3 is missing from those of fusing sutures. In the suture mesenchyme, TGFβs are expressed at very low levels until and unless they fuse, at which time, high levels of TGFβ1 and β2 are found [55, 56]. These patterns suggest that the β1 and β2 forms promote suture ossification while β3 maintains patency, and indeed, experimental manipulation of the levels of these factors supports this hypothesis. Addition of purified TGFβ2 or neutralizing antibodies against TGFβ3 to ex vivo calvarial cultures increases cell proliferation and suture ossification. The converse experiment, adding TGFβ3 or antibodies against TGFβ2, decreases proliferation and maintains suture patency [57, 58].

All three TGFβ proteins confer their effects on target cells by binding to the type II receptor, TgfβrII [54] (fig. 6). The liganded receptor is an active serine/threonine kinase that binds to and phosphorylates the type I receptor. Type I and II receptors are dimers, and so the activated Tgfβr signaling complex is a tetramer. Heterozygosity of either receptor causes craniosynostosis in humans as a part of Marfan Syndrome related disorders [59, 60], while conditional deletion of TgfβrII in the cranial neural crest of mice leads to agenesis of calvarial bones [61]. These findings punctuate the requirement for intact TGFβ signaling in cranial development.

The traditional TGFβ receptor signaling pathway is via the cytoplasmic Smads 2 and 3, which bind to and are phosphorylated by the receptor complex. These then dimerize with the co-Smad, Smad4, and enter the nucleus to bind DNA and activate transcription [62]. Smad2 appears to be the central Tgfβr mediator in cranofacial development [63]. Though simple on its face, studies in recent years have uncovered alternate Tgfβr signaling pathways and multiple nodes of intersection with other cytokine and growth factor receptor pathways.

Studies of the signaling pathways activated by TGFβs in the developing calvarium have revealed that the differences in biological effect of the different TGFβ ligands derive from differential activation of the above pathways. TGFβ2 promotion of suture closure was shown to proceed through Erk activation [64, 65], while TGFβ3 functions through Smad2 activation. This is an example of pathway discrimination at the receptor level. At the post-transcriptional level, TGFβ2 also increases expression of Erk1/2 while inhibiting expression of the receptor Smads 2 and 3. The presence of more intermediates in common with the Fgfr pathway may also potentiate abilities of the FGFs to induce proliferation and mineralization. Thus, TGFβ2 tips the long-term balance of the cell toward suture obliteration. Conversely, blockage of Erk1/2 phosphorylation rescues Smad2/3 expression [65] and favors the primary TGFβ3 signaling pathway to preserve suture patency. The key unknown in TGFβ signaling is how the 3 ligands bind the same Tgfβr I and II complex in the same cells but cause differential activation of downstream effectors.

Integration of Signaling and Concluding Remarks

The signaling pathways between Eph/ephrin, FGF and TGFβ receptors are clearly so interwoven as to be inextricable in the control of osteoblast function. Our treatment of these pathways here, simplified though it is, allows us to glimpse how their crosstalk may function to regulate bone synthesis. For example, the combination of MAPK activation from Ephs, Fgfr1, and TGFβ2 activation of Tgfβr in the inner OB layer of the calvarial bones might tip intracellular signaling over a threshold of differentiation and stimulate bone synthesis, whereas the combination of Fgfr2, and TGFβ3 Smad signaling predominance in the outer pre-OB layer might not reach the differentiation threshold but instead favor proliferation.

Though somewhat speculative, this exercise highlights the importance of a full understanding of molecular signaling in the calvarial bone growth centers. Not only is continued elucidation of the pathways downstream of each receptor critical, but also the higher order interactions of cross talk between receptor classes. Our current, primitive level of understanding is already allowing development of rudimentary treatments of bone growth defects such as anti-TGFβ2 treatment of calvarial defects in animal models [66, 67]. A true, in depth picture will facilitate far more targeted and effective treatments for clinical bone disorders in the future.

References

1 Chai Y, Jiang X, Ito Y, Bringas P Jr, Han J, et al: Fate of the mammalian cranial neural crest during tooth and mandibular morphogenesis. Development 2000; 127:1671–1679.

2 Jiang X, Iseki S, Maxson RE, Sucov HM, Morriss-Kay GM: Tissue origins and interactions in the mammalian skull vault. Dev Biol 2002;241:106–116.

3 Opperman LA, Passarelli RW, Morgan EP, Reintjes M, Ogle RC: Cranial sutures require tissue interactions with dura mater to resist osseous obliteration in vitro. J Bone Miner Res 1995;10:1978–1987.

4 Opperman LA, Sweeney TM, Redmon J, Persing JA, Ogle RC: Tissue interactions with underlying dura mater inhibit osseous obliteration of developing cranial sutures. Dev Dyn 1993;198:312–322.

5 Xiao G, Wang D, Benson MD, Karsenty G, Franceschi RT: Role of the alpha2-integrin in osteoblast-specific gene expression and activation of the Osf2 transcription factor. J Biol Chem 1998; 273:32988–32994.

6 Franceschi RT, Ge C, Xiao G, Roca H, Jiang D: Transcriptional regulation of osteoblasts. Ann N Y Acad Sci 2007; 1116:196–207.

7 Zhou G, Zheng Q, Engin F, Munivez E, Chen Y, et al: Dominance of SOX9 function over RUNX2 during skeletogenesis. Proc Natl Acad Sci USA 2006;103: 19004–19009.

8 Ducy P, Zhang R, Geoffroy V, Ridall AL, Karsenty G: Osf2/Cbfa1: a transcriptional activator of osteoblast differentiation. Cell 1997;89:747–754.

9 Komori T, Yagi H, Nomura S, Yamaguchi A, Sasaki K, et al: Targeted disruption of Cbfa1 results in a complete lack of bone formation owing to maturational arrest of osteoblasts. Cell 1997;89:755–764.

10 Otto F, Thornell AP, Crompton T, Denzel A, Gilmour KC: *Cbfa1*, a candidate gene for cleidocranial dysplasia syndrome, is essential for osteoblast differentiation and bone development. Cell 1997;89: 765–771.

11 Ducy P, Karsenty G: Two distinct osteoblast-specific cis-acting elements control expression of a mouse osteocalcin gene. Mol Cell Biol 1995;15:1858–1869.

12 Xiao G, Jiang D, Thomas P, Benson MD, Guan K, Karsenty G, Franceschi RT: MAPK pathways activate and phosphorylate the osteoblast-specific transcription factor, Cbfa1. J Biol Chem 2000;275: 4453–4459.

13 Bialek P, Kern B, Yang X, Schrock M, Sosic D, et al: A twist code determines the onset of osteoblast differentiation. Dev Cell 2004;6:423–435.

14 el Ghouzzi V, Le Merrer M, Perrin-Schmitt F, Lajeunie E, Benit P, et al: Mutations of the TWIST gene in the Saethre-Chotzen syndrome. Nat Genet 1997;15:42–46.

15 Howard TD, Paznekas WA, Green ED, Chiang LC, Ma N, et al: Mutations in *TWIST*, a basic helix-loop-helix transcription factor, in Saethre-Chotzen syndrome. Nat Genet 1997;15:36–41.

16 Satokata I, Ma L, Ohshima H, Bei M, Woo I, et al: Msx2 deficiency in mice causes pleiotropic defects in bone growth and ectodermal organ formation. Nat Genet 2000;24:391–395.

17 Jabs EW, Müller U, Li X, Ma L, Luo W, et al: A mutation in the homeodomain of the human *MSX2* gene in a family affected with autosomal dominant craniosynostosis. Cell 1993;75:443–450.

18 Wilkie AO, Tang Z, Elanko N, Walsh S, Twigg SR, et al: Functional haploinsufficiency of the human homeobox gene *MSX2* causes defects in skull ossification. Nat Genet 2000;24:387–390.

19 Merrill AE, Bochukova EG, Brugger SM, Ishii M, Pilz DT, et al: Cell mixing at a neural crest-mesoderm boundary and deficient ephrin-Eph signaling in the pathogenesis of craniosynostosis. Hum Mol Genet 2006;15:1319–1328.
20 Himanen JP, Saha N, Nikolov DB: Cell-cell signaling via Eph receptors and ephrins. Curr Opin Cell Biol 2007;19:534–542.
21 Pasquale EB: Eph receptor signalling casts a wide net on cell behaviour. Nat Rev Mol Cell Biol 2005;6:462–475.
22 Pasquale EB: Eph-ephrin bidirectional signaling in physiology and disease. Cell 2008;133:38–52.
23 Twigg SR, Kan R, Babbs C, Bochukova EG, Robertson SP, et al: Mutations of ephrin-B1 *(EFNB1)*, a marker of tissue boundary formation, cause craniofrontonasal syndrome. Proc Natl Acad Sci USA 2004;101:8652–8657.
24 Davy A, Aubin J, Soriano P: Ephrin-B1 forward and reverse signaling are required during mouse development. Genes Dev 2004;18:572–583.
25 Davy A, Soriano P: Ephrin signaling in vivo: look both ways. Dev Dyn 2005;232:1–10.
26 Cowan CA, Henkemeyer M: The SH2/SH3 adaptor Grb4 transduces B-ephrin reverse signals. Nature 2001;413:174–179.
27 Cowan CA, Yokoyama N, Saxena A, Chumley MJ, Silvany RE, et al: Ephrin-B2 reverse signaling is required for axon pathfinding and cardiac valve formation but not early vascular development. Dev Biol 2004;271:263–271.
28 Xu NJ, Henkemeyer M: Ephrin-B3 reverse signaling through Grb4 and cytoskeletal regulators mediates axon pruning. Nat Neurosci 2009;12:268–276.
29 Ting MC, Wu NL, Roybal PG, Sun J, Liu L, Yen Y, Maxson RE Jr: EphA4 as an effector of Twist1 in the guidance of osteogenic precursor cells during calvarial bone growth and in craniosynostosis. Development 2009;136:855–864.
30 Zhao C, Irie N, Takada Y, Shimoda K, Miyamoto T, et al: Bidirectional ephrinB2-EphB4 signaling controls bone homeostasis. Cell Metab 2006;4:111–121.
31 Boyd AW, Lackmann M: Signals from Eph and ephrin proteins: a developmental tool kit. Sci STKE 2001:re20.
32 Beg AA, Sommer JE, Martin JH, Scheiffele P: alpha2-Chimaerin is an essential EphA4 effector in the assembly of neuronal locomotor circuits. Neuron 2007;55:768–778.
33 Cowan CW, Shao YR, Sahin M, Shamah SM, Lin MZ, et al: Vav family GEFs link activated Ephs to endocytosis and axon guidance. Neuron 2005;46:205–217.
34 Shamah SM, Lin MZ, Goldberg JL, Estrach S, Sahin M, et al: EphA receptors regulate growth cone dynamics through the novel guanine nucleotide exchange factor ephexin. Cell 2001;105:233–244.
35 Zhou L, Martinez SJ, Haber M, Jones EV, Bouvier D, et al: EphA4 signaling regulates phospholipase Cgamma1 activation, cofilin membrane association, and dendritic spine morphology. J Neurosci 2007;27:5127–5138.
36 Koga T, Matsui Y, Asagiri M, Kodama T, de Crombrugghe B, Nakashima K, Takayanagi H: NFAT and Osterix cooperatively regulate bone formation. Nat Med 2005;11:880–885.
37 Ornitz DM, Xu J, Colvin JS, McEwen DG, MacArthur CA, et al: Receptor specificity of the fibroblast growth factor family. J Biol Chem 1996;271:15292–15297.
38 Turner N, Grose R: Fibroblast growth factor signalling: from development to cancer. Nat Rev Cancer 10:116–129.
39 Wilkie AO: Bad bones, absent smell, selfish testes: the pleiotropic consequences of human FGF receptor mutations. Cytokine Growth Factor Rev 2005;16:187–203.
40 Iseki S, Wilkie AO, Heath JK, Ishimaru T, Eto K, Morriss-Kay GM: Fgfr2 and osteopontin domains in the developing skull vault are mutually exclusive and can be altered by locally applied FGF2. Development 1997;124:3375–3384.
41 Iseki S, Wilkie AO, Morriss-Kay GM: Fgfr1 and Fgfr2 have distinct differentiation- and proliferation-related roles in the developing mouse skull vault. Development 1999;126:5611–5620.
42 Yu K, Xu J, Liu Z, Sosic D, Shao J, et al: Conditional inactivation of FGF receptor 2 reveals an essential role for FGF signaling in the regulation of osteoblast function and bone growth. Development 2003;130:3063–3074.
43 Jacob AL, Smith C, Partanen J, Ornitz DM: Fibroblast growth factor receptor 1 signaling in the osteo-chondrogenic cell lineage regulates sequential steps of osteoblast maturation. Dev Biol 2006;296:315–328.
44 Eswarakumar VP, Schlessinger J: Skeletal overgrowth is mediated by deficiency in a specific isoform of fibroblast growth factor receptor 3. Proc Natl Acad Sci USA 2007;104:3937–3942.
45 Su N, Sun Q, Li C, Lu X, Qi H, et al: Gain-of-function mutation in FGFR3 in mice leads to decreased bone mass by affecting both osteoblastogenesis and osteoclastogenesis. Hum Mol Genet 2010;19:1199–1210.
46 Gotoh N: Regulation of growth factor signaling by FRS2 family docking/scaffold adaptor proteins. Cancer Sci 2008;99:1319–1325.
47 Kouhara H, Hadari YR, Spivak-Kroizman T, Schilling J, Bar-Sagi D, Lax I, Schlessinger J: A lipid-anchored Grb2-binding protein that links FGF-receptor activation to the Ras/MAPK signaling pathway. Cell 1997;89:693–702.
48 Mohammadi M, Honegger AM, Rotin D, Fischer R, Bellot F, et al: A tyrosine-phosphorylated carboxy-terminal peptide of the fibroblast growth factor receptor (Flg) is a binding site for the SH2 domain of phospholipase C-gamma 1. Mol Cell Biol 1991;11:5068–5078.
49 Zhou W, Feng X, Wu Y, Benge J, Zhang Z, Chen Z: FGF-receptor substrate 2 functions as a molecular sensor integrating external regulatory signals into the FGF pathway. Cell Res 2009;19:1165–1177.
50 Fukai J, Yokote H, Yamanaka R, Arao T, Nishio K, Itakura T: EphA4 promotes cell proliferation and migration through a novel EphA4-FGFR1 signaling pathway in the human glioma U251 cell line. Mol Cancer Ther 2008;7:2768–2778.
51 Xian W, Schwertfeger KL, Rosen JM: Distinct roles of fibroblast growth factor receptor 1 and 2 in regulating cell survival and epithelial-mesenchymal transition. Mol Endocrinol 2007;21:987–1000.
52 de Caestecker M: The transforming growth factor-beta superfamily of receptors. Cytokine Growth Factor Rev 2004;15:1–11.
53 Moustakas A, Heldin CH: The regulation of TGFbeta signal transduction. Development 2009;136:3699–3714.
54 Wharton K, Derynck R: TGFbeta family signaling: novel insights in development and disease. Development 2009;136:3691–3697.

55 Opperman LA, Nolen AA, Ogle RC: TGF-beta 1, TGF-beta 2, and TGF-beta 3 exhibit distinct patterns of expression during cranial suture formation and obliteration in vivo and in vitro. J Bone Miner Res 1997;12:301–310.
56 Roth DA, Longaker MT, McCarthy JG, Rosen DM, McMullen HF, et al: Studies in cranial suture biology: Part I. Increased immunoreactivity for TGF-beta isoforms (beta 1, beta 2, and beta 3) during rat cranial suture fusion. J Bone Miner Res 1997;12:311–321.
57 Opperman LA, Adab K, Gakunga PT: Transforming growth factor-beta 2 and TGF-beta 3 regulate fetal rat cranial suture morphogenesis by regulating rates of cell proliferation and apoptosis. Dev Dyn 2000;219:237–247.
58 Opperman LA, Chhabra A, Cho RW, Ogle RC: Cranial suture obliteration is induced by removal of transforming growth factor (TGF)-beta 3 activity and prevented by removal of TGF-beta 2 activity from fetal rat calvaria in vitro. J Craniofac Genet Dev Biol 1999;19:164–173.
59 Loeys BL, Chen J, Neptune ER, Judge DP, Podowski M, et al: A syndrome of altered cardiovascular, craniofacial, neurocognitive and skeletal development caused by mutations in *TGFBR1* or *TGFBR2*. Nat Genet 2005;37:275–281.
60 Mizuguchi T, Matsumoto N: Recent progress in genetics of Marfan syndrome and Marfan-associated disorders. J Hum Genet 2007;52:1–12.
61 Ito Y, Yeo JY, Chytil A, Han J, Bringas P Jr, et al: Conditional inactivation of Tgfbr2 in cranial neural crest causes cleft palate and calvaria defects. Development 2003;130:5269–5280.
62 Shi Y, Massague J: Mechanisms of TGF-beta signaling from cell membrane to the nucleus. Cell 2003;113:685–700.
63 Weinstein M, Yang X, Deng C: Functions of mammalian Smad genes as revealed by targeted gene disruption in mice. Cytokine Growth Factor Rev 2000;11:49–58.
64 Kim HJ, Lee MH, Park HS, Park MH, Lee SW, et al: Erk pathway and activator protein 1 play crucial roles in FGF2-stimulated premature cranial suture closure. Dev Dyn 2003;227:335–346.
65 Opperman LA, Fernandez CR, So S, Rawlins JT: Erk1/2 signaling is required for Tgf-beta 2-induced suture closure. Dev Dyn 2006;235:1292–1299.
66 Mooney MP, Losken HW, Moursi AM, Bradley J, Azari K, et al: Anti-TGF-beta2 antibody therapy inhibits postoperative resynostosis in craniosynostotic rabbits. Plast Reconstr Surg 2007;119:1200–1212; discussion 1213–1235.
67 Mooney MP, Losken HW, Moursi AM, Shand JM, Cooper GM, et al: Postoperative anti-Tgf-beta2 antibody therapy improves intracranial volume and craniofacial growth in craniosynostotic rabbits. J Craniofac Surg 2007;18:336–346; discussion 347–349.

Lynne A. Opperman
Texas A&M Health Science Center
Baylor College of Dentistry
3302 Gaston Ave., Dallas TX, 75246 (USA)
Tel. +1 214 828 8134, Fax +1 214 874 4538, E-Mail lopperman@bcd.tamhsc.edu

Muenke M, Kress W, Collmann H, Solomon BD (eds): Craniosynostoses: Molecular Genetics, Principles of Diagnosis, and Treatment.
Monogr Hum Genet. Basel, Karger, 2011, vol 19, pp 28–44

Signal Transduction Pathways and Their Impairment in Syndromic Craniosynostosis

J.J. Connerney[a] · D.B. Spicer[b]

[a]Department of Biology, Boston University, Boston, Mass., [b]Center for Molecular Medicine, Maine Medical Center Research Institute, Scarborough, Me., USA

Abstract

The cranial sutures act as the growth centers for the flat bones of the skull. They regulate the growth of these bones, but also prevent their premature fusion, known as craniosynostosis, to allow for the growth of the brain. In the past 15 years or so, many of the signaling pathways and transcription factors that regulate cranial suture formation and patency have been identified, largely through the identification of genes that are mutated in syndromic forms of craniosynostosis. While many such genes have been identified as being important in these processes, exactly how these pathways integrate with one another to regulate the formation and morphogenesis of the craniofacial structures is only starting to be understood. In the past few years, functional differences between tissues within the sutures have emerged as critical regulators of suture patency, and several recent studies have begun to determine how changes to this signaling affect these tissues to alter their function and result in craniosynostosis. Here, we review the current literature on the regulation of normal suture growth and patency, and on the events that occur due to changes to these pathways resulting in craniosynostosis.

The skull is composed of 22 separate bones, which are categorized into 2 components, the neurocranium and the viscerocranium. The neurocranium includes the skull vault, which covers the brain and sensory organs, while the viscerocranium comprises the bones of the face. The majority of the cranial bones, especially those of the neurocranium, are known as flat bones and arise from intramembranous ossification, the direct formation of bone from mesenchymal cell precursors. These flat bones of the cranium and face remain separated by openings termed sutures that allow for deformation of the skull during childbirth and absorption of mechanical trauma in childhood. The sutures also function as the growth centers of these bones, allowing growth of the skull during fetal and postnatal development in concert with the expanding brain. With the exception of the metopic suture, which closes during the 2nd or 3rd year of life, the rest of the cranial sutures slowly become more fibrous and interdigitated and eventually ossify during the 2nd or 3rd decade of life. In the mouse, all of the cranial sutures remain patent except for the posterior interfrontal suture, which is equivalent to the metopic suture in humans, and fuses during the first few weeks after birth.

The development of the head and facial structures is a complex interplay between many different signaling pathways, transcription factors, and tissue interactions, and the bones and mesenchyme of the head are derived from both the mesoderm and the cranial neural crest. Because of this complexity, it is not surprising that craniofacial abnormalities are among the most common features of all birth defects. One of the most common classes of craniofacial defects is craniosynostosis, which is the premature fusion of 1 or more of the cranial sutures and occurs in about 1 in 2,500 births. This abnormal fusion of the calvarial bones results in craniofacial dysmorphisms that are accompanied by associated phenotypes such as hypertelorism, mid-face hypoplasia, intracranial hypertension, deafness, respiratory obstruction, and mental retardation. Often, limb abnormalities are also associated with many craniosynostosis syndromes, indicating that similar signaling pathways likely mediate limb development and cranial suture formation and patency. Non-syndromic forms of craniosynostosis are most common, however the identification of mutated genes in the syndromic forms has helped identify many of the signaling pathways and transcription factors that are involved in the formation of the sutures and the regulation of their patency. While many such genes have been identified as being important in these processes, exactly how these pathways and transcription factors integrate with one another to regulate the formation and morphogenesis of the craniofacial structures is only starting to be understood.

Suture Anatomy

The skull vault is composed of paired frontal and parietal bones, the occipital bone (equivalent to the interparietal bone in the mouse), and the membranous portions of the sphenoid and temporal bones (fig. 1). These membranous bones arise from 1 or more mesenchymal condensations that form near the skull base and expand towards the apex of the cranium. Sutures form when these bones appose one another, and fontanels occur where 2 or more sutures meet. The sagittal and metopic sutures (or interfrontal suture in the mouse) form at the midline where the paired parietal or frontal bones approximate each other, respectively. These bones meet in a butt end as opposed to the overlapping nature of the coronal suture, which forms between the frontal and parietal bones. Lineage analysis in the mouse has determined that the coronal suture is at an interface between the neural crest and mesoderm (fig. 2) [1, 2]. The majority of the bones anterior to the coronal suture, including the frontal bone, are derived from the neural crest, while the parietal bone and the suture mesenchyme of the coronal suture are mesodermally derived. The overlap between the frontal and parietal bone primordia is established at E9, with the mesoderm lying external to the neural crest. The initial mesenchymal condensations for the frontal and parietal bones are formed relatively close to one another and maintain this relationship. As these bones expand towards the midline, the coronal suture forms in zipper-like fashion.

There are primarily 4 tissues that contribute to the regulation of the growth of the calvaria bones, suture formation, and suture patency (fig. 1). At the leading edge of the growing calvaria bones are the osteogenic fronts, which are the growth centers for these bones, somewhat equivalent to the growth plates of long bones. These are comprised of highly proliferative cells that express osteogenic markers such as Runx2 and alkaline phosphatase and lay down new bone matrix. The opposing osteogenic fronts are separated by the sutural mesenchyme, which is primarily composed of non-proliferative cells and a fibrous extracellular matrix. The calvaria bones and sutures reside between the periosteal and meningeal membranes, known as the pericranium and dura mater, respectively. There have been numerous studies aimed at determining the roles of these different tissues in the regulation of suture growth and patency. We will focus on recent studies and a few other key findings here, but the reader is referred to several other reviews for a more complete discussion of this topic [3–5].

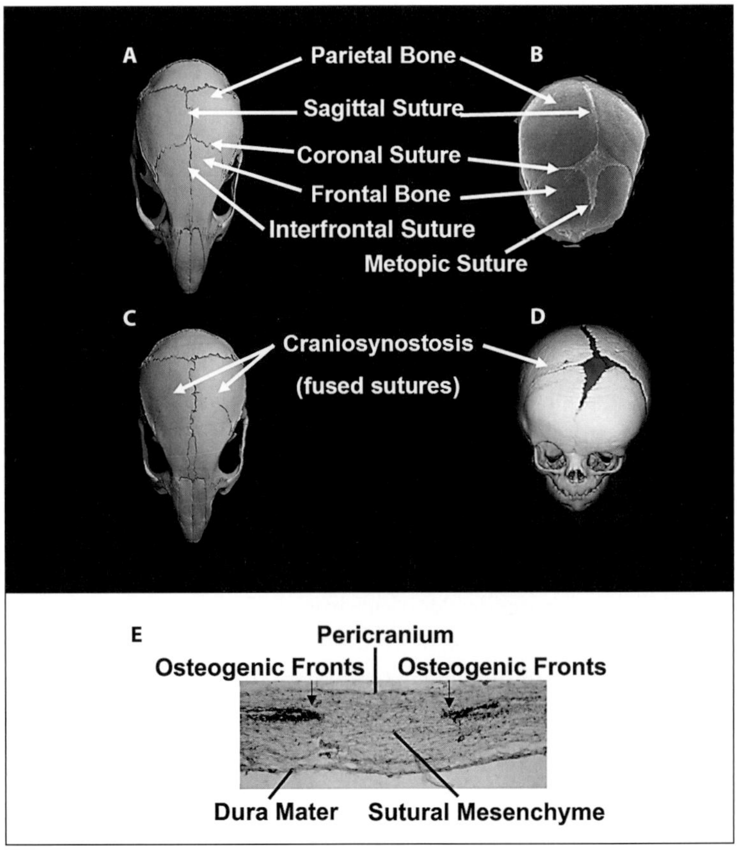

Fig. 1. Skull and suture anatomy. **A**, **B** Normal mouse (**A**) and human (**B**) skulls with the cranial bones and sutures labeled. **C** Twist$^{+/-}$ mouse skull showing fused coronal sutures near the midline. **D** Saethre-Chotzen syndrome patient with fused right coronal suture. **E** Section through sagittal suture of P1 mouse stained for alkaline phosphatase expression to outline the osteogenic fronts. The osteogenic fronts, sutural mesenchyme, dura mater, and pericranium are labeled.

Dura Mater

The dura mater is the meningeal layer that lines the brain and is thus situated between the brain and the calvaria, and changes in the dura mater have long been thought to play a role in regulating suture growth and patency. Many studies, both clinical and experimental, have demonstrated that the dura mater is critical for calvarial growth [3–5]. Several different genetic models have also shown that growth of the calvaria during embryogenesis does not occur in the absence of the dura mater. The most definitive lineage analysis of the different cranial components in the mouse has been done by genetically labeling the neural crest cells before they emigrate from the dorsal aspect of the neural tube and brain, and thus, all neural crest cells are permanently labeled in these mice [1]. Some of the same authors recently extended this with a nice study directly comparing the cranial development of mice with either the neural crest or the cranial mesoderm labeled (fig. 2A, B) [2]. These analyses used double transgenic mice containing the *R26R* reporter transgene, which constitutively expresses β-galactosidase following Cre-mediated recombination, and either the *Wnt1-Cre* transgene, which expresses Cre recombinase in the dorsal neural tube and brain, or *Mesp1-Cre*, which expresses Cre in the progenitors of the cranial

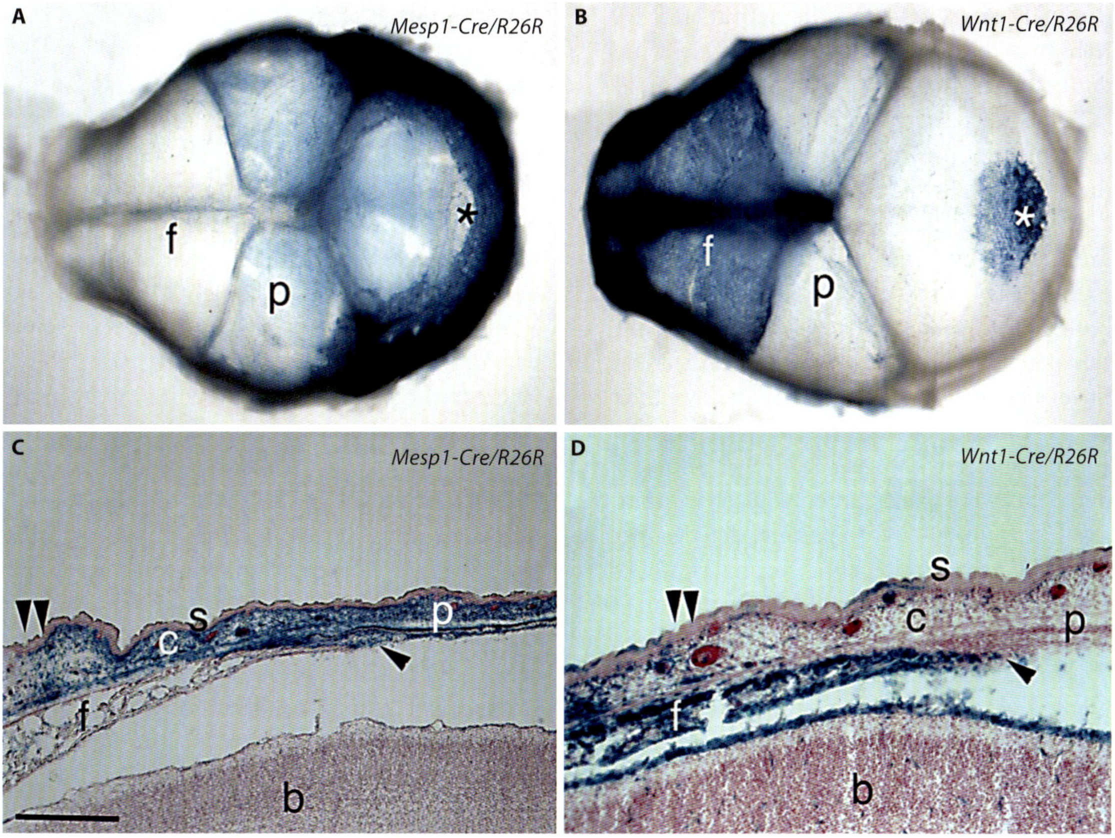

Fig. 2. Mesoderm and neural crest derivation of the skull. **A**, **B** Whole mount X-gal staining of skull vaults at E17.5, brain and the skin removed: reciprocal staining patterns are present in *Wnt1-Cre/R26R* and *Mesp1-Cre/R26R* skulls. **A** The parietal (p) and the lateral parts of the interparietal (asterisk) bones are of mesodermal origin; mesoderm-derived meninges underlie the interparietal bone, showing as a light blue-stained area. **B** The frontal (f) bones and medial part of the interparietal bone (asterisk) are of neural crest origin; faint X-gal staining of the parietal bone is due to underlying neural crest-derived meninges. **C**, **D** Reciprocal patterns of X-gal staining of horizontal sections of the coronal suture (arrowhead) flanked by frontal (f) and parietal (p) bones: the neural crest-mesoderm boundary (double arrowheads) in the dermal connective tissue layer (c) is rostral to that of the skeletogenic layer. b = Brain, s = skin. Reprinted from [2] with permission from Elsevier.

mesoderm. As discussed above, these studies determined that the coronal suture is at an interface between neural crest and mesoderm-derived tissues. They also found that the dura mater under the parietal bone is derived from the neural crest (fig. 2). Many studies have used a similar strategy of using the *Wnt1-Cre* transgene to knockout genes specifically in the neural crest, and several of these conditional knockouts have resulted in defects in the formation or the complete ablation of the mesenchymal tissues derived from the neural crest, collectively known as the ectomesenchyme. For instance, there is a complete loss of the ectomesenchyme following deletion of either *β-catenin* or *Twist1* from the neural crest [6, 7]. In both of these cases, the parietal bone, which is derived from the mesoderm and therefore contained a normal genotype in these mice, did not grow because the underlying dura mater did not form.

While these studies indicate a requirement for the dura mater in calvaria growth, many experiments have provided evidence that it also plays both positive and negative roles in regulating suture patency. Opperman et al. demonstrated that the dura mater was required to maintain the patency of the coronal suture in rats. In these studies, coronal suture complexes from E19 or postnatal day 1 rats were transplanted with or without the associated dura mater to parietal defects of adult rats [8]. They found that the coronal suture complexes that included the dura mater remained patent for up to 3 weeks. However, there was abnormal fusion of the sutures that were transplanted without the dura, suggesting that there is an inhibitory factor secreted by the dura mater that prevents fusion. In contrast, several studies from the Longaker lab have identified an activity of the dura mater that promotes the fusion of the interfrontal suture [9]. The significance of these findings is that they demonstrate that there are regional differences in the dura mater that can act to either promote or inhibit suture fusion. The Longaker lab directly demonstrated this when they excised a rectangular-shaped strip of the contiguous sagittal and interfrontal sutures from day 8 rats, while leaving the underlying dura mater intact. The strip was then rotated 180° and reimplanted into the calvarial defect. They found that after 3 weeks the sagittal suture that was now over the interfrontal dura mater had fused while the interfrontal suture over the sagittal dura mater had remained patent [10]. Collectively, these and other experiments indicate that the dura mater plays an active role in regulating suture patency, but it is still unclear how these regional differences within the dura mater are created.

Pericranium

The pericranium, which overlies the calvaria and cranial sutures, also influences the growth of the calvaria bones but seems to play a lesser role in regulating suture patency. In rodents, only the endocranial side of the interfrontal suture normally fuses, leaving the ectocranial portion open. Moss found that periosteal stripping of this suture consistently promoted the fusion of the ectocranial part of the interfrontal suture, suggesting that a factor in the pericranium is required to keep the sutures patent. However, periosteal stripping over the sagittal suture promoted suture fusion in only 25% of the animals and stripping the pericranium over the coronal suture never led to suture fusion [11]. The role of the pericranium in suture patency was revisited by Opperman et al. in studies where the coronal sutures of fetal and neonatal rats with or without the periostium were transplanted to a calvaria defect of an adult rat, much the same as they did when studying the role of the dura mater, and they found that removal of the periostium did not induce coronal suture fusion [12]. Therefore, as with the dura mater, there are likely regional differences within the pericranium that produce signals that either positively or negatively affect calvaria growth and suture patency.

Osteogenic Fronts and Suture Mesenchyme

While signals from the membranes encasing the sutures play significant roles in regulating the growth and patency of the sutures, the differential response to these signals within the suture mesenchyme and osteogenic fronts also plays a role in this regulation. This is primarily mediated through the differential expression of receptors and positive and negative components of these signaling pathways. In the last several years, distinct functional differences between the osteogenic fronts and the sutural mesenchyme have emerged. In an elegant study by Lana-Elola et al.

using a combination of cell transplantation and cell labeling experiments to determine the contribution of these 2 cell populations to the growth of the parietal bones, they found that only cells within the osteogenic fronts became incorporated within the growing bones. When cells just outside the osteogenic fronts were labeled only a few of these cells were incorporated into the bone, and no cells labeled in the mid-suture did so [13]. This finding is consistent with the lineage mapping experiments using the *Wnt1-Cre;R26R* and *Mesp1-Cre;R26R* mice. Those experiments showed that the frontal bone and osteogenic fronts associated with the frontal bone are derived from the neural crest while the parietal bone, its associated osteogenic front, and the sutural mesenchyme are all mesodermally-derived [1, 2]. Furthermore, by E15.5 the frontal bone has grown up under dermal connective tissue that is mesodermally derived (fig. 2C, D) [2]. Because no labeled cells are incorporated into the frontal bone of the *Mesp1-Cre;R26R* mice, these findings demonstrate that normal growth of these bones occurs primarily, or perhaps exclusively, by proliferation and differentiation of cells within the osteogenic fronts with no recruitment of cells from the sutural mesenchyme. The mid-sutural mesenchyme, however, does have osteogenic potential as these cells can undergo osteogenic differentiation in culture [14], and when an excised piece of mesenchyme from the middle of the sagittal suture was transplanted to the osteogenic fronts some of those cells were incorporated into the growing parietal bone [13]. The converse experiment of transplanting the osteogenic fronts to the mid-suture to see if they would form bone there has not been done, so it is unclear whether the mid-suture lacks an osteogenic promoting signal, or if the cellular, or extracellular environment of the mid-suture is inhibitory to osteogenic differentiation.

This boundary between the osteogenic fronts and sutural mesenchyme may play a crucial role in regulating suture patency. This was first suggested by Merrill et al. when they observed abnormal mixing of sutural mesenchyme cells with the osteogenic fronts in *Twist1*$^{+/-}$ mice, which develop coronal synostosis [15]. This cell mixing was demonstrated using the *Wnt1-Cre;R26R* transgenes on the *Twist1*$^{+/-}$ background. Because this method of cell labeling specifically labels neural crest cells, the genesis of this boundary between the frontal bone osteogenic fronts and the sutural mesenchyme was first interpreted to be due to the differential derivation between these cell populations, and that *Twist1* haploinsufficiency affected 1 or both of these lineages to disrupt the boundary. However, a more recent study from the same group labeled progenitor cells of the parietal bones to demonstrate that a similar boundary existed between the osteogenic fronts of the parietal bone and the sutural mesenchyme, and this boundary was also disrupted in *Twist1*$^{+/-}$ mice [16]. Because the parietal bone and sutural mesenchyme are both derived from the mesoderm, the functional boundary that is defective in the sutures of *Twist1*$^{+/-}$ mice is likely the boundary between osteogenic and non-osteogenic cells determined by the cell labeling studies by Lana-Elola et al. [13] instead of a boundary between the neural crest and mesoderm per se.

Therefore, properties of the sutural mesenchyme may be important regulators of suture patency and these properties may be imposed upon these cells by the underlying dura mater. Indeed, James et al. found that sutural mesenchyme cells isolated from the sagittal and interfrontal sutures had different proliferative and differentiation capabilities. Cells from the interfrontal suture, which normally fuses, proliferated and differentiated to a greater degree than cells from the sagittal suture, which normally remains patent [14]. Furthermore, interfrontal sutural cells had a greater response to FGF2 than cells from the sagittal suture [14], and FGF2 was expressed at higher levels in the dura mater of fusing versus non-fusing sutures [17]. However, the factors regulating suture patency may change as sutures mature. For instance, Kim et al. demonstrated that removal of the dura mater at embryonic stages led to abnormal closure of the sagittal suture, but this did not occur if the dura mater was removed at postnatal stages [18]. There also seems to be natural mixing of cells as the sutures mature, even in sutures that do not fuse. Gagan et al. examined the sutures of *Wnt1-Cre;R26R* mice postnatally and found that cells from the dura mater became incorporated within the sagittal sutures and the calvaria bones. By postnatal day 30 there was a significant contribution of neural crest cells to the parietal bone, and conversely, the dura mater was largely made up of mesodermally-derived cells at this time [19]. Interestingly, they also found that a significant number of osteoclasts were labeled by the *Wnt1-Cre;R26R* transgene postnatally. This is surprising because osteoclasts are usually derived from hematopoietic precursors and not the neural crest. A potential caveat to this conclusion, however, is that the *Wnt1-Cre;R26R* transgenic model does not just label neural crest cells, but will label any cell that at one time expressed *Wnt1*. During embryogenesis *Wnt1* expression is restricted to the dorsal neural tube and brain, and therefore any labeled cell outside of these locations is likely to be a neural crest cell that has migrated from the neural tube. The expression of *Wnt1* postnatally, however, has not been thoroughly characterized and thus the designation of neural crest derivation based upon the presence of the *Wnt1-Cre;R26R* label needs to be done with caution at these later time points.

Genes Associated with Syndromic Craniosynostosis

The regulation of the growth and patency of the cranial sutures, therefore, is mediated by an integrated response to signaling from and within the dura mater, pericranium, osteogenic fronts, and sutural mesenchyme, as well as forces from adjacent tissues such as the brain. In order to identify the mechanisms that promote craniosynostosis we need to understand how changes to this signaling affect each of these tissues to alter their function. Through the identification of gene mutations associated with syndromic forms of craniosynostosis, as well as from gene knockout models in mice that include craniosynostosis as part of the phenotype, the FGF, BMP, TGFβ, Ephrin, and Wnt pathways have all been linked with this anomaly. There is also some evidence that the shh and notch pathways may be involved as well [20, 21]. Thus the mechanisms regulating suture patency are likely quite complex and involve the integration of all of these pathways. Numerous studies in many different systems have documented interactions between many if not all of these pathways, and many of these interactions can be positive or negative depending on what other signaling is concurrently occurring. This complexity could account for the significant amount of phenotypic variability that is observed within craniosynostosis syndromes, even between family members containing the same mutation. In fact, identical mutations in *FGFR2* are associated with different syndromes (Crouzon, Pfeiffer, and Apert syndromes) [22, 23] and mutations to *FGFR1* and *FGFR2* are both associated with the same syndrome (Pfeiffer syndrome) [23]. Below we will introduce the signaling pathways and transcription factors that are altered in syndromic craniosynostosis and will discuss how these pathways may integrate with one another to regulate suture patency and fusion. The genetics of craniosynostosis has recently been extensively reviewed by Passos-Bueno et al., and we refer the reader there for a more detailed description of that and for the primary references [23].

Fibroblast Growth Factor (FGF) Receptors

Genes for 22 highly conserved FGF ligands and 5 FGF receptors (FGFR) have been identified in mammals. FGFRs have 3 extracellular immunoglobulin-like domains, a single hydrophobic membrane-spanning segment, and a split cytoplasmic tyrosine kinase domain. Alternative mRNA splicing of the third Ig domain (IgIII) results in IgIIIb and IgIIIc isoforms, which have different ligand binding specificities. FGFR5, also known as FGFRL1, lacks the split cytoplasmic tyrosine kinase domain and hence the function of FGFRL1 is still unclear, although a mutation within this gene has recently been implicated in craniosynostosis [24]. Signaling by FGFRs requires the formation of a complex involving 2 FGF molecules bound to an FGFR dimer. FGFs have an initial low affinity for FGFRs, however the presence of heparin sulfate proteoglycans (HSP) stabilizes this interaction and promotes a more stable 2:2 FGF:FGFR complex. The high affinity of FGFs to HSPs is also thought to restrict the diffusion of FGFs through tissues [25]. FGF signaling is involved in many processes during embryonic development and in the adult organism, including the regulation of cell proliferation, differentiation, and migration, and it plays a critical role in skeletal biology. Approximately 20% of all cases of craniosynostosis are due to mutations in *FGFR1*, *FGFR2*, or *FGFR3*, and these mutations are found in at least 6 syndromes of craniosynostosis, including Apert, Crouzon, Pfeiffer, Muenke, Jackson-Weiss, and Beare-Stevenson syndromes [23]. Bicoronal craniosynostosis or cloverleaf skull, distinctive facial features, and limb abnormalities most often characterize all of these syndromes. Furthermore, mutations in *FGFR2* and *FGFR3* have been identified in some patients with non-syndromic craniosynostosis suggesting that this may be a common pathway associated with many forms of suture fusion [23].

Mutations to *FGFR1–3* that result in craniosynostosis are all gain-of-function mutations that act dominantly. The mutations confer either ligand-dependent or ligand-independent activation upon the receptor by several different mechanisms, including increased affinity for FGF proteins, loss of FGF-binding specificity, ectopic FGFR splice form expression, and ligand-independent dimerization and activation of the receptor. As noted above, while there are some genotype-phenotype correlations there is also considerable phenotypic variability with different genes associated with the same phenotype as well as the same mutation being found in multiple syndromes, which is exemplified by 1 case where a mother and daughter with the same *FGFR2* mutation presented with clinical features of Crouzon and Pfeiffer syndromes, respectively [26]. This phenotypic variability suggests the presence of genetic modifiers and functional redundancy between receptors.

Activating mutations in *FGFR2* account for approximately 90% of all cases of syndromic craniosynostosis, including Apert, Crouzon, Pfeiffer, Jackson-Weiss, and Beare-Stevenson syndromes [23]. The majority of mutations result in missense amino acid substitutions, and approximately 20% of these either create or destroy cysteine residues. These mutations disrupt intramolecular disulfide bonds, generally in the IgIII domain, and create unpaired cysteines that can form intermolecular disulfide bonds between receptor molecule dimers leading to constitutive activation. These types of ligand-independent activating mutations are found in more severe forms of Pfeiffer and Crouzon syndrome. Mutations that affect splicing of the exons encoding the IgIII domain account for about 10% of Pfeiffer patients, and these cases have more severe limb abnormalities. This same domain was affected in 2 Apert syndrome patients that had *Alu*-element insertions upstream of the exon encoding IgIIIc. All of these mutations result in ectopic, or enhanced expression of the *FGFR2IIIb* isoform, which allows for a different set of FGF ligands, which only bind to FGFR2IIIb, to activate FGF signaling in the normal *FGFR2IIIc* expressing tissue [23]. A similar outcome is achieved by 2 of the most common mutations in the IgII-IgIII linker region that account for the majority of Apert syndrome cases, Ser252Trp and Pro253Arg. These mutations result in enhanced ligand affinity, especially to FGF2 and FGF9, as well as some loss of ligand specificity. The Ser252Trp mutation, which accounts for about 66% of Apert cases, is associated with a more severe phenotype that often includes cleft palate. Homologous mutations to the *FGFR2*(Pro253Arg) mutation are also found in *FGFR1* and *FGFR3*. The *FGFR1*(Pro252Arg) mutation accounts for ~5% of Pfeiffer syndrome cases, which tend to have a milder phenotype than the cases caused by *FGFR2* mutations. The homologous mutation in *FGFR3*, Pro250Arg, is found in 6–8% of all craniosynostosis patients and causes Muenke syndrome, which is the most common form of syndromic craniosynostosis. In general, these homologous mutations in *FGFR1* and *FGFR3* result in milder phenotypes than the *FGFR2*(Pro253Arg) mutation associated with Apert syndrome [23]. This is most likely due to the different relative expression patterns and expression levels of the receptors within the sutures and elsewhere than to distinct differences in receptor signaling, and this will be discussed further below.

TWIST1

Haploinsufficiency of *TWIST1* is associated with Saethre-Chotzen syndrome (SCS), which is one of the most common autosomal dominant disorders of craniosynostosis, occurring in 1 in 25,000 to 1 in 50,000 live births [27]. The most frequent clinical phenotypes include abnormal head shape due to premature closure of the coronal suture, hypertelorism, and mid-face deficiency. Typical limb abnormalities include soft tissue syndactyly. More than 100 different mutations have been identified within the *TWIST1* gene, suggesting the SCS phenotype is due to haploinsufficiency of *TWIST1* [23]. This is also indicated by the fact that $Twist1^{+/-}$ mice present with a similar phenotype, including premature closure of the coronal suture and limb abnormalities, and thus represent a useful model for SCS [28]. Mutations in *FGFR2* and *FGFR3* have been reported in some patients that have phenotypes consistent with SCS, indicating that haploinsufficiency of *TWIST1* gives a similar phenotype as activation of FGFR signaling [23].

MSX2

Boston-type craniosynostosis results from a mutation in *MSX2*, a highly conserved homeobox gene on the long arm of chromosome 5. This autosomal dominant disorder is characterized by synostosis of the coronal suture and presents with variable phenotypes that include fronto-orbital recession, frontal bossing and turribrachycephaly. The mutation is a C to A transversion resulting in a substitution of a histidine for a proline (Pro148His) within the DNA-binding region of the protein. This increases the DNA-binding affinity of the protein resulting in enhanced protein activity [3]. In the last few years several patients with craniosynostosis have been identified who have an extra copy of *MSX2*, further supporting that *MSX2* gain-of-function promotes craniosynostosis ([29] and references within). Conversely, mutations that result in *MSX2* haploinsufficiency cause ossification deficiencies and parietal foramina [3].

Eph/Ephrin Signaling

The Eph receptors are one of the largest receptor tyrosine kinase (RTK) families. The ligands of these RTK's are the ephrins which are divided into 2 subclasses. The A-subclass: ephrinA1–ephrinA5 which are anchored to the membrane by a glycosylphosphatidylinositol (GPI) linkage; and the B-subclass: ephrinB1–ephrinB3 which have a transmembrane domain with a short cytoplasmic region. Eph/ephrin signaling is important in the regulation of cell migration and in the establishment of tissue boundaries during embryonic development. The interaction between the Eph receptor with its corresponding ephrin ligand causes a simultaneous activation of downstream signaling in both the receptor- and ligand-expressing cells.

Loss-of-function mutations in *EFNB1* cause craniofrontonasal dysplasia. This is an X-linked dominant disorder that predominantly and more severely affects females. These patients present with coronal synostosis with brachycephaly, hypertelorism, downslanting palpebral fissures, clefting of the nasal tip, cleft lip and palate, abnormal clavicles and raised scapulae [23] (see Chapter 10). Mutations within the *EFNA4* gene have also been found in several patients with non-syndromic craniosynostosis [15].

TGFβ Signaling

Mutations in *TGFBR1* and *TGFBR2* result in craniofacial defects resembling marfanoid craniosynostosis [30]. These are the first mutations in this pathway directly linking it with craniosynostosis in humans, and this finding supports several studies by Opperman and colleagues, which have implicated TGFβ signaling in the regulation of suture patency (e.g. [31]). TGFβ2 and TGFβ3 have opposing effects on suture patency. Addition of TGFβ2 to patent sutures will promote fusion, while neutralizing antibodies to TGFβ2 will prevent synostosis of fusing sutures. The opposite is true for TGFβ3, which acts by downregulating the expression of *TGFBR1* [31].

Integration of Pathways and Mechanisms of Craniosynostosis

How these different signaling pathways and transcription factors integrate with each other to alter the function of the sutural tissues and promote craniosynostosis is not clearly understood. Is there an underlying mechanism that is common to both syndromic and non-syndromic forms of craniosynostosis, or are there separate means to achieve the same outcome? The fact that *FGFR* mutations are found in the vast majority of syndromic cases and have been identified in some cases of non-syndromic craniosynostosis would suggest that at least FGF signaling is central to this process.

Approximately 20% of all cases of craniosynostosis are due to alterations in one of the FGF receptor genes, which result in a gain-of-function mutation through different mechanisms [23]. Several mouse models with increased FGF signaling support this. The *Bey* (bulgy-eye) mouse mutant that contains an intragenic retroviral insertion between the *Fgf3* and *Fgf4* genes that increases the expression of these genes develops synostosis of several sutures [32]. Similarly, the *Eks* (Elbow-knee-synostosis) mouse mutant develops coronal synostosis due to a gain-of-function mutation in the *Fgf9* gene [33]. Additionally, a mouse mutant was developed to study the function of *FGFR2IIIc* by deleting exon 9 of *Fgfr2* [34]. This effectively eliminated transcripts encoding FGFR2IIIc but also resulted in the ectopic expression of *Fgfr2IIIb*, and these mice develop coronal synostosis. As a further indication that this was a gain-of function phenotype, heterozygous loss of *Fgf10*, one of the FGFR2IIIb-specific ligands, prevented craniosynostosis in these mice [35]. However, decreased FGF receptor expression is also associated with craniosynostosis. Mice containing a point mutation that prevented the translation of the *Fgfr2IIIc* isoform and did not affect *Fgfr2IIIb* expression also developed craniosynostosis [36]. These mice had a deficiency in ossification and delayed formation of the midline sutures with a shift towards less proliferation and premature differentiation. This resulted in synostosis of several sutures in the skull base and the coronal suture. Somewhat surprisingly, mice where *Fgfr2* was deleted using *Dermo1-Cre*, which results in *Fgfr2* deletion in osteoblast and chondrocyte progenitor cells, were phenotypically normal at birth and only later developed growth retardation and a dome-shaped skull, indicating that *Fgfr2* is not required for osteoblast proliferation or differentiation during early skull formation [37]. Therefore, tight control of FGF signaling is essential for normal suture formation and patency.

Fgfr1, Fgfr2, and *Fgfr3* are all expressed in the sutures. *Fgfr1* is expressed in the differentiating osteoblasts that are associated with the edge of the osteoid. *Fgfr2* is highly expressed in the proliferating cells in the osteogenic fronts just outside of the *Fgfr1* domain, and is expressed at much lower levels in the sutural mesenchyme. *Fgfr3* expression is similar to *Fgfr2* except at much lower levels [38–41]. Rice et al. defined these expression domains further by determining the expression patterns of the IIIb and IIIc isoforms of each of these receptors [42]. In many areas of the embryo the IIIb and IIIc FGF receptor isoforms are associated with epithelial and mesenchymal expression patterns, respectively, while the FGF ligands that specifically interact with each of these receptors are expressed in the reciprocal domain. In the mesenchymal tissues of the sutures, however, some of the genes associated with epithelial expression are also present. The expression domains of the IIIc isoforms of all 3 FGF receptors correspond to the previously defined expression domains described above. *Fgfr1IIIb* and *Fgfr3IIIb* are not expressed in the sutures, however *Fgfr2IIIb*, which is usually associated with epithelial expression, is expressed in a similar pattern as *Fgfr2IIIc* in the osteogenic fronts and sutural mesenchyme, only at lower levels. Importantly, as analyzed by RT-PCR, the expression of all of the FGF ligands except *Fgf4* and *Fgf8* was detected in sutural tissues [43]. *Fgf2* and *Fgf9* are probably the most abundantly expressed FGF ligands in the sutures and both are highly expressed in the sutural mesenchyme and underlying dura mater, with low levels in the osteogenic fronts [17, 18, 42]. FGF2 can activate all FGF receptors while FGF9 only activates the IIIc isoforms of all 3 FGF receptors, as well as FGFR3IIIb [25]. Therefore, similar to the paracrine signaling between the epithelial and mesenchymal tissues in other parts of the embryo, these expression patterns suggest that FGF ligands from the mid-suture act in a paracrine manner to regulate the growth of the osteogenic fronts. The *Eks* mouse mutant gives some insight into this. These mice contain a mutation in *Fgf9* that prevents FGF9 homodimerization. FGF9 monomers have a lower affinity for heparin than the dimeric FGF9 molecules and thus have increased diffusion through developing tissues leading to ectopic FGF9 signaling [33]. Therefore, the osteogenic fronts would receive a higher concentration of the mutant FGF9 protein, which would lead to enhanced proliferation and differentiation. This is essentially the complementary mechanism that occurs due to the *FGFR3*(Pro250Arg) mutation that enhances the binding affinity of FGFR3 for FGF9 and causes Muenke syndrome [44]. In that case, the increased affinity would allow FGFR3(Pro250Arg) to respond to lower levels of FGF9, thus expanding the area of activation.

In line with their expression patterns, *Fgfr2* is associated with osteoblast proliferation while *Fgfr1* is associated with promoting early osteoblast differentiation. Whether there is a functional difference in the signaling by these receptors or if the difference is in the stage of differentiation that the cells expressing the different receptors are in is still unclear. Early osteogenic differentiation is correlated with downregulation of *Fgfr2* expression, which can be seen both in vivo and in vitro. Decreased expression of FGFR2 was observed in the sutures of patients with Apert and Pfeiffer syndromes who had activating mutations in *FGFR2* [45]. In addition, calvaria osteoblasts isolated from *Fgfr2*(Ser252Trp) mice, which model Apert syndrome, had an increased capacity for proliferation and also differentiated better than controls. This increased differentiation correlated with the downregulation of *Fgfr2* expression [46]. However, when wild type osteoblasts were transfected with constitutively expressing constructs for either *Fgfr2*(Ser252Trp) or *Fgfr2*(Cys352Tyr), a mutation found in Crouzon syndrome, the osteoblasts were inhibited from differentiating [47], demonstrating the necessity of this negative FGFR2 autoregulation for the promotion of differentiation. In contrast, expression of FGFR1 has been associated with the promotion of differentiation by directly inducing the expression of *Runx2* [48]. *Runx2* encodes an early marker of osteogenic differentiation that is required for osteoblast differentiation and can promote osteogenic differentiation when expressed in mesenchymal stem cells [49]. *Fgfr1*(Pro250Arg) mice, a model of Pfeiffer syndrome, have increased expression of *Runx2* in their sutures and transfection of 10T1/2 fibroblasts with an *Fgfr1*(Pro250Arg) expression plasmid induced the expression of *Runx2* [48]. However, while *Runx2* may be induced, addition of FGF to these cells or to other osteoblast cell lines, which express high levels of endogenous *Fgfr1*, prevents their differentiation [50], indicating that this regulation is complex. The expression of *Runx2* within the sutures is also much broader than *Fgfr1* expression, and extends throughout the osteogenic fronts encompassing the expression domains of both *Fgfr1* and *Fgfr2* [41], suggesting there may be other components to this regulation.

The promotion of early but not late osteoblast differentiation by FGF can be recapitulated in the sutures by the addition of FGF-soaked beads. FGF2 beads placed on the coronal sutures of E15.5 mice decreased the expression of *Fgfr2* and *Fgfr3* while increasing the expression of *Fgfr1* and *Spp1* (osteopontin), but later differentiation and mineralization was inhibited [38, 39]. FGF4 beads had a similar effect on late differentiation when placed on the parietal bone, inhibiting the expression of the late osteogenic marker *Bsp* [42]. Interestingly, the placement of FGF4 or FGF2 beads on the osteogenic fronts of the sagittal suture in E15.5 calvaria explant cultures promoted suture closure, while placement of the beads in the mid-suture resulted in increased proliferation but did not promote suture closure [18, 51]. The differential response of these 2 cell populations to the FGF beads is very similar to the differential response of cranial neural crest cells to low and high doses of FGF. FGF signaling is required for the osteogenic differentiation of cranial neural crest cells, which form much of the skull, but low levels of FGF induce cell proliferation and inhibit differentiation while high levels of FGF do the opposite [52]. The differential expression of the FGF receptors in the sutures, low in the mid-suture and high in the osteogenic fronts, may mediate the differential response to the FGF beads by generating low and high amounts of signaling in these respective locations resulting in differing outcomes. Consistent with this hypothesis, *Twist1*$^{+/-}$ mice have increased expression of *Fgfr2* in the sutural mesenchyme [42, 51, 53], and when FGF2 beads were placed on the mid-suture of these mice in calvaria explant cultures the FGF beads promoted suture closure [51].

The role of bone morphogenetic protein (BMP) in the regulation of suture formation and patency is still unclear. As their name implies, BMPs can promote osteogenic differentiation, but only in the right context. There are no mutations to this pathway that result in craniosynostosis, but that may be due to the requirement of this pathway for many earlier developmental processes, which results in loss of viability of mice with mutations in this pathway. Many studies have shown that inhibition of BMP signaling inhibits osteogenic differentiation. Furthermore, addition of the BMP inhibitor noggin to either naturally fusing or pathogenically fusing sutures can prevent synostosis from occurring [54]. However, BMP beads placed on the osteogenic fronts or on the mid-suture did not promote suture closure in calvaria explant cultures as observed when FGF beads were used [18]. This suggests that BMP signaling is necessary but not sufficient to promote suture closure.

FGF signaling seems to integrate with BMP signaling to mediate differential gene regulation within the sutures. BMP signaling induces the expression of *Msx2* [18] as well as the expression of the helix-loop-helix (HLH) inhibitor *Id1* [42] and the BMP inhibitor *noggin (Nog)* [17, 55]. However, BMP signaling is most active in the osteogenic fronts [16–18, 51] where *Id1* and *noggin* are most highly expressed [17, 42, 46, 53], while *Msx2* is predominantly expressed in the mid suture mesenchyme [18], suggesting that there may be different mechanisms of induction for these genes. Indeed, Rice et al. found that the presence of the *Foxc1* transcription factor was required for BMP induction of *Msx2* but not for the induction of *noggin*. Consistent with such a role, *Foxc1* is expressed in a similar domain as *Msx2* in the sutural mesenchyme and dura mater but not in the osteogenic fronts, and *Foxc1*$^{-/-}$ mice have low expression of *Msx2* [56].

Interestingly, *Foxc1* expression is regulated by FGF signaling [55]. The edge of *Foxc1* expression, just outside the osteogenic fronts [56], corresponds to the boundary between osteogenic and non-osteogenic cells in the suture, discussed previously in this review, which is also the border between high and low FGF signaling. Because increased *MSX2* expression, which is regulated by FOXC1, results in craniosynostosis [23, 29], maintenance of this border in gene expression seems critical in maintaining suture patency. This is indicated in *Twist1*$^{+/-}$ mice, where this boundary is disrupted and *Msx2* expression is increased, but craniosynostosis is prevented in *Twist1*$^{+/-}$; *Msx2*$^{+/-}$ mice [15].

The Eph/Ephrin signaling pathway also seems to play an important, although still unclear role in this process. Mutations in *EFNB1* (ephrin-B1) are associated with craniofrontonasal syndrome, which includes craniosynostosis [23], and mutations in *EFNA4* (ephrin-A4) have been identified in several patients with non-syndromic craniosynostosis [15]. Whether mutation of these different members of this pathway promotes craniosynostosis using the same mechanism is not known. The genes encoding the ephrin-A2 and ephrin-A4 ligands and the EphA4 receptor are all expressed in the developing frontal bone and within the sutures, and their expression decreases or is altered in *Twist1*$^{+/-}$ mice correlating with the loss of the osteogenic/non-osteogenic boundary [15]. However, none of the *ephrin* or *Eph* genes analyzed in that study were expressed in a pattern to suggest that they suffice for the formation or maintenance of this boundary [15]. Recently, Ting et al. demonstrated that *EphA4*$^{-/-}$ mice developed a similar phenotype as the *Twist1*$^{+/-}$ mice, including the disruption of this same boundary and the later development of craniosynostosis. Furthermore, the double heterozygous *EphA4*$^{+/-}$;*Twist1*$^{+/-}$ mice had a more severe suture phenotype than *Twist*$^{+/-}$ mice. This study observed defects in cell migration in the *EphA4*$^{-/-}$ mice that were suggested to affect cell recruitment to the forming bones [16]. Mutations in X-linked *EFNB1* affect female patients more severely than males, which is thought to be due to chimeric loss-of-function from random X inactivation [23]. A study by Davy et al. found that this mosaic loss of *ephrin-B1* resulted in defective gap junction formation and aberrant osteoblast differentiation [57] (see Chapter 10).

From the above discussion it is evident that suture formation and patency are regulated by many different signaling pathways and that there is substantial cross-talk between these pathways. As a result, it is difficult to draw a linear pathway for the regulation of these processes. The experimental evidence indicates that the genes that are most often associated with craniosynostosis, *FGFR1–3*, *TWIST1*, and *MSX2*, are central in this regulation. *Twist1* seems to be upstream of both *Msx2* and FGF signaling since the expression of *Msx2* and *Fgfr2* is expanded in the sutures of *Twist1*$^{+/-}$ mice [15, 42, 51, 53], although *Twist1* may be downstream of FGF signaling as well. FGF beads induced *Twist1* expression in calvaria explant cultures [42], however *Twist1* expression was relatively normal or slightly decreased in the sutures of *Fgfr2*(Ser252Trp) mice [46]. In the limbs, FGF induction of *Twist1* is indirect [58], suggesting that this regulation in the sutures may be more complex as well.

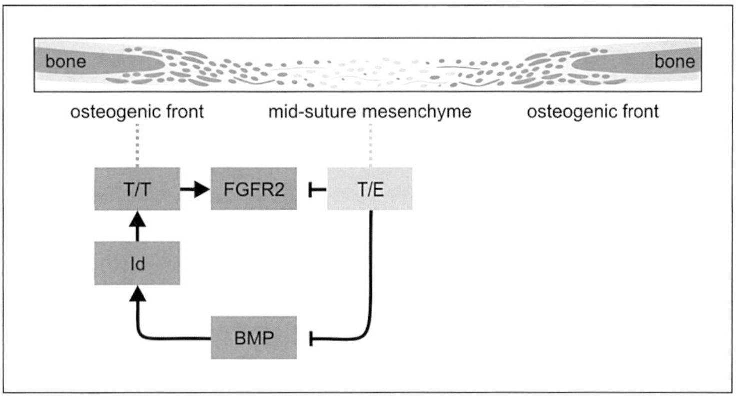

Fig. 3. Twist1 complexes define FGF activity within the suture. Twist1 homodimers (T/T) induce Fgfr2 expression in the osteogenic fronts while Twist1/E protein heterodimers (T/E) inhibit its expression in the mid-suture. This dual control helps to define a distinct border of high and low Fgfr2 expression. The T/T domain is defined by Id expression, which is induced by canonical BMP signaling. T/E dimers inhibit the BMP-Smad pathway [60] helping to restrict Id expression. When Twist levels decrease in *Twist1* haploinsufficiency, BMP activity and Id expression are increased, enhancing T/T formation and Fgfr2 expression [51, 53].

Twist1 has both positive and negative effects on *Fgfr2* expression depending on whether it interacts with itself to form homodimers or interacts with ubiquitously expressed bHLH E proteins to form heterodimers (fig. 3) [51, 53]. This dual regulation helps define the border of high and low FGF signaling between the osteogenic fronts and suture mesenchyme. The ratio between the Twist1 dimers is regulated by the HLH Id proteins, which in turn are induced by BMP signaling. This ratio is disrupted in *Twist1*$^{+/-}$ mice resulting in an increase in FGF and BMP signaling throughout the sutures. Decreasing Id levels, by crossing *Twist1*$^{+/-}$ mice with *Id1*$^{-/-}$ mice, prevented craniosynostosis [51, 53], which may be part of the mechanism of how administration of noggin can prevent suture fusion [54].

Finally, is the disruption of this osteogenic/non-osteogenic boundary necessary or sufficient for craniosynostosis? The formation of this boundary seems to be equivalent to the formation of a functional suture, where the boundary prevents the progression of the osteogenic fronts into the sutural space. The models where this has been best characterized, *Twist1*$^{+/-}$, *EphA4*$^{+/-}$, and *Fgfr2*(Ser252Trp) mice, indicate that this boundary really never forms at the base of the coronal sutures that are predisposed to fusion in these models [15, 16, 46]. However, as the calvaria extend apically in these mice a relatively normal coronal suture does form [46, 51, 53]. Fusion of the coronal sutures in *Twist1*$^{+/-}$ mice occurs at different places along the suture and is not confined or even more prevalent at the lateral base of the suture where boundary disruption is most often observed (fig. 1) [15, 16, 46]. This suggests that while boundary disruption may be required for synostosis, it may not necessarily be a predictor of where or if synostosis will occur. Because fusion often initiates near the midline, it also suggests that abnormal signaling can disrupt a seemingly normally functioning boundary. This latter point was demonstrated by Shukla et al. who found that administration of FGF inhibitors in utero can prevent craniosynostosis in *Fgfr2*(Ser252Trp) mice, but they also showed that removal of these inhibitors after birth can initiate craniosynostosis at that time [59], demonstrating that disruption of suture integrity can occur in presumably normally functioning sutures. Conversely, boundary disruption during embryonic development does not seem to be sufficient for craniosynostosis to occur since inhibition of FGF signaling after birth was sufficient to prevent craniosynostosis in *Twist1*$^{+/-}$ mice [51], which is promising for therapeutic interventions. In many of these models, enhanced growth and differentiation of the osteogenic fronts is associated with craniosynostosis. However, in a model where Twist1 homodimers were overexpressed in the sutures, there was abnormal growth and differentiation of the calvaria bones that resulted in a large overlap of the frontal and parietal bones forming the coronal suture, but there was no synostosis of these bones [51]. Thus, increased proliferation and differentiation is not sufficient to promote craniosynostosis, which may indicate that the process of craniosynostosis can be broken down into at least 2 distinct events. One involves the breakdown of the osteogenic/non-osteogenic boundary allowing the progression of the osteogenic fronts, and the other is the actual bony fusion, of which much less is known. Understanding these separable processes may open new therapeutic strategies to manage the growth and fusion of these bones.

References

1 Jiang X, Iseki S, Maxson RE, Sucov HM, Morriss-Kay GM: Tissue origins and interactions in the mammalian skull vault. Dev Biol 2002;241:106–116.

2 Yoshida T, Vivatbutsiri P, Morriss-Kay G, Saga Y, Iseki S: Cell lineage in mammalian craniofacial mesenchyme. Mech Dev 2008;125:797–808.

3 Lenton KA, Nacamuli RP, Wan DC, Helms JA, Longaker MT: Cranial suture biology. Curr Top Dev Biol 2005;66:287–328.

4 Rice DP: Developmental anatomy of craniofacial sutures. Front Oral Biol 2008;12:1–21.

5 Cohen MM Jr: Sutural biology and the correlates of craniosynostosis. Am J Med Genet 1993;47:581–616.

6 Bildsoe H, Loebel DA, Jones VJ, Chen YT, Behringer RR, Tam PP: Requirement for *Twist1* in frontonasal and skull vault development in the mouse embryo. Dev Biol 2009;331:176–188.

7 Brault V, Moore R, Kutsch S, Ishibashi M, Rowitch DH, et al: Inactivation of the beta-catenin gene by *Wnt1-Cre*-mediated deletion results in dramatic brain malformation and failure of craniofacial development. Development 2001;128:1253–1264.

8 Opperman LA, Sweeney TM, Redmon J, Persing JA, Ogle RC: Tissue interactions with underlying dura mater inhibit osseous obliteration of developing cranial sutures. Dev Dyn 1993;198:312–322.

9 Roth DA, Bradley JP, Levine JP, McMullen HF, McCarthy JG, Longaker MT: Studies in cranial suture biology: part II. Role of the dura in cranial suture fusion. Plast Reconstr Surg 1996;97:693–699.

10 Levine JP, Bradley JP, Roth DA, McCarthy JG, Longaker MT: Studies in cranial suture biology: regional dura mater determines overlying suture biology. Plast Reconstr Surg 1998;101:1441–1447.

11 Moss ML: Inhibition and stimulation of sutural fusion in the rat calvaria. Anat Rec 1960;136:457–467.

12 Opperman LA, Persing JA, Sheen R, Ogle RC: In the absence of periosteum, transplanted fetal and neonatal rat coronal sutures resist osseous obliteration. J Craniofac Surg 1994;5:327–332.

13 Lana-Elola E, Rice R, Grigoriadis AE, Rice DP: Cell fate specification during calvarial bone and suture development. Dev Biol 2007;311:335–346.

14 James AW, Xu Y, Wang R, Longaker MT: Proliferation, osteogenic differentiation, and FGF-2 modulation of posterofrontal/sagittal suture-derived mesenchymal cells in vitro. Plast Reconstr Surg 2008; 122:53–63.

15 Merrill AE, Bochukova EG, Brugger SM, Ishii M, Pilz DT, et al: Cell mixing at a neural crest-mesoderm boundary and deficient ephrin-Eph signaling in the pathogenesis of craniosynostosis. Hum Mol Genet 2006;15:1319–1328.

16 Ting MC, Wu NL, Roybal PG, Sun J, Liu L, et al: *EphA4* as an effector of *Twist1* in the guidance of osteogenic precursor cells during calvarial bone growth and in craniosynostosis. Development 2009; 136:855–864.

17 Warren SM, Brunet LJ, Harland RM, Economides AN, Longaker MT: The BMP antagonist noggin regulates cranial suture fusion. Nature 2003;422:625–629.

18 Kim HJ, Rice DP, Kettunen PJ, Thesleff I: FGF-, BMP- and Shh-mediated signalling pathways in the regulation of cranial suture morphogenesis and calvarial bone development. Development 1998; 125:1241–1251.

19 Gagan JR, Tholpady SS, Ogle RC: Cellular dynamics and tissue interactions of the dura mater during head development. Birth Defects Res C Embryo Today 2007;81:297–304.
20 Kamath BM, Stolle C, Bason L, Colliton RP, Piccoli DA, et al: Craniosynostosis in Alagille syndrome. Am J Med Genet 2002;112:176–180.
21 Jenkins D, Seelow D, Jehee FS, Perlyn CA, Alonso LG, et al: *RAB23* mutations in Carpenter syndrome imply an unexpected role for hedgehog signaling in cranial-suture development and obesity. Am J Hum Genet 2007;80:1162–1170.
22 Piccione M, Antona V, Niceta M, Fabiano C, Martines M, et al: Q289P mutation in the *FGFR2* gene: first report in a patient with type 1 Pfeiffer syndrome. Eur J Pediatr 2009;168:1135–1139.
23 Passos-Bueno MR, Serti Eacute AE, Jehee FS, Fanganiello R, Yeh E: Genetics of craniosynostosis: genes, syndromes, mutations and genotype-phenotype correlations. Front Oral Biol 2008;12:107–143.
24 Rieckmann T, Zhuang L, Fluck CE, Trueb B: Characterization of the first FGFRL1 mutation identified in a craniosynostosis patient. Biochim Biophys Acta 2009;1792:112–121.
25 Ornitz DM: FGFs, heparan sulfate and FGFRs: complex interactions essential for development. Bioessays 2000;22: 108–112.
26 Hollway GE, Suthers GK, Haan EA, Thompson E, David DJ, et al: Mutation detection in *FGFR2* craniosynostosis syndromes. Hum Genet 1997;99:251–255.
27 el Ghouzzi V, Le Merrer M, Perrin-Schmitt F, Lajeunie E, Benit P, et al: Mutations of the *TWIST* gene in the Saethre-Chotzen syndrome. Nat Genet 1997;15:42–46.
28 Carver EA, Oram KF, Gridley T: Craniosynostosis in *Twist* heterozygous mice: A model for Saethre-Chotzen syndrome. Anat Rec 2002;268:90–92.
29 Kariminejad A, Kariminejad R, Tzschach A, Ullmann R, Ahmed A, et al: Craniosynostosis in a patient with 2q37.3 deletion 5q34 duplication: association of extra copy of *MSX2* with craniosynostosis. Am J Med Genet A 2009;149A:1544–1549.
30 Loeys BL, Chen J, Neptune ER, Judge DP, Podowski M, et al: A syndrome of altered cardiovascular, craniofacial, neurocognitive and skeletal development caused by mutations in *TGFBR1* or *TGFBR2*. Nat Genet 2005;37:275–281.
31 Rawlins JT, Opperman LA: Tgf-beta regulation of suture morphogenesis and growth. Front Oral Biol 2008;12:178–196.
32 Carlton MB, Colledge WH, Evans MJ: Crouzon-like craniofacial dysmorphology in the mouse is caused by an insertional mutation at the *Fgf3/Fgf4* locus. Dev Dyn 1998;212:242–249.
33 Harada M, Murakami H, Okawa A, Okimoto N, Hiraoka S, et al: FGF9 monomer/dimer equilibrium regulates extracellular matrix affinity and tissue diffusion. Nat Genet 2009;41:289–298.
34 Hajihosseini MK, Wilson S, De Moerlooze L, Dickson C: A splicing switch and gain-of-function mutation in *FgfR2-IIIc* hemizygotes causes Apert/Pfeiffer-syndrome-like phenotypes. Proc Natl Acad Sci USA 2001;98:3855–3860.
35 Hajihosseini MK, Duarte R, Pegrum J, Donjacour A, Lana-Elola E, et al: Evidence that Fgf10 contributes to the skeletal and visceral defects of an Apert syndrome mouse model. Dev Dyn 2009;238: 376–385.
36 Eswarakumar VP, Monsonego-Ornan E, Pines M, Antonopoulou I, Morriss-Kay GM, Lonai P: The *IIIc* alternative of *Fgfr2* is a positive regulator of bone formation. Development 2002;129:3783–3793.
37 Yu K, Xu J, Liu Z, Sosic D, Shao J, et al: Conditional inactivation of FGF receptor 2 reveals an essential role for FGF signaling in the regulation of osteoblast function and bone growth. Development 2003;130:3063–3074.
38 Iseki S, Wilkie AO, Heath JK, Ishimaru T, Eto K, Morriss-Kay GM: *Fgfr2* and *osteopontin* domains in the developing skull vault are mutually exclusive and can be altered by locally applied FGF2. Development 1997;124:3375–3384.
39 Iseki S, Wilkie AO, Morriss-Kay GM: *Fgfr1* and *Fgfr2* have distinct differentiation- and proliferation-related roles in the developing mouse skull vault. Development 1999;126:5611–5620.
40 Johnson D, Iseki S, Wilkie AO, Morriss-Kay GM: Expression patterns of *Twist* and *Fgfr1, -2* and *-3* in the developing mouse coronal suture suggest a key role for *Twist* in suture initiation and biogenesis. Mech Dev 2000;91:341–345.
41 Yoshida T, Phylactou LA, Uney JB, Ishikawa I, Eto K, Iseki S: Twist is required for establishment of the mouse coronal suture. J Anat 2005;206:437–444.
42 Rice DP, Aberg T, Chan Y, Tang Z, Kettunen PJ, et al: Integration of FGF and TWIST in calvarial bone and suture development. Development 2000;127: 1845–1855.
43 Hajihosseini MK, Heath JK: Expression patterns of fibroblast growth factors-18 and -20 in mouse embryos is suggestive of novel roles in calvarial and limb development. Mech Dev 2002;113:79–83.
44 Ibrahimi OA, Zhang F, Eliseenkova AV, Linhardt RJ, Mohammadi M: Proline to arginine mutations in FGF receptors 1 and 3 result in Pfeiffer and Muenke craniosynostosis syndromes through enhancement of FGF binding affinity. Hum Mol Genet 2004;13:69–78.
45 Britto JA, Moore RL, Evans RD, Hayward RD, Jones BM: Negative autoregulation of fibroblast growth factor receptor 2 expression characterizing cranial development in cases of Apert (P253R mutation) and Pfeiffer (C278F mutation) syndromes and suggesting a basis for differences in their cranial phenotypes. J Neurosurg 2001;95:660–673.
46 Holmes G, Rothschild G, Roy UB, Deng CX, Mansukhani A, Basilico C: Early onset of craniosynostosis in an Apert mouse model reveals critical features of this pathology. Dev Biol 2009;328:273–284.
47 Raucci A, Bellosta P, Grassi R, Basilico C, Mansukhani A: Osteoblast proliferation or differentiation is regulated by relative strengths of opposing signaling pathways. J Cell Physiol 2008;215:442–451.
48 Zhou YX, Xu X, Chen L, Li C, Brodie SG, Deng CX: A Pro250Arg substitution in mouse Fgfr1 causes increased expression of Cbfa1 and premature fusion of calvarial sutures. Hum Mol Genet 2000;9: 2001–2008.
49 Ducy P, Zhang R, Geoffroy V, Ridall AL, Karsenty G: Osf2/Cbfa1: a transcriptional activator of osteoblast differentiation. Cell 1997;89:747–754.

50 Mansukhani A, Bellosta P, Sahni M, Basilico C: Signaling by fibroblast growth factors (FGF) and fibroblast growth factor receptor 2 (FGFR2)-activating mutations blocks mineralization and induces apoptosis in osteoblasts. J Cell Biol 2000;149:1297–1308.
51 Connerney J, Andreeva V, Leshem Y, Mercado M, Dowell K, et al: Twist1 homodimers enhance FGF responsiveness of the cranial sutures and promote suture closure. Dev Biol 2008;318:323–334.
52 Sarkar S, Petiot A, Copp A, Ferretti P, Thorogood P: FGF2 promotes skeletogenic differentiation of cranial neural crest cells. Development 2001;128:2143–2152.
53 Connerney J, Andreeva V, Leshem Y, Muentener C, Mercado MA, Spicer DB: Twist1 dimer selection regulates cranial suture patterning and fusion. Dev Dyn 2006;235:1345–1357.
54 Wan DC, Kwan MD, Lorenz HP, Longaker MT: Current treatment of craniosynostosis and future therapeutic directions. Front Oral Biol 2008;12:209–230.
55 Rice R, Rice DP, Thesleff I: Foxc1 integrates Fgf and Bmp signalling independently of twist or noggin during calvarial bone development. Dev Dyn 2005;233:847–852.
56 Rice R, Rice DP, Olsen BR, Thesleff I: Progression of calvarial bone development requires Foxc1 regulation of Msx2 and Alx4. Dev Biol 2003;262:75–87.
57 Davy A, Bush JO, Soriano P: Inhibition of gap junction communication at ectopic Eph/ephrin boundaries underlies craniofrontonasal syndrome. PLoS Biol 2006;4;e315.
58 Isaac A, Cohn MJ, Ashby P, Ataliotis P, Spicer DB, et al: FGF and genes encoding transcription factors in early limb specification. Mech Dev 2000;93:41–48.
59 Shukla V, Coumoul X, Wang RH, Kim HS, Deng CX: RNA interference and inhibition of MEK-ERK signaling prevent abnormal skeletal phenotypes in a mouse model of craniosynostosis. Nat Genet 2007;39:1145–1150.
60 Hayashi M, Nimura K, Kashiwagi K, Harada T, Takaoka K, et al: Comparative roles of Twist-1 and Id1 in transcriptional regulation by BMP signaling. J Cell Sci 2007;120:1350–1357.

Douglas B. Spicer
Center for Molecular Medicine
Maine Medical Center Research Institute
81 Research Drive, Scarborough, ME, 04074 (USA)
Tel. +1 207 885 8150, Fax +1 207 885 8179, E-Mail spiced@mmc.org

Muenke M, Kress W, Collmann H, Solomon BD (eds): Craniosynostoses: Molecular Genetics, Principles of Diagnosis, and Treatment.
Monogr Hum Genet. Basel, Karger, 2011, vol 19, pp 45–57

The Molecular Bases for FGF Receptor Activation in Craniosynostosis and Dwarfism Syndromes

A. Beenken · M. Mohammadi

New York University School of Medicine, Department of Pharmacology, New York, N.Y., USA

Abstract

Many craniosynostosis and dwarfism syndromes are attributable to gain-of-function mutations in *FGFR1*, *FGFR2*, and *FGFR3*. The molecular bases by which these pathogenic mutations over-activate FGFRs have been characterized extensively through the use of X-ray crystallography and biochemical techniques. Analyses of gain-of-function mutations in the tyrosine kinase domain of FGFR have led to the discovery of a novel autoinhibitory molecular brake at the kinase hinge/interlobe region that is released by different mutations to varying degrees, leading to a range of ligand-independent activation. Most of the ectodomain mutations confer ligand-independent gain-of-function by facilitating covalent receptor dimerization through disulfide bridge formation. A few ectodomain mutations are ligand-dependent, the prime example being the Apert syndrome (AS) mutations, FGFR2c p.S252W and FGFR2c p.P253R. These mutations introduce additional contacts between the mutated FGFR and FGF to increase the affinity of the mutated FGFR for both its cognate FGFs and for FGFs that are outside the normal specificity profile of wild type FGFR. Interestingly, surface plasmon resonance (SPR) data suggest that for a given ligand-dependent mutation, the severity of the craniofacial phenotype correlates with a generalized gain in binding of the mutant FGFR to all FGFs present in the cranial suture, while a specific gain in binding of the mutant FGFR to FGF10 accounts for the severity of syndactyly.

Fibroblast growth factor (FGF) signaling plays pleiotropic roles in human development and metabolism. The FGF family of ligands is grouped into 6 subfamilies on the basis of phylogeny and sequence homology: The paracrine subfamilies include the FGF1 subfamily comprising FGF1, 2; the FGF7 subfamily comprising FGF3, 7, 10, 22; the FGF4 subfamily comprising FGF4, 5, 6; the FGF8 subfamily comprising FGF8, 17, 18; and the FGF9 subfamily comprising FGF9, 16, 20. The endocrine-acting FGF19 subfamily comprises FGF19, 21, 23 [1, 2]. The paracrine FGFs play central roles in tissue patterning and organogenesis [3], while the endocrine FGFs regulate a variety of metabolic processes, including glucose homeostasis, bile acid synthesis, and phosphate and vitamin D homeostasis [4–8].

The FGFR consists of 3 extracellular immunoglobulin-like domains (D1, D2, and D3), a transmembrane domain, and an intracellular bipartite tyrosine kinase domain [9]. D2, D3 and the D2-D3 linker mediate binding of FGFR to FGF [10–12], while the D1 domain and D1-D2 linker play autoinhibitory roles in FGFR signaling [13, 14]. There are 4 *FGFR* genes in mammals, and tissue-specific alternative splicing of the D3 domain in *FGFR1–3* yields epithelial 'b' and mesenchymal 'c' isoforms [15–17]. Ligands expressed in the epithelium such as those of the FGF8 and FGF9 families activate mesenchymally expressed FGFRc isoforms, while FGF7 subfamily ligands expressed in the mesenchyme activate FGFRb isoforms in the epithelium. This leads to the establishment of an epithelial-mesenchymal signaling loop that guides embryogenesis [18–22].

FGF-FGFR signaling occurs in a heparan sulfate (HS) dependent fashion [23–26]. Crystallographic studies have yielded 2 different models to explain how HS promotes FGF-FGFR binding and dimerization. The symmetric model proposed by Mohammadi and colleagues displays a 2:2:2 FGF:FGFR:HS stoichiometry in which multivalent protein-protein contacts between the 2 FGF-FGFR halves are the main driving force of dimerization and HS solely acts to facilitate these protein-protein contacts [27]. In contrast, the asymmetric model put forth by Blundell and colleagues displays a 2:2:1 FGF:FGFR:HS stoichiometry in which a single HS chain bridges 2 FGFs in *trans* and each FGF interacts with only 1 FGFR. In contrast to the symmetric model, there are no direct protein-protein contacts between the 2 FGF-FGFR halves in this model. In other words, the asymmetric dimer is held together solely by the ability of HS to dimerize FGFs, and consequently this mode of dimerization is strictly HS-dependent [28]. Another key difference between the 2 models pertains to the isomerization state of the FGFR-invariant proline located in the D2-D3 linker. In the symmetric model, this proline (p.P253 in FGFR2) adopts a *trans* conformation, whereas in the asymmetric model it is found in a *cis* conformation. Blundell and coworkers have proposed that the *cis* and *trans* conformations of the linker residue represent the active and inactive states of the receptor respectively, and that HS promotes *trans* to *cis* conversion.

FGF- and HS-mediated dimerization of FGFRs juxtaposes the cytoplasmic kinase domains, allowing them to transphosphorylate each other on activation loop (A-loop) tyrosines to upregulate FGFR kinase activity. A-loop phosphorylation is followed by transphosphorylation of tyrosines in the C-tail, kinase insert, and juxtamembrane region. The phosphorylated tyrosines and surrounding sequences recruit downstream intracellular signaling molecules including PLCγ and CRKL to facilitate their phosphorylation by the activated FGFR kinase. PLCγ activation leads to PIP2 hydrolysis and PKC activation [29], whereas CRKL links FGFR activation to the RAC1/CDC42 pathway [30]. In contrast, FRS2α, the FGFR substrate that links FGFR activation to the MAPK pathway [31], associates constitutively with the intracellular juxtamembrane region of FGFR and requires only A-loop tyrosine phosphorylation for activation.

Gain-of-Function Mutations in FGFR1–3 in Skeletal Syndromes

Gain-of-function mutations in FGFR1–3 are responsible for many forms of human craniosynostosis and dwarfism syndromes. Generally speaking, the mechanisms by which these mutations impart gain of function to the diseased FGFRs can be divided into those that are ligand-independent and those that are ligand-dependent.

A. Ligand-Independent Gain-of-Function Mutations. Among the syndromes associated with ligand-independent gain-of-function mutations are Crouzon syndrome, Pfeiffer syndrome, Antley-Bixler syndrome, thanatophoric dysplasia types I and II, and Jackson-Weiss syndrome [32]. Ligand-independent gain-of-function mutations in the intracellular tyrosine kinase domain map to the key regulatory regions of the kinase domain including the A-loop, αC helix, and kinase hinge/interlobe region. These mutations elevate the intrinsic enzymatic activity of the kinase domain, thereby bypassing the need for FGF-FGFR dimerization to activate the tyrosine kinase domain via A-loop tyrosine phosphorylation. Structural studies carried out in our laboratory have shown that these mutations disengage an autoinhibitory molecular brake at the kinase hinge/interlobe region that serves to suppress the kinase activity of the tyrosine kinase domain in the absence of FGF and HS [33].

The ligand-independent gain-of-function mutations in the extracellular domain of FGFR map to the D2-D3 linker, D3 domain, and the extracellular juxtamembrane region of receptor. The majority of these mutations introduce an unpaired cysteine that then leads to the formation of disulfide-linked FGFR dimers, thereby bypassing the need for FGF- and HS-dependent FGFR dimerization [34–36]. An unpaired cysteine can be created through 3 mechanisms: (1) substitution of a non-cysteine residue for either of the 2 cysteines that form the intramolecular disulfide bridge within the D3 domain [37–40], (2) mutations that destabilize the D3 fold and interfere with the ability of the cysteine pair within D3 to form an intramolecular disulfide bridge, freeing up the cysteines for intermolecular disulfide formation between FGFRs [41], and (3) mutation of a non-cysteine residue on the surface of D3 or in the extracellular juxtamembrane region into a cysteine [42–44]. Interestingly, the degree of FGFR activation by disulfide bridge formation is sensitive to the location where the free cysteine appears on the surface of D3 or in the extracellular juxtamembrane region [45]. Based on this observation, we infer that there may be differences in the orientations of the FGFR ectodomains within these disulfide-linked dimers that probably translate into differences in the juxtapositioning of the intracellular tyrosine kinase domains and their signaling properties.

B. Ligand-Dependent Gain-of-Function Mutations. Ligand-dependent gain-of-function mutations are associated with Muenke syndrome (MS), Pfeiffer syndrome (PS), and Apert syndrome (AS). The mutations causing these syndromes are of paternal origin and impart a selective growth advantage to male germ line cells, explaining why the incidence of the syndromes correlates with advanced age in the father [46–49] (see Chapter 6). A p.P250R mutation in FGFR3c is responsible for Muenke syndrome [50], a craniosynostosis disorder that exhibits no syndactyly (see Chapter 8). PS has a variety of clinical presentations, and the milder PS type I resulting from a p.P252R mutation in FGFR1c is primarily characterized by craniosynostosis as well [51]. The p.S252W and p.P253R mutations underlying AS map to the D2-D3 linker region of FGFR2 and account for 99% of AS cases [52] (see Chapter 7). Since AS mutations map to the region preceding the alternatively spliced D3, they are manifested in both isoforms of FGFR. Although both AS mutations lead to craniosynostosis and syndactyly, p.S252W is associated with more severe craniofacial features, while p.P253R is associated with more severe syndactyly [53–55]. Structural and biochemical data show that these ligand-dependent mutations act by increasing ligand binding affinity as well as by overriding the ligand binding specificity of the affected receptors [56–60]. Extensive surface plasmon resonance (SPR)-based binding studies have also shed light onto the molecular bases of these phenotypic differences associated with different ligand-dependent mutations [57–59]. These SPR studies, along with structural studies of diseased FGFRs in complex with FGFs, have played an instrumental role in dissecting the correct mode of FGF-FGFR dimerization [57, 58, 61].

Structural and Biochemical Analysis of Mutations Leading to Ligand-Dependent Gain of Function

Structural Characterization of Apert Syndrome Mutations

The first glimpse of how ligand-dependent mutations confer gain of function to FGFRs was provided by the crystal structures of FGF2 in complex with FGFR2c mutants harboring either the p.S252W or p.P253R AS mutation [57]. Both structures showed that AS mutations introduce additional contacts between the ligand and receptor (fig. 1A, D).

The AS mutations did not alter the overall conformation of FGFR2c as evidenced by the fact that superimposition of the αC traces of the entire D2-D3 binding domain of the p.S252W and p.P253R FGFR2c mutants onto wild type FGFR2c yields root mean square (RMS) deviations of less than 0.4 Å. This observation negates the previous proposal that AS mutations induce conformational changes in receptor structure that enhance ligand binding affinity [56, 60]. Notably, to provide physiological

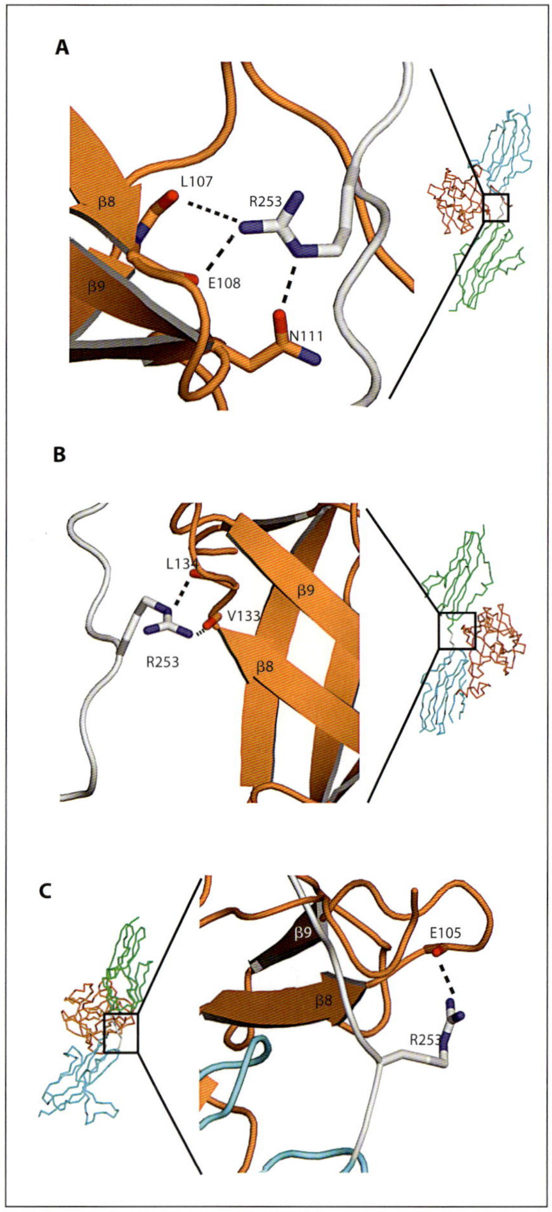

Fig. 1. Ligand-dependent gain-of-function mutations in the D2-D3 linker of the FGFR ectodomain. **A** The FGF2-FGFR2c p.P253R structure (PDB ID: 1IIL) [57] shows that the p.R253 residue engages in 3 new hydrogen bonds: 2 with backbone oxygens of p.L107 and p.E108, and a third with p.N111's side chain amide. Ligand is depicted in orange, FGFR D2 domain in green, FGFR linker in grey, and FGFR D3 domain in cyan. Nitrogen atoms are depicted in blue, and oxygen atoms in red. Hydrogen bonds are indicated by dashed lines. A subsequent structure of FGF2-FGFR1c p.P252R, a mutation found in PS, demonstrated exactly the same new contacts [59]. **B** p.R253 in the FGF8-FGFR2c p.P253R complex (PDB ID: 2FDB) [62] engages in hydrogen bonds with the backbone carbonyls of p.V133 and p.L134 in FGF8. **C** In FGF1-FGFR2b p.P253R, p.R253 makes only 1 hydrogen bond with the backbone carbonyl oxygen of p.E105, which is consistent with the nominal gain in binding of FGF1 to FGFR2b p.P253R relative to wild type seen with SPR [58].

support for the asymmetric model, Blundell and colleagues had also suggested that the p.S252W AS mutation confers gain of function by facilitating a *trans*-to-*cis* conversion of the D2-D3 linker p.P253 of FGFR2 [28]. However, the observation that p.P253 remains in a *trans* conformation in the FGF2-FGFR2c p.S252W crystal structure strongly disputes this proposition and provides support for the symmetric model of FGF-FGFR dimerization in normal physiology (fig. 1D).

In the FGF2-FGFR2c p.P253R structure (fig. 1A), the substituted arginine residue makes

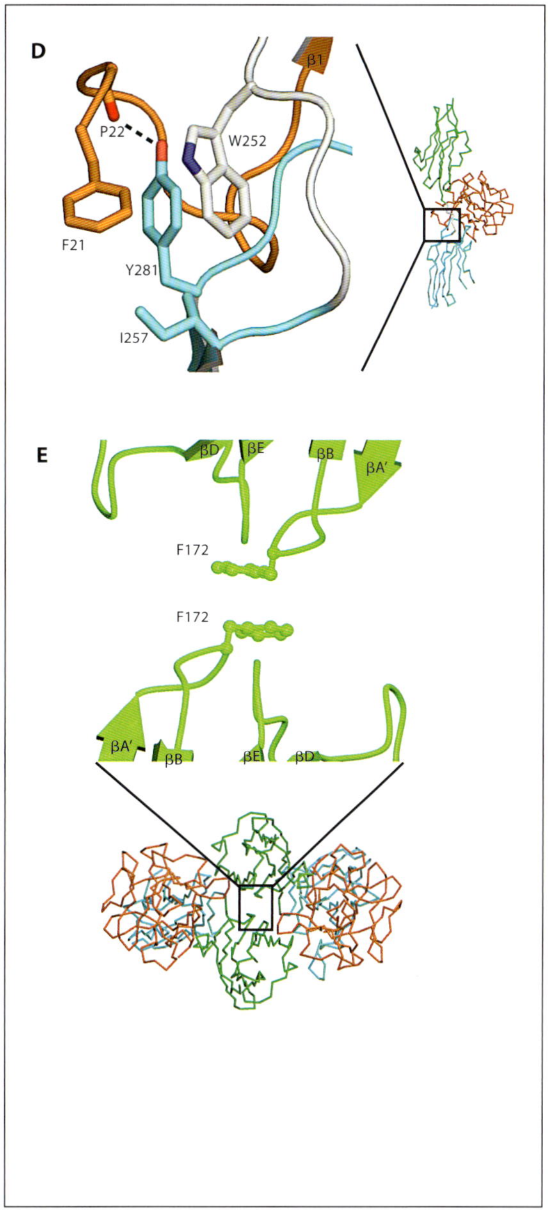

Fig. 1. D The FGF2-FGFR2c p.S252W structure (PDB ID: 1II4) [57] shows that p.W252 engages in a hydrophobic patch with p.Y281 and p.I257 of receptor that interacts with p.F21 of FGF2. Among the additional new contacts observed in this structure are a hydrogen bond between a backbone atom of FGF2 p.P22 and the side chain hydroxyl group of p.Y281. In the FGF10-FGFR2b p.S252W structure (not shown), similar contacts are seen as in FGF2, except in this case p.W252 engages hydrophobically with p.L73 in the αN helix of FGF10. The nearest approach of that contact is only 4.2 Å, which accounts for the modest increase in binding to FGF10 of FGFR2b p.S252W relative to wild type as observed with SPR [58]. **E** In the FGF10-FGFR2b p.A172F structure, p.F172 of one receptor packs against p.F172 of the second receptor, leading to a total of 187 $Å^2$ of surface area buried, compared to only 76 $Å^2$ in the wild type dimer.

additional hydrogen bonds primarily with backbone atoms in the FGF core, suggesting that the mutation would enhance binding of the mutant receptor to all FGFs. Indeed, subsequent structures of FGF8b with FGFR2c p.P253R (fig. 1B) [62], of FGF1 with FGFR2b p.P253R (fig. 1C), and of FGF2 with FGFR1c p.P252R [59], also showed that the arginine residue introduced into the mutant FGFR engages in additional hydrogen bonds with FGF ligand that are reminiscent of those seen in the FGF2-FGFR2c p.P253R structure. This strongly suggests that the structural mechanism by which the proline-to-arginine mutation in the D2-D3 linker confers ligand-dependent gain of function is universal to FGFR1–3 (fig. 1A–C). Moreover, the conserved nature of the additional contacts seen between ligand and backbone atoms of the mutant receptor indicates that the proline-to-arginine mutation should increase affinity of the receptor towards all FGFs.

In contrast, the substituted tryptophan in the FGF2-FGFR2c p.S252W structure makes hydrophobic contacts with p.F21 in the N-terminus of FGF2 (fig. 1D), the most divergent region of FGFs. This led to an initial hypothesis that the S252W mutation would enhance the affinity of the diseased FGFR2 only to those FGFs possessing a hydrophobic residue at the position analogous to p.F21 of FGF2 [57]. However, subsequent biochemical findings showed that p.S252W FGFR2c does in fact bind to nearly all FGFs with enhanced affinity [58, 59]. Furthermore, a crystal structure of FGF10 in complex with FGFR2b p.S252W exhibited the surprising result that the substituted tryptophan in the FGF10-FGFR2b p.S252W structure made additional hydrophobic contacts with p.L73 of FGF10, a residue that is located 2 residues downstream from the location analogous to p.F21 of FGF2 [58]. These findings indicate that the N-termini of FGFs that lack a hydrophobic residue at the position analogous to p.F21 in FGF2 may nonetheless still adopt conformations that are compatible with the formation of hydrophobic contacts with the substituted p.W252 in mutant FGFR2.

Taken together, these structural findings suggest that both the p.P253R and p.S252W mutations should increase the affinity of mutated FGFR2 to all FGFs, even to those outside the normal specificity profile of FGFR2b or FGFR2c. In other words, the AS mutations should breach the specificity barrier established by alternative splicing in the D3 domain, enabling autocrine signaling wherein mesenchymally expressed FGFR2c can bind and become activated by mesenchymally expressed FGFs such as those in the FGF7 subfamily, and epithelially expressed FGFR2b can bind and become activated by epithelially expressed FGFs such as those in the FGF8 and FGF9 subfamilies.

Consistent with the idea that AS mutations lead to pathogenesis by enabling illegitimate autocrine FGFR2 signaling is the fact that rare cases of AS have been associated with de novo Alu-element insertions that led to ectopic expression of FGFR2b in mesenchymal tissue [52]. It was suggested that the abnormal expression patterns seen in these rare forms of AS would allow for pathological autocrine FGF10-FGFR2b signaling loops to take place. Indeed, the severity of pathology in these cases correlated with the level of ectopic FGFR2b expression. Genetic studies in mice also corroborate this hypothesis, as mice with a genetically altered splicing switch of 'c' to 'b' that resulted in 'b' isoform expression in mesenchymal tissue also exhibited AS-like phenotypes [63].

Molecular Basis for the Craniofacial and Syndactyly Phenotypes in Patients with Apert, Muenke, and Pfeiffer Syndrome Mutations

Comprehensive SPR experiments were undertaken to gain insight into the underlying molecular basis for the observed differences in the severity of syndactyly and craniofacial phenotypes associated with AS mutations. An opportunity for understanding the molecular basis for these phenotypic differences was provided by a patient harboring a compound p.S252L/p.A315S mutation in FGFR2c that segregated in *cis*. Interestingly, this patient presented with syndactyly but lacked craniosynostosis [64]. SPR-based binding studies showed that the p.S252L/p.A315S mutation caused a gain in binding of mutated FGFR2c to FGF10 but not to other FGFs expressed in the cranial sutures. This data is consistent with a model in which craniosynostosis arises from generalized activation of mutated FGFRs by multiple FGFs in the cranial sutures, while illegitimate activation of mutated FGFR2c specifically by FGF10 is responsible for syndactyly. This finding was corroborated by a case of a PS patient harboring an unusual p.D321A mutation that presented with syndactyly [65]. SPR experiments

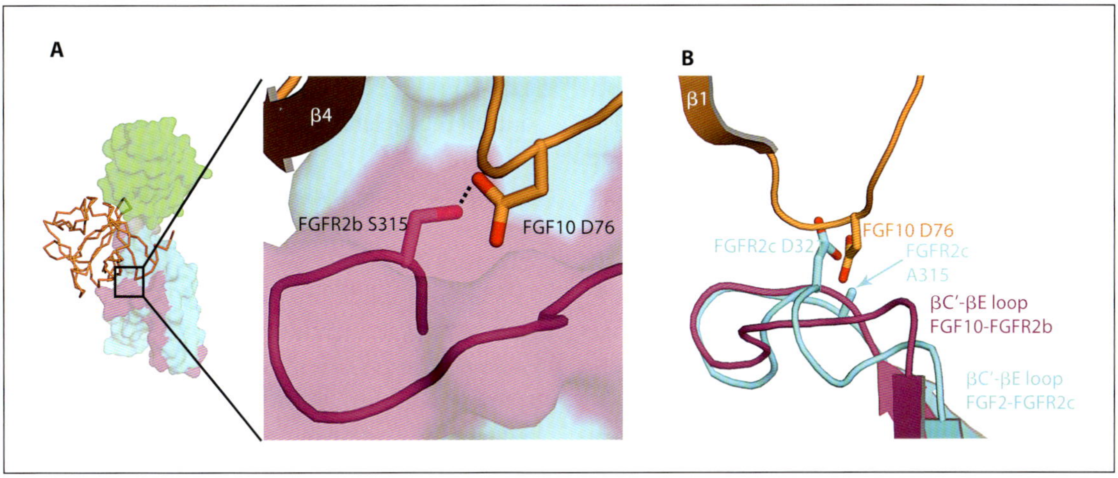

Fig. 2. Ligand-dependent gain-of-function mutations in the βC'-βE loop of D3 of the FGFR ectodomain. **A** The contact between p.S315 in FGFR2b and p.D76 in FGF10 is shown from the FGF10-FGFR2b structure (PDB ID: 1NUN) [66]. The p.A315S mutation in FGFR2c would introduce this contact between FGF10 and FGFR2c and thus increase binding between ligand and receptor. FGFR2b is rendered as a surface, with the alternatively spliced portion of D3 colored in purple and the unspliced portion in cyan. **B** The FGF10-FGFR2b complex has been superimposed onto that of FGF2-FGFR2c (PDB ID: 1EV2) [10], revealing the clash and electrostatic repulsion that would take place between FGF10 p.D76 and FGFR2c p.D321 were FGF10 to attempt to bind to FGFR2c. It is predicted that the p.D321A mutation in FGFR2c would resolve this clash and enable illegitimate binding of FGF10 to FGFR2c [58]. The position of the p.A315 in FGFR2c that is mutated to serine in the p.S252L/p.A315S mutant is indicated with an arrow.

showed that the p.D321A mutation likewise enabled the mutated FGFR2c to bind FGF10. However, in contrast to the p.S252L/p.A315S double mutation, p.D321A also allowed binding of the mutated FGFR2c to other FGFs expressed in the cranial sutures [58]. This broad activation of FGFs by FGFR2c p.D321A is consistent with the craniosynostosis observed in this patient's presentation.

The ability of the p.S252L/p.A315S double mutation and the p.D321A mutation to allow illegitimate binding of FGFR2c to FGF10 is consistent with published crystal structures of FGF-FGFR complexes. p.S252L is predicted to introduce novel hydrophobic contacts reminiscent of those seen in the FGF2-FGFR2c p.S252W structure, while p.A315S introduces a 'b' splice isoform-specific residue into the βC'-βE loop of FGFR2c. In the FGF10-FGFR2b structure [66], p.S315 hydrogen bonds with p.D76 of FGF10, a residue also conserved in FGF7 and FGF22, two other members of the FGF7 subfamily. Notably, this is the most specific interaction observed between FGF10 and FGFR2b (fig. 2A). By introducing p.S315 into FGFR2c, the p.S252L/p.A315S mutation now likely enables this new illegitimate contact between FGFR2c and FGF10. On the other hand, FGFR2c p.D321A confers illegitimate binding of FGF10 to the mutated FGFR2c by eliminating a major steric and electrostatic repulsion between p.D321 in the FGFR2c βC'-βE loop and p.D76 of FGF10. (fig. 2B) Importantly, molecular investigations of the p.S252L/p.A315S and p.D321A FGFR2 mutations provide unbiased support for the symmetric model of FGF-FGFR dimerization. In the symmetric FGF-FGFR dimerization model, the βC'-βE loop is critical in determining ligand binding specificity, whereas in the asymmetric model this loop has no such role.

Notably the p.P252R mutation in FGFR1c responsible for PS type I and the p.P250R mutation in FGFR3c responsible for Muenke syndrome [50] (the analogous mutations to FGFR2c p.P253R) do not impart FGF10 binding to the mutated FGFR1c or FGFR3c but do impart a general increase of binding of the mutant receptors to their cognate ligands [59]. These data are in accord with the model that illegitimate autocrine signaling by FGF10 through FGFR2c P253R is what accounts for syndactyly, since PS type I is only variably associated with syndactyly and MS is never associated with syndactyly. Furthermore, the increased binding of these PS and MS mutants towards many of their cognate ligands is consistent with the presentation of craniosynostosis in these patients. Interestingly, the lack of FGF10 binding to FGFR1c p.P252R and FGFR3c p.P250R can be explained structurally by the need for residues in D2 of FGFR2 that are lacking in FGFR1 and FGFR3 and are critical for FGF10 binding [66].

Gathering all the evidence together then, distinct mechanisms appear to underlie craniofacial and limb pathology in AS. The craniofacial phenotypes seen in AS result from the over-activation of FGFR2 by the wide spectrum of FGFs expressed in the cranial sutures. On the other hand, syndactyly primarily results from illegitimate autocrine activation of mesenchymal FGFR2c by FGF10. Subsequent genetic experiments have helped confirm these results, showing that knockdown of FGF10 in mice carrying AS mutations can rescue some of the skeletal abnormalities of the AS mouse model [67].

In light of all these evidences, the molecular bases for the different phenotypic profiles seen in patients with the FGFR2c p.S252W and FGFR2c p.P253R AS mutations can now be understood. The more severe craniofacial phenotype associated with the p.S252W mutation arises primarily from an increased affinity of mutant FGFR to all FGFs in the cranial suture, while the more severe syndactyly associated with the p.P253R mutation arises primarily from an autocrine signaling loop between FGF10 and mutant FGFR2c. It is still important to keep in mind however, that craniosynostosis and syndactyly are associated with both of the classic AS mutations and that both mutations lead to a generalized increase in affinity towards FGFs as well as to autocrine signaling across the FGF-FGFR specificity barrier.

Structural Characterization of p.A172F Mutation in FGFR2 Responsible for Pfeiffer Syndrome

The crystal structure of FGF10 in complex with FGFR2b containing the p.A172F mutation found in a PS patient revealed yet another example of how

Fig. 3. Ligand-independent gain-of-function mutations in the intracellular kinase domain of FGFR2. **A** Overall structure of the unphosphorylated kinase (PDB ID: 2PSQ) [33]. The N- and C-lobe, the β4, β5, and β8 strands, the αC helix, and the hinge and activation loop (A-loop) are all labeled for ease of reference for the following figures. The hinge/interlobe region where the molecular brake resides and the region of the activation loop are boxed. The N-lobe is colored light brown, the activation loop is colored blue, the β4-αC loop is colored orange, the β8 strand is colored cyan, and the hinge is colored purple. **B** A close-up view of the molecular brake in the hinge/interlobe region of the unphosphorylated kinase. The intricate network of hydrogen bonds between a triad of residues in the hinge, β4-αC loop, and β8 strand with backbone atoms in the β4-αC loop keep the kinase in an autoinhibited state. Each of the 3 residues in the triad is targeted in mutations leading to pathology in humans. **C** p.E565A kinase (PDB ID: 2Q0B) [33]. In crystal structures of the mutant kinases, it was observed that the network of hydrogen bonds that constituted the autoinhibitory molecular brake was dissociated. The p.E565A mutation is one such example of a mutation in FGFR2 that disengages the autoinhibitory brake. The loss of these hydrogen bonds allowed the N-lobe to rotate towards the C-lobe at the same pivot point as observed in A-loop tyrosine phosphorylated wild type FGFR2. This rotation of the N-lobe causes a significant rearrangement of the A-loop that brings the catalytic domains into proper alignment for activation of the kinase (not shown). **D** p.K526E kinase (PDB ID: 2PZP) [33]. This mutation in the αC helix causes ligand-independent activation by creating new hydrogen bonds between p.E526 and p.R664 in the A-loop that facilitate the rotation of the N-lobe toward the C-lobe and disengage p.N549 from interacting with residues in the αC-β4 loop. The unphosphorylated kinase is colored pink, and the p.K526E mutant kinase is colored turquoise. **E** p.K659N kinase (PDB ID: 2PVY) [33]. This mutation of an A-loop residue drives

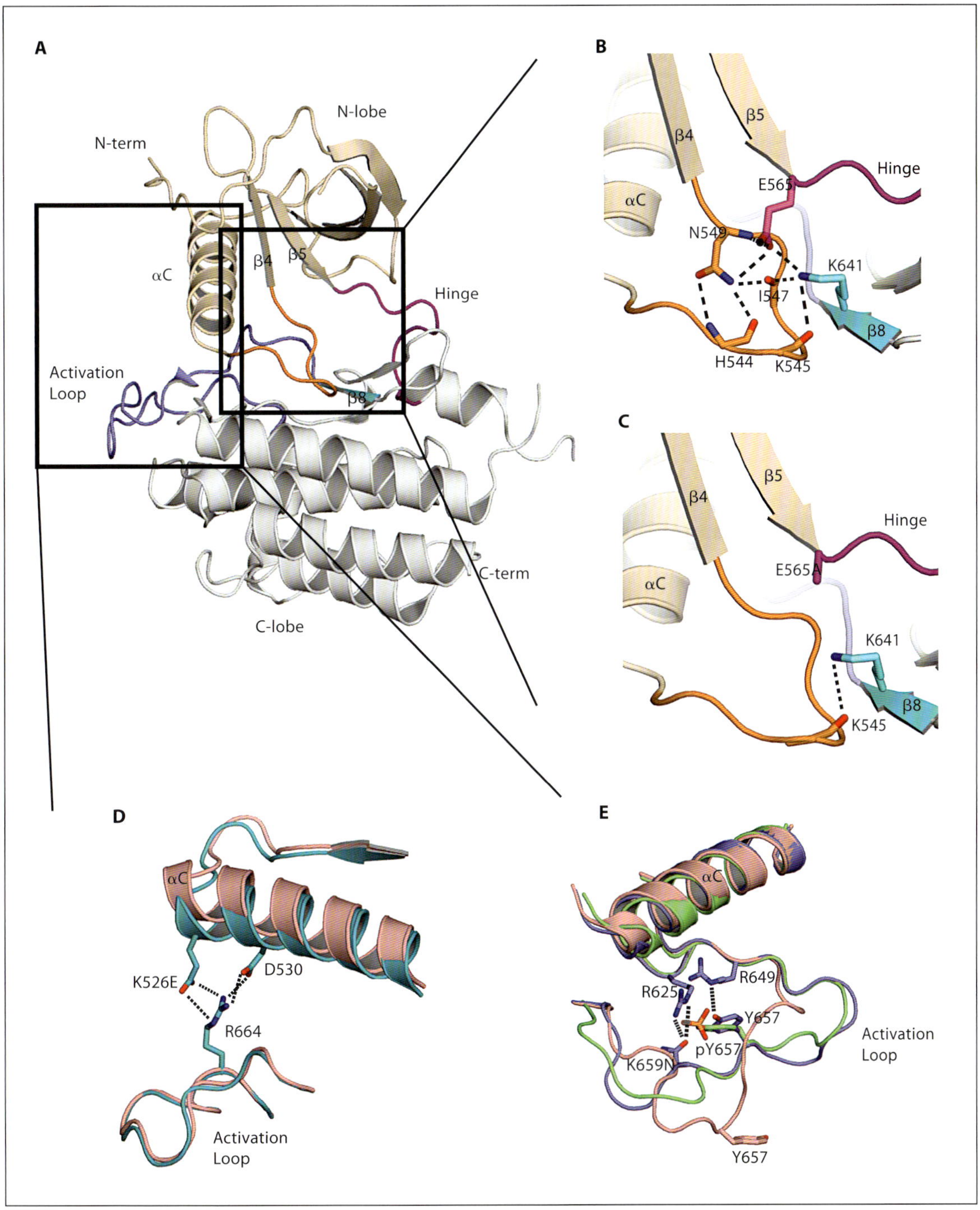

the active conformation of the A-loop even though p.Y657 of the A-loop remains unphosphorylated. In this structure, p.N659 forms 2 hydrogen bonds with p.R625 in the catalytic loop, and p.Y657 hydrogen bonds the side chain of p.R649. These new hydrogen bonds cause rotation of the N-lobe towards the C-lobe and disengage p.N549 from its interactions with backbone atoms in the αC-β4 loop. In the figure, the A-loop of the unphosphorylated kinase is in pink, the A-loop of the phosphorylated kinase is in green, and the A-loop of the p.K659N mutant kinase is in blue.

pathogenic mutations override the normal mechanism of FGFR activation. The p.A172F mutation maps onto a region on D2 of receptor that participates in direct receptor-receptor contacts according to the symmetric dimerization model. In the structure of the FGF10-FGFR2b p.A172F complex, the introduced phenylalanine residue fortifies the direct FGFR-FGFR interface, enabling the ligand to more easily induce receptor dimerization (fig. 1E) [61]. Importantly the structural study of FGF10-FGFR2b p.A172F also provided unbiased evidence in favor of the symmetric model of FGF-FGFR dimerization, as direct receptor-receptor interactions are a unique feature of the symmetric model.

Structural and Biochemical Analysis of Mutations Leading to Ligand-Independent Gain of Function

Mutations in the Intracellular Kinase Domain of FGFR2

Numerous mutations leading to craniosynostosis and dwarfism syndromes map to the kinase domain, and steady state kinetics analyses of mutant receptors have shown that they impart different degrees of constitutive receptor activation [33]. Comparison of the crystal structures of unphosphorylated wild type FGFR2 kinase in the resting state, activated A-loop phosphorylated wild type FGFR2 kinase, and 7 unphosphorylated mutant FGFR2 kinases each harboring a distinct pathogenic mutation led to the identification of a novel autoinhibitory network of hydrogen bonds at the kinase hinge/interlobe region that suppresses the ability of kinase to adopt an active conformation. This network, termed the molecular brake, is mediated by a triad of residues (p.N549 in the loop between αC helix and β4 strand, p.E565 in the hinge region, and p.K641 in the β8 strand) (fig. 3A, B), and in normal physiology it dissociates when the A-loop tyrosine is phosphorylated. Each of the 3 constituents of the brake is subject to mutation in craniosynostosis and dwarfism syndromes. Crystallographic studies of p.N549H, p.N549T, p.E565G, p.E565A, and p.K641R in FGFR2 show that these mutations cause varying degrees of ligand-independent gain of function by directly loosening this molecular brake (fig. 3C). The crystal structures of FGFR2 p.K526E and FGFR2 p.K659N show that the autoinhibitory brake can also be loosened by long-range allosteric effects (fig. 3D, E). This brake is conserved in other receptor tyrosine kinases (RTKs), including VEGFR2, c-KIT, CSF1R, and TEK [33], suggesting that it is a general feature of RTK regulation.

Conclusion

Crystallographic and biochemical characterization of FGFR ectodomains and kinase domains harboring gain-of-function mutations responsible for human skeletal disorders have shown how these mutations override the physiological mechanisms of FGFR regulation. These studies underscore the power of applying structural biology to understanding the molecular mechanism of human disease.

Several problems remain in the field for structural biologists to address. First, to elucidate the mechanism whereby ligand-dependent mutations enable FGFR2c to illegitimately signal in response to FGF10, a crystal structure needs to be solved of FGF10 bound to FGFR2c p.P253R, FGFR2c p.S252W, or FGFR2c p.S252L/p.A315S. Second, crystal structures of pathological dimers arising from disulfide bridges linking FGFR ectodomains would be informative and likely even provide new understanding into the mechanism of FGF-FGFR dimerization in normal physiology. Such crystal structures would allow for the investigation of how different orientations of the receptor ectodomain impact the function of the intracellular kinase.

Since many of the germline mutations in FGFRs associated with skeletal disorders also occur as somatic mutations in cancer, structural studies of FGFRs harboring these mutations should facilitate drug discovery not only for the treatment of craniosynostosis and dwarfism syndromes but also for cancer. Mutation of FGFR2 p.S252W associated with AS is also found to be mutated somatically in endometrial cancers [68]. Mutation of p.N549 in FGFR2 leads to PS [69], and mutation of the analogous asparagine in other tyrosine kinase family members has been associated with glioblastomas (FGFR1, PDGFRα) [70], rhabdomyosarcomas (FGFR4) [71], and gastrointestinal tumors (PDGFRα) [72, 73]. Mutation of K650 in FGFR3 responsible for severe achondroplasia with developmental delay and acanthosis nigricans (SADDAN) and thanatophoric dysplasia types I and II (TDI, TDII) [74], is seen frequently in bladder and cervical cancers [75, 76], and multiple myeloma [77, 78]. Continued investigation of the structural biology of these mutations will be relevant to wide-ranging areas of human pathophysiology.

Acknowledgements

This work was supported by NIH-NIDCR 2R01 DE013686 (to M.M.). A.B. was partially supported by the training grant in Pharmacological Sciences (NIH-NIGMS 2T32 GM066704).

References

1 Itoh N, Ornitz DM: Evolution of the *Fgf* and *Fgfr* gene families. Trends Genet 2004;20:563–569.

2 Popovici C, Roubin R, Coulier F, Birnbaum D: An evolutionary history of the FGF superfamily. Bioessays 2005;27: 849–857.

3 Beenken A, Mohammadi M: The FGF family: biology, pathophysiology and therapy. Nat Rev Drug Discov 2009;8: 235–253.

4 Fu L, John LM, Adams SH, Yu XX, Tomlinson E, et al: Fibroblast growth factor 19 increases metabolic rate and reverses dietary and leptin-deficient diabetes. Endocrinology 2004;145:2594–2603.

5 Kharitonenkov A, Shiyanova TL, Koester A, Ford AM, Micanovic R, et al: FGF-21 as a novel metabolic regulator. J Clin Invest 2005;115:1627–1635.

6 Kuro-o M: Klotho as a regulator of fibroblast growth factor signaling and phosphate/calcium metabolism. Curr Opin Nephrol Hypertens 2006;15:437–441.

7 Tomlinson E, Fu L, John L, Hultgren B, Huang X, et al: Transgenic mice expressing human fibroblast growth factor-19 display increased metabolic rate and decreased adiposity. Endocrinology 2002;143:1741–1747.

8 Yu C, Wang F, Kan M, Jin C, Jones RB, et al: Elevated cholesterol metabolism and bile acid synthesis in mice lacking membrane tyrosine kinase receptor FGFR4. J Biol Chem 2000;275:15482–15489.

9 Lee PL, Johnson DE, Cousens LS, Fried VA, Williams LT: Purification and complementary DNA cloning of a receptor for basic fibroblast growth factor. Science 1989;245:57–60.

10 Plotnikov AN, Hubbard SR, Schlessinger J, Mohammadi M: Crystal structures of two FGF-FGFR complexes reveal the determinants of ligand-receptor specificity. Cell 2000;101:413–424.

11 Plotnikov AN, Schlessinger J, Hubbard SR, Mohammadi M: Structural basis for FGF receptor dimerization and activation. Cell 1999;98:641–650.

12 Stauber DJ, DiGabriele AD, Hendrickson WA: Structural interactions of fibroblast growth factor receptor with its ligands. Proc Natl Acad Sci USA 2000;97:49–54.

13 Olsen SK, Ibrahimi OA, Raucci A, Zhang F, Eliseenkova AV, et al: Insights into the molecular basis for fibroblast growth factor receptor autoinhibition and ligand-binding promiscuity. Proc Natl Acad Sci USA 2004;101:935–940.

14 Wang F, Kan M, Yan G, Xu J, McKeehan WL: Alternately spliced NH2-terminal immunoglobulin-like loop I in the ectodomain of the fibroblast growth factor (FGF) receptor 1 lowers affinity for both heparin and FGF-1. J Biol Chem 1995; 270:10231–10235.

15 Johnson DE, Lu J, Chen H, Werner S, Williams LT: The human fibroblast growth factor receptor genes: a common structural arrangement underlies the mechanisms for generating receptor forms that differ in their third immunoglobulin domain. Mol Cell Biol 1991;11:4627–4634.

16 Miki T, Bottaro DP, Fleming TP, Smith CL, Burgess WH, et al: Determination of ligand-binding specificity by alternative splicing: two distinct growth factor receptors encoded by a single gene. Proc Natl Acad Sci USA 1992;89:246–250.

17 Orr-Urtreger A, Bedford MT, Burakova T, Arman E, Zimmer Y, et al: Developmental localization of the splicing alternatives of fibroblast growth factor receptor-2 (FGFR2). Dev Biol 1993;158: 475–486.

18 Hogan BL, Yingling JM: Epithelial/mesenchymal interactions and branching morphogenesis of the lung. Curr Opin Genet Dev 1998;8:481–486.

19 Jin C, Wang F, Wu X, Yu C, Luo Y, McKeehan WL: Directionally specific paracrine communication mediated by epithelial FGF9 to stromal FGFR3 in two-compartment premalignant prostate tumors. Cancer Res 2004;64:4555–4562.

20 Pirvola U, Zhang X, Mantela J, Ornitz DM, Ylikoski J: Fgf9 signaling regulates inner ear morphogenesis through epithelial-mesenchymal interactions. Dev Biol 2004;273:350–360.

21 Xu X, Weinstein M, Li C, Naski M, Cohen RI, et al: Fibroblast growth factor receptor 2 (FGFR2)-mediated reciprocal regulation loop between FGF8 and FGF10 is essential for limb induction. Development 1998;125:753–765.

22 Zhang X, Stappenbeck TS, White AC, Lavine KJ, Gordon JI, Ornitz DM: Reciprocal epithelial-mesenchymal FGF signaling is required for cecal development. Development 2006;133:173–180.

23 Lin X, Buff EM, Perrimon N, Michelson AM: Heparan sulfate proteoglycans are essential for FGF receptor signaling during *Drosophila* embryonic development. Development 1999;126:3715–3723.
24 Ornitz DM, Yayon A, Flanagan JG, Svahn CM, Levi E, Leder P: Heparin is required for cell-free binding of basic fibroblast growth factor to a soluble receptor and for mitogenesis in whole cells. Mol Cell Biol 1992;12:240–247.
25 Rapraeger AC, Krufka A, Olwin BB: Requirement of heparan sulfate for bFGF-mediated fibroblast growth and myoblast differentiation. Science 1991; 252:1705–1708.
26 Yayon A, Klagsbrun M, Esko JD, Leder P, Ornitz DM: Cell surface, heparin-like molecules are required for binding of basic fibroblast growth factor to its high affinity receptor. Cell 1991;64:841–848.
27 Schlessinger J, Plotnikov AN, Ibrahimi OA, Eliseenkova AV, Yeh BK, et al: Crystal structure of a ternary FGF-FGFR-heparin complex reveals a dual role for heparin in FGFR binding and dimerization. Mol Cell 2000;6:743–750.
28 Pellegrini L, Burke DF, von Delft F, Mulloy B, Blundell TL: Crystal structure of fibroblast growth factor receptor ectodomain bound to ligand and heparin. Nature 2000;407:1029–1034.
29 Huang J, Mohammadi M, Rodrigues GA, Schlessinger J: Reduced activation of RAF-1 and MAP kinase by a fibroblast growth factor receptor mutant deficient in stimulation of phosphatidylinositol hydrolysis. J Biol Chem 1995;270:5065–5072.
30 Seo JH, Suenaga A, Hatakeyama M, Taiji M, Imamoto A: Structural and functional basis of a role for CRKL in a fibroblast growth factor 8-induced feed-forward loop. Mol Cell Biol 2009;29: 3076–3087.
31 Kouhara H, Hadari YR, Spivak-Kroizman T, Schilling J, Bar-Sagi D, et al: A lipid-anchored Grb2-binding protein that links FGF-receptor activation to the Ras/MAPK signaling pathway. Cell 1997; 89:693–702.
32 Wilkie AO: Bad bones, absent smell, selfish testes: the pleiotropic consequences of human FGF receptor mutations. Cytokine Growth Factor Rev 2005; 16:187–203.
33 Chen H, Ma J, Li W, Eliseenkova AV, Xu C, et al: A molecular brake in the kinase hinge region regulates the activity of receptor tyrosine kinases. Mol Cell 2007; 27:717–730.
34 Galvin BD, Hart KC, Meyer AN, Webster MK, Donoghue DJ: Constitutive receptor activation by Crouzon syndrome mutations in fibroblast growth factor receptor (FGFR)2 and FGFR2/Neu chimeras. Proc Natl Acad Sci USA 1996;93:7894–7899.
35 Neilson KM, Friesel R: Ligand-independent activation of fibroblast growth factor receptors by point mutations in the extracellular, transmembrane, and kinase domains. J Biol Chem 1996;271:25049–25057.
36 Neilson KM, Friesel RE: Constitutive activation of fibroblast growth factor receptor-2 by a point mutation associated with Crouzon syndrome. J Biol Chem 1995;270:26037–26040.
37 Meyers GA, Day D, Goldberg R, Daentl DL, Przylepa KA, et al: FGFR2 exon IIIa and IIIc mutations in Crouzon, Jackson-Weiss, and Pfeiffer syndromes: evidence for missense changes, insertions, and a deletion due to alternative RNA splicing. Am J Hum Genet 1996;58:491–498.
38 Oldridge M, Wilkie AO, Slaney SF, Poole MD, Pulleyn LJ, et al: Mutations in the third immunoglobulin domain of the fibroblast growth factor receptor-2 gene in Crouzon syndrome. Hum Mol Genet 1995;4:1077–1082.
39 Park WJ, Meyers GA, Li X, Theda C, Day D, et al: Novel *FGFR2* mutations in Crouzon and Jackson-Weiss syndromes show allelic heterogeneity and phenotypic variability. Hum Mol Genet 1995; 4:1229–1233.
40 Wilkie AO, Morriss-Kay GM, Jones EY, Heath JK: Functions of fibroblast growth factors and their receptors. Curr Biol 1995;5:500–507.
41 Robertson SC, Meyer AN, Hart KC, Galvin BD, Webster MK, Donoghue DJ: Activating mutations in the extracellular domain of the fibroblast growth factor receptor 2 function by disruption of the disulfide bond in the third immunoglobulin-like domain. Proc Natl Acad Sci USA 1998;95:4567–4572.
42 Jabs EW, Li X, Scott AF, Meyers G, Chen W, et al: Jackson-Weiss and Crouzon syndromes are allelic with mutations in fibroblast growth factor receptor 2. Nat Genet 1994;8:275–279.
43 Przylepa KA, Paznekas W, Zhang M, Golabi M, Bias W, et al: Fibroblast growth factor receptor 2 mutations in Beare-Stevenson cutis gyrata syndrome. Nat Genet 1996;13:492–494.
44 Pulleyn LJ, Reardon W, Wilkes D, Rutland P, Jones BM, et al: Spectrum of craniosynostosis phenotypes associated with novel mutations at the fibroblast growth factor receptor 2 locus. Eur J Hum Genet 1996;4:283–291.
45 Adar R, Monsonego-Ornan E, David P, Yayon A: Differential activation of cysteine-substitution mutants of fibroblast growth factor receptor 3 is determined by cysteine localization. J Bone Miner Res 2002;17:860–868.
46 Glaser RL, Broman KW, Schulman RL, Eskenazi B, Wyrobek AJ, Jabs EW: The paternal-age effect in Apert syndrome is due, in part, to the increased frequency of mutations in sperm. Am J Hum Genet 2003;73:939–947.
47 Glaser RL, Jiang W, Boyadjiev SA, Tran AK, Zachary AA, et al: Paternal origin of FGFR2 mutations in sporadic cases of Crouzon syndrome and Pfeiffer syndrome. Am J Hum Genet 2000;66:768–777.
48 Goriely A, McVean GA, Rojmyr M, Ingemarsson B, Wilkie AO: Evidence for selective advantage of pathogenic *FGFR2* mutations in the male germ line. Science 2003;301:643–646.
49 Rannan-Eliya SV, Taylor IB, De Heer IM, Van Den Ouweland AM, Wall SA, Wilkie AO: Paternal origin of *FGFR3* mutations in Muenke-type craniosynostosis. Hum Genet 2004;115:200–207.
50 Passos-Bueno MR, Wilcox WR, Jabs EW, Sertie AL, Alonso LG, Kitoh H: Clinical spectrum of fibroblast growth factor receptor mutations. Hum Mutat 1999;14:115–125.
51 Muenke M, Schell U, Hehr A, Robin NH, Losken HW, et al: A common mutation in the fibroblast growth factor receptor 1 gene in Pfeiffer syndrome. Nat Genet 1994;8:269–274.
52 Oldridge M, Zackai EH, McDonald-McGinn DM, Iseki S, Morriss-Kay GM, et al: De novo Alu-element insertions in *FGFR2* identify a distinct pathological basis for Apert syndrome. Am J Hum Genet 1999;64:446–461.
53 Lajeunie E, Cameron R, El Ghouzzi V, de Parseval N, Journeau P, et al: Clinical variability in patients with Apert's syndrome. J Neurosurg 1999;90:443–447.
54 Slaney SF, Oldridge M, Hurst JA, Morriss-Kay GM, Hall CM, et al: Differential effects of FGFR2 mutations on syndactyly and cleft palate in Apert syndrome. Am J Hum Genet 1996;58:923–932.

55 von Gernet S, Golla A, Ehrenfels Y, Schuffenhauer S, Fairley JD: Genotype-phenotype analysis in Apert syndrome suggests opposite effects of the two recurrent mutations on syndactyly and outcome of craniofacial surgery. Clin Genet 2000;57:137–139.
56 Anderson J, Burns HD, Enriquez-Harris P, Wilkie AO, Heath JK: Apert syndrome mutations in fibroblast growth factor receptor 2 exhibit increased affinity for FGF ligand. Hum Mol Genet 1998;7: 1475–1483.
57 Ibrahimi OA, Eliseenkova AV, Plotnikov AN, Yu K, Ornitz DM, Mohammadi M: Structural basis for fibroblast growth factor receptor 2 activation in Apert syndrome. Proc Natl Acad Sci USA 2001;98: 7182–7187.
58 Ibrahimi OA, Zhang F, Eliseenkova AV, Itoh N, Linhardt RJ, Mohammadi M: Biochemical analysis of pathogenic ligand-dependent FGFR2 mutations suggests distinct pathophysiological mechanisms for craniofacial and limb abnormalities. Hum Mol Genet 2004;13: 2313–2324.
59 Ibrahimi OA, Zhang F, Eliseenkova AV, Linhardt RJ, Mohammadi M: Proline to arginine mutations in FGF receptors 1 and 3 result in Pfeiffer and Muenke craniosynostosis syndromes through enhancement of FGF binding affinity. Hum Mol Genet 2004;13:69–78.
60 Yu K, Herr AB, Waksman G, Ornitz DM: Loss of fibroblast growth factor receptor 2 ligand-binding specificity in Apert syndrome. Proc Natl Acad Sci USA 2000; 97:14536–14541.
61 Ibrahimi OA, Yeh BK, Eliseenkova AV, Zhang F, Olsen SK, et al: Analysis of mutations in fibroblast growth factor (FGF) and a pathogenic mutation in FGF receptor (FGFR) provides direct evidence for the symmetric two-end model for FGFR dimerization. Mol Cell Biol 2005;25:671–684.
62 Olsen SK, Li JY, Bromleigh C, Eliseenkova AV, Ibrahimi OA, et al: Structural basis by which alternative splicing modulates the organizer activity of FGF8 in the brain. Genes Dev 2006;20:185–198.
63 Hajihosseini MK, Wilson S, De Moerlooze L, Dickson C: A splicing switch and gain-of-function mutation in *FgfR2-IIIc* hemizygotes causes Apert/Pfeiffer-syndrome-like phenotypes. Proc Natl Acad Sci USA 2001;98:3855–3860.
64 Wilkie AO, Patey SJ, Kan SH, van den Ouweland AM, Hamel BC: FGFs, their receptors, and human limb malformations: clinical and molecular correlations. Am J Med Genet 2002;112:266–278.
65 Nagase T, Nagase M, Hirose S, Ohmori K: Mutations in fibroblast growth factor receptor 2 gene and craniosynostotic syndromes in Japanese children. J Craniofac Surg 1998;9:162–170.
66 Yeh BK, Igarashi M, Eliseenkova AV, Plotnikov AN, Sher I, et al: Structural basis by which alternative splicing confers specificity in fibroblast growth factor receptors. Proc Natl Acad Sci USA 2003;100:2266–2271.
67 Hajihosseini MK, Duarte R, Pegrum J, Donjacour A, Lana-Elola E, et al: Evidence that Fgf10 contributes to the skeletal and visceral defects of an Apert syndrome mouse model. Dev Dyn 2009;238: 376–385.
68 Pollock PM, Gartside MG, Dejeza LC, Powell MA, Mallon MA, et al: Frequent activating FGFR2 mutations in endometrial carcinomas parallel germline mutations associated with craniosynostosis and skeletal dysplasia syndromes. Oncogene 2007;26:7158–7162.
69 Kan SH, Elanko N, Johnson D, Cornejo-Roldan L, Cook J, et al: Genomic screening of fibroblast growth-factor receptor 2 reveals a wide spectrum of mutations in patients with syndromic craniosynostosis. Am J Hum Genet 2002;70:472–486.
70 Rand V, Huang J, Stockwell T, Ferriera S, Buzko O, et al: Sequence survey of receptor tyrosine kinases reveals mutations in glioblastomas. Proc Natl Acad Sci USA 2005;102:14344–14349.
71 Taylor JG 6th, Cheuk AT, Tsang PS, Chung JY, Song YK, et al: Identification of *FGFR4*-activating mutations in human rhabdomyosarcomas that promote metastasis in xenotransplanted models. J Clin Invest 2009;119:3395–3407.
72 Corless CL, Schroeder A, Griffith D, Town A, McGreevey L, et al: *PDGFRA* mutations in gastrointestinal stromal tumors: frequency, spectrum and in vitro sensitivity to imatinib. J Clin Oncol 2005;23:5357–5364.
73 Medeiros F, Corless CL, Duensing A, Hornick JL, Oliveira AM, et al: KIT-negative gastrointestinal stromal tumors: proof of concept and therapeutic implications. Am J Surg Pathol 2004;28:889–894.
74 Bellus GA, Spector EB, Speiser PW, Weaver CA, Garber AT, et al: Distinct missense mutations of the FGFR3 Lys650 codon modulate receptor kinase activation and the severity of the skeletal dysplasia phenotype. Am J Hum Genet 2000;67:1411–1421.
75 Cappellen D, De Oliveira C, Ricol D, de Medina S, Bourdin J, et al: Frequent activating mutations of FGFR3 in human bladder and cervix carcinomas. Nat Genet 1999;23:18–20.
76 van Rhijn BW, van Tilborg AA, Lurkin I, Bonaventure J, de Vries A, et al: Novel fibroblast growth factor receptor 3 *(FGFR3)* mutations in bladder cancer previously identified in non-lethal skeletal disorders. Eur J Hum Genet 2002;10: 819–824.
77 Chesi M, Nardini E, Brents LA, Schröck E, Ried T, et al: Frequent translocation t(4;14)(p16.3;q32.3) in multiple myeloma is associated with increased expression and activating mutations of fibroblast growth factor receptor 3. Nat Genet 1997;16:260–264.
78 Richelda R, Ronchetti D, Baldini L, Cro L, Viggiano L, et al: A novel chromosomal translocation t(4;14)(p16.3;q32) in multiple myeloma involves the fibroblast growth-factor receptor 3 gene. Blood 1997;90:4062–4070.

Moosa Mohammadi
New York University School of Medicine, Department of Pharmacology
550 First Avenue, MSB #424/431/414
New York, NY, 10016 (USA)
Tel. +1 212 263 2907, Fax +1 212 263 7133, E-Mail Moosa.Mohammadi@nyumc.org

Muenke M, Kress W, Collmann H, Solomon BD (eds): Craniosynostoses: Molecular Genetics, Principles of Diagnosis, and Treatment.
Monogr Hum Genet. Basel, Karger, 2011, vol 19, pp 58–66

Recurrent Germline Mutations in the *FGFR2/3* Genes, High Mutation Frequency, Paternal Skewing and Age-Dependence

N. Arnheim · P. Calabrese

Molecular and Computational Biology Program, University of Southern California, Los Angeles, Calif., USA

Abstract

FGFR-associated bone dysplasias and craniosynostosis can have an astonishingly high frequency of recurrent nucleotide substitutions, which are paternally derived and age-dependent. There is increased probability for these point mutations to occur in the paternal germline in an age-dependent manner, which has been demonstrated both in semen and in slices of testes. The process is driven by a selective advantage of spermatogonial cells in adults. This has been demonstrated experimentally as the 2 recurrent mutations associated with Apert syndrome cluster in small distinct areas of the testes of normal tissue donors and by sperm analysis.

Specific Human Germline Nucleotide Substitutions Predominantly Come from Men and Increase with Age

Studies of the parental origin of sporadic cases of autosomal and sex-linked diseases have revealed many examples where the spontaneous mutations arose primarily in the male parents' germline [reviewed in 1–4]. In addition, comparisons between DNA sequences on the sex chromosomes and autosomes in different primate species [reviewed in 1] suggests that human males have on average a ~3–7 times greater neutral mutation frequency than females [1, 4–6].

Besides a male mutation bias, studies of some diseases show, that de novo mutations are more likely to occur as the male parent ages [2, 7–11]. This paternal age effect (PAE) was discovered using epidemiological data in sporadic cases of diseases [7–10, 12]. Achondroplasia is the most common form of short-limbed dwarfism and an example of a condition that exhibits both a strong male bias and a PAE [7–10, 12]. The same is true for Apert syndrome and perhaps also for Muenke syndrome and hypochondroplasia, though PAE in these latter conditions is less well-defined. These conditions result from mutations in the *FGFR2* or *FGFR3* genes.

Models to Explain Male Bias and the Paternal Age Effect

Both male-biased mutation and the PAE are typically explained by noting a fundamental difference in how gametes are formed in males and females [2, 7, 8, 10, 11, 13, 14]. In females, oogonia undergo their last premeiotic cell division during fetal development. Up until puberty, male germ cell progenitors experience approximately the same number of cell generations as female germ cells. However, after puberty, self-renewing spermatogonial cell divisions continue throughout a man's life so that sperm produced by spermatogonia from an older man have experienced many more cell generations than sperm of a younger man [2, 7–11, 13, 15, 16]. Therefore, since each cell division in the self-renewing spermatogonial cell lineage presents an additional opportunity for mutation during DNA replication, it is expected that as men age the number of mutations in their germline will increase.

Human Germline Nucleotide Substitution Mutations Vary Markedly in Frequency

Historically, studies using epidemiological data have revealed that certain genes have much higher disease mutation frequencies than other genes [8]. Thus, for some, a direct estimate of the disease mutation frequency can be made, whereas new mutations for other diseases are too infrequent to allow for an accurate direct estimate.

Before the gene mapping and DNA sequencing era, it was assumed that genetic diseases with a high de novo frequency resulted from the presence of a relatively large number of nucleotide sites in the gene that could cause the disease if mutated. We now know that this is not necessarily true. For example new mutations in the fibroblast growth factor receptor 3 gene (*FGFR3*) produce offspring with achondroplasia (MIM100800) at a birth frequency of 10^{-4}–10^{-5}. In comparison, the expected average overall frequency of mutations per nucleotide site in humans is $\sim 10^{-8}$ [17, 18]. It was assumed that many sites within the achondroplasia gene were targets for disease-causing mutations. Thus, imagine the surprise when it was discovered that virtually all of the sporadic cases of achondroplasia occur at the same *FGFR3* nucleotide (c.1138G>A) [19–21]. The most intuitive explanation was that this nucleotide site must be a mutation 'hot spot' and the mutation rate per cell division at this nucleotide site was significantly greater than the genome average. This discrepancy between the frequency of affected individuals born and the expected mutation frequency is now known for a number of other genes (see below).

Confirmation of High Nucleotide Substitution Germline Mutation Frequencies, Mutation Hot Spot versus Germline Selection Model

In 2002, we showed that it was possible to make experimental estimates of human disease nucleotide substitution mutation frequencies at the common achondroplasia site based solely on DNA analysis of sperm cells from normal individuals [22]. Soon afterwards, other studies using similar approaches involving mutations in sperm [23–25] examined Apert syndrome (MIM101200). Similar to achondroplasia, virtually all new Apert syndrome cases arise from new mutations, and there is an unexpectedly high frequency at 2 nucleotide sites (c.755C>G or c.758C>G) in the *FGFR2* gene. Apert syndrome also shows a marked PAE and a male mutation-bias. In general, all these studies [23–25] demonstrated a high frequency of de novo disease mutations in sperm from normal individuals, suggesting the presence of mutation hot spots.

The above mentioned studies on achondroplasia and Apert syndrome also suggested an alternative interpretation to the hot spot model. This interpretation speculates that selection can act to increase the sperm mutation frequency. Several studies explicitly suggested that diploid premeiotic germ cells that undergo a de novo Apert mutation gain a selective advantage over non-mutant premeiotic germ cells, thereby increasing the frequency of mutant sperm in the testis [22, 24–26].

Germline selection may extend to females. For example, trisomy 21 carrying oocytes have been

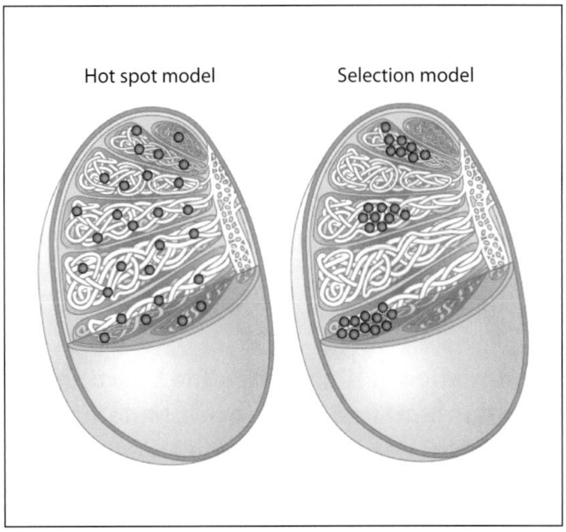

Fig. 1. Circles represent mutant testis cells (taken from [3]).

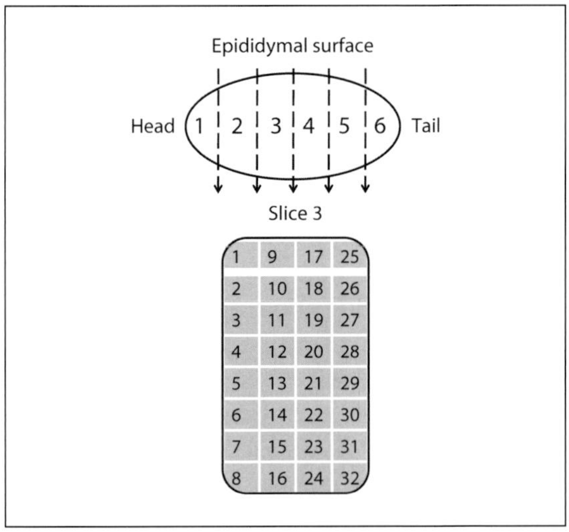

Fig. 2. Testis dissection scheme modified from [30].

suggested to have a selective survival advantage over normal oocytes as women age, at least partially explaining the increased frequency of Down syndrome in women of advanced maternal age [27, 28].

Testing the Mutation Hot Spot versus Germline Selection Model

In human testes, there is a population of premeiotic self-renewing A pale spermatogonial cells (SrAp cells), which divide continuously throughout a man's life. The SrAp cells lie uniformly scattered along the basal membrane of the seminiferous tubules that are in turn uniformly distributed throughout the testis. If a nucleotide site has a mutation rate per cell division that is much higher than average (the site is a mutation hot spot), then the mutant SrAp (and their meiotic and postmeiotic descendents) will be found uniformly distributed throughout the testis. However, if the elevated mutation frequency is due rather to a selective advantage conferred on SrAp cells harboring this mutation, then the mutants will be clustered (fig. 1, [3]).

Experimental Analysis

We studied the spatial distribution of the Apert syndrome c.755C>G and c.758C>G mutations within the testes of normal tissue donors. Each testis was cut into six slices and each slice further divided into a 4×8 grid of ~equal size pieces for a total of 192 pieces (fig. 2, [29, 30]) thereby giving an address that defines the position of every piece relative to one another. The DNA was purified from each piece and quantitated. The number of mutants in each piece was estimated using a modified PCR assay (called PAP [31]). A dilution was found at which no more than a single mutant molecule (on average) is expected in any DNA sample. The number of samples containing a mutation is counted and the mutation frequency is estimated from the total number of genome equivalents tested in each sample and the dilution factor.

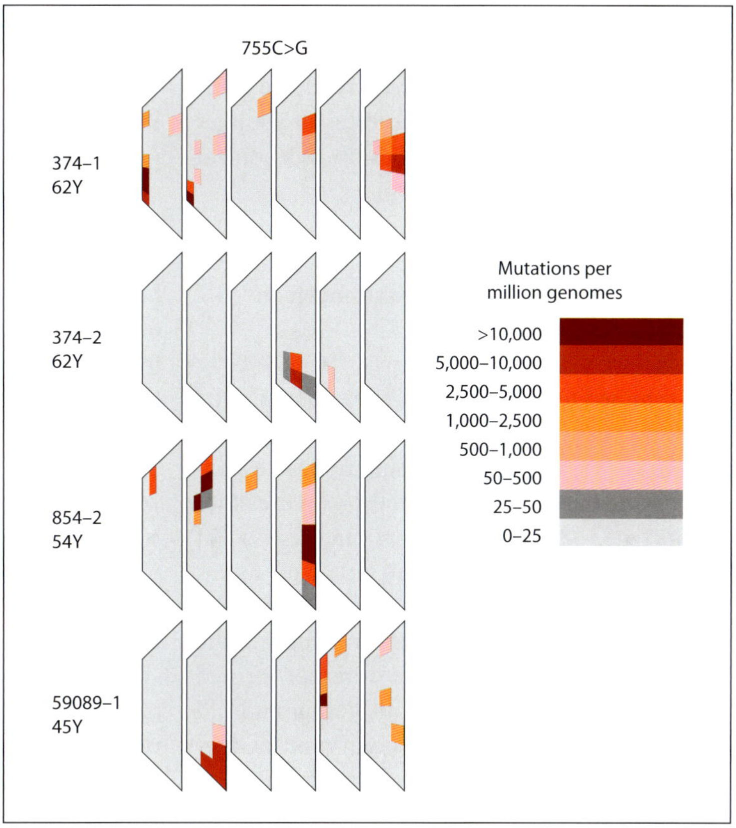

Fig. 3. Distribution of 755C>G and 758C>G mutations in 4 testes from older donors modified from [29]. From left to right are slices 1–6. Each slice is a 4×8 matrix of ~equal sized pieces.

The c.755C>G and c.758C>G Apert syndrome mutations in 4 testes from older donors (62, 54, and 45 years old) and in the testes of younger donors (described later) was analyzed [29, 30]. In the 4 older donors' testes, the results were similar for the 2 mutations (see fig. 3, [29, 30]). To cite an example, in 1 testis of a 62-year-old man (374–1), the c.755C>G mutation frequencies of individual pieces varied by several orders of magnitude, ranging from $<10^{-6}$ (no mutants found among 1 million genomes tested) to as high as 0.027 with an average frequency of 3.8×10^{-4}. This average value was close to that observed for an epididymal sperm sample taken from the proximal vas deferens of the same testis (4.5×10^{-4}). All the testes (fig. 3) are characterized by a very small number of pieces with 10^3 to $>10^4$ fold higher mutation frequencies than the remaining pieces. As a measure of this clustering, the minimum number of pieces (among a total of 192) required to contain 95% of the mutant genomes in the testes ranges from 0.3% to 8%. According to a uniform spatial distribution, many more pieces, which together contain 95% of the genomes, would have been needed. In many cases, several of the pieces with high mutation frequencies appeared to form foci adjacent to one another in 1 slice or between slices. Since we studied both the c.755C>G and c.758C>G mutations in the same testis pieces, we were also able to study whether these 2 hotspots significantly overlapped. They did not, which is expected if the different mutations arose independently.

Our results appeared to reject the hot spot model: the mutations cluster within the testis and are not distributed uniformly. Next, we compared these data to those from testes of younger donors and to the testis distribution of a control mutation.

Apert Syndrome Mutation Frequencies in Young Testis Donors

We examined testes from 2 younger donors, aged 19 and 23 years [29], and more recently a 21- and 36-year-old for the c.755G>C mutation. These results differed dramatically from those in the older donors (aged 45, 54, and 62 years). In the testes of the younger donors, there were either no mutation clusters or the clusters had much lower frequencies ($\sim 10^{-7}$). This observation supports the idea that the mutation clusters were not formed during testes development (both young and old donors went through the same embryonic and fetal development), but rather grew in the testes as men aged.

Testis Distribution of a C to G Transversion Mutation at a Control CpG Site

We also analyzed a completely unrelated site (the C of a CpG site in an intron of the *CAV1* gene) for C to G mutations [30]. Unlike the c.755C>G Apert syndrome mutation (also at a CpG site), there was a narrow range of frequencies in the individual pieces ($<4 \times 10^{-6}$ to 2×10^{-5}) in both testes of the 62-year-old donor. The control site mutation frequency is 2 orders of magnitude less than at the 2 Apert sites. The lack of any foci with very high mutation frequencies suggests that clustering is unusual in the human testis and that something is fundamentally different between the control CpG site and either of the Apert-associated mutation sites.

By Including Selection, Computational Analysis Explains the Testis Data

We created a mathematical model of human germline development [29, 30] to test the hot spot model. This model (see fig. 1) predicted a uniform distribution of mutations, unlike the data (see fig. 3), and we were therefore able to reject the hot spot model [29, 30]. Our testis experiments on Apert syndrome along with studies examining Apert mutations in sperm [24, 25] suggest that there must be an alternative explanation to the hot spot model for the high frequency of mutation. Germline selection is one possibility [22, 24, 26]. The form of selection we considered [29, 30] is that both Apert mutations promote rare symmetric divisions of SrAp cells in the adult testis. Since these new SrAp cells should remain close to their progenitors, these rare symmetric divisions enable mutation clusters to form and grow locally (similar to a tumor), increasing the overall mutation frequency in the testis. Interestingly, studies on *FGFR2* in endometrial carcinomas revealed a high frequency of tumors with the c.755C>G mutation [32].

To examine our selection idea we modified our mathematical model of human germline development [29, 30]. The modified model contained a selection parameter p: at each adult-phase generation, a mutated SrAp divides symmetrically with probability p and divides asymmetrically with probability 1–p (after a symmetric division, each daughter SrAp reverts to asymmetric divisions until the next rare symmetric division). A similar model was independently proposed by Crow [33].

We inferred the selection parameter and the mutation rate per cell division by fitting both the overall testis mutation frequency and the minimum number of pieces that together contain 95% of the mutant genomes. The inferred probability value of the selection parameter was approximately 0.01 (on average 1 of every hundred divisions is symmetric). With this parameter value the distribution of frequencies in the testis pieces now matches the data. In the computer simulations, foci of high mutation frequency emerge and, as in the testis data, these foci often intersect several adjacent testis pieces. Moreover, simulations with the inferred mutation rate per cell division match the observed mutation frequencies of the testes (10^{-4}–10^{-5}); however, simulations with this same mutation rate, but setting the selection parameter to zero so that there is no selection and all adult phase generations are asymmetric predicted a much lower testis mutation frequency in the range expected for CpG sites in the studies on neutral and other disease mutations [17, 18]. We conclude that the new Apert syndrome mutation frequency is so high because of selection, not because of recurrent nucleotide substitution.

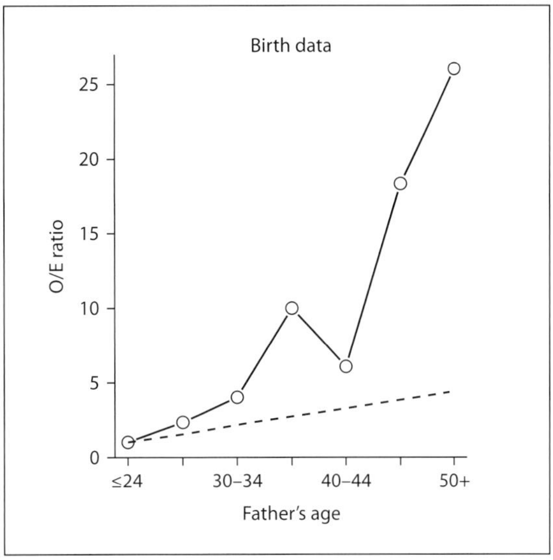

Fig. 4. The solid line is the observed/expected (O/E) ratio for Apert syndrome as a function of the father's age, normalized to be one for the youngest age category. The dashed line shows the increase expected due to the number of germline divisions (taken from [34]).

The Parental Age Effect of Apert Syndrome Occurrence Revisited

Figure 4 [34] shows the birth data [9] for Apert syndrome. The solid line is the observed/expected (O/E) birth ratio as a function of the father's age. The 'observed' numerator is the number of affected births to fathers in that age category, and the 'expected' denominator is proportional to the total number of births in the population (the vast majority of which do not have the disease) to fathers in that age category.

Recently, for achondroplasia and Apert syndrome, several studies [23, 24, 35] tested whether the increase in the birth incidence with the father's age (fig. 4) is consistent with the increase in the sperm mutation frequency of normal donors (not affected, nor known fathers of affected children) varying in age. If true then the O/E ratio is an estimate of the sperm mutation frequency. Previously in achondroplasia, we had shown that though the frequency of the causal mutation in sperm increased on average with the age of the donor, this increase was not sufficient to explain the increase in the birth data. This led us speculate that perhaps the mutated sperm were more likely to fertilize an egg than the non-mutated sperm. For Apert syndrome, 1 study had suggested that the increase in the birth data was consistent with the increase in the sperm data [24], while another study [23] had determined the 2 increases were not consistent (the 2 studies collected sperm samples from different individuals).

We recently [34] carried out an experiment on sperm where we measured the frequency of both the c.755C>G and c.758C>G mutations in 314 normal donors, more than double the number in either of the 2 previous studies, and with an assay at least 25 times more sensitive. The donors ranged in age from 18 to 78 years. Figure 5a and b [34] shows that, on average, the frequency of the 2 mutations increases with the age of the donor. The ratio of the average c.755C>G sperm mutation frequency to the average c.758C>G frequency is 1.99 (note the different Y axis scales in fig. 5), which is expected since in clinical studies two

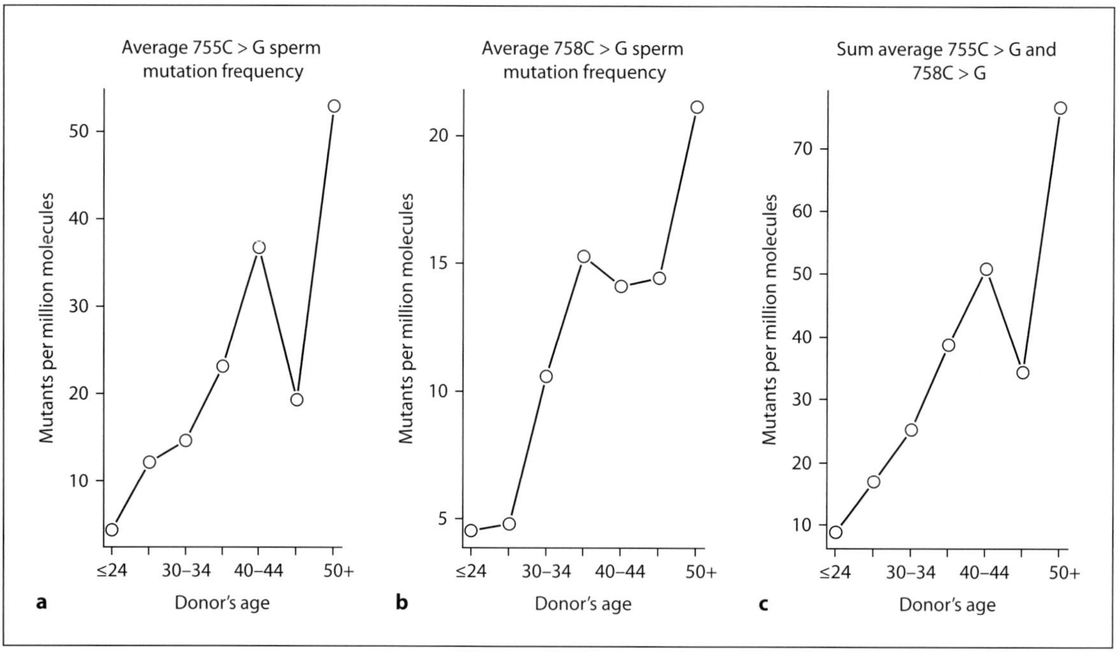

Fig. 5. The average Apert sperm mutation frequencies (taken from [34]).

thirds of cases are caused by the c.755C>G mutation and the remaining one third by the c.758C>G mutation [36]. Since either 1 of the 2 mutations is sufficient to cause Apert syndrome, we also show the average of the sum of these 2 mutations' frequencies (fig. 5c). Statistical analysis showed us that we could not reject the hypothesis that the birth data is consistent with the sperm data.

Perhaps the most striking visual property of figure 5 is the non-monotonic increase in frequency. For the birth data, the O/E ratio is lower for the 40–44 than the 35–39 and 45–49 age categories. The birth data [9] is a compilation of 3 studies published in 1960 [37], 1975 [38], and 1987 [9]. This decrease in the O/E ratio for the 40–44 age group is present in all 3 studies at the same age category. For the sperm data, the sum of the 2 mutation frequencies is lower for the 45–49 age category than the 40–44 and 50+ age categories. The dip in the sperm data is 5 years later than in the birth data [34]. Statistical analysis has supported the dips in both the birth data and the sperm data [9, 34]. A possible explanation of these dips is the introduction of fresh, usually quiescent, reserve population of A dark (Ad) spermatogonia at middle age that appear to replace SrAp cells that die (see [34]). As for the different ages of the dips in the birth and the sperm data, the birth data is from 3 studies that were published between 20 and 50 years ago, while the sperm donors were recruited much more recently. There is some evidence that contemporary youths begin puberty at younger ages [39, 40] and that there has been a decrease in sperm quality over the last 50 years [41]. The effects of these or other possible generational changes (such as environmental exposures) are unclear, but it is conceivable that they could influence the difference in timing of the non-monotonic increase in the birth and sperm data.

Why Does the Sperm Mutation Frequency Go up with Age?

The standard explanation for the PAE is that the replication of premeiotic cells throughout a male's life leads to an accumulation of more mutations in the germline of older individuals, increasing the mutation frequency in their sperm. This explanation, however, expects a linear increase with age (see fig. 4). Risch et al. [9] examined the birth data for several paternal age effect diseases and found that some showed a linear increase, but that others, such as Apert syndrome, featured an exponential increase. The dashed line in figure 4 shows the linear increase expected due to the number of germline cell generations. This dashed line was calculated simply by counting the average number of cell generations for fathers in each age category, using the estimate that SrAp divide every 16 days [42]. The O/E ratio (solid line), in figure 4, has a 26-fold increase from the youngest age category to the oldest, while the expected increase due to the number of germline divisions has only a 4-fold increase. The results shown in figure 4 argue that the standard explanation for the paternal age effect is not sufficient to explain the birth data for Apert syndrome. The germline selection model we introduced to explain the clustering of mutations in the testes could also contribute to the greater than linear increase in mutation frequencies observed in both the birth data and the sperm data. However, the details are not well understood and await further investigations.

References

1 Li WH, Yi S, Makova K: Male-driven evolution. Curr Opin Genet Dev 2002;12:650–656.
2 Glaser RL, Jabs EW: Dear old dad. Sci Aging Knowledge Environ 2004;re1.
3 Arnheim N, Calabrese P: Understanding what determines the frequency and pattern of human germline mutations. Nat Rev Genet 2009;10:478–488.
4 Ellegren H: Characteristics, causes and evolutionary consequences of male-biased mutation. Proc Biol Sci 2007;274:1–10.
5 Makova KD, Li WH: Strong male-driven evolution of DNA sequences in humans and apes. Nature 2002;416:624–626.
6 Chimpanzee Sequencing and Analysis Consortium: Initial sequence of the chimpanzee genome and comparison with the human genome. Nature 2005;437:69–87.
7 Vogel F, Rathenberg R: Spontaneous mutation in man. Adv Hum Genet 1975;5:223–318.
8 Vogel F, Motulsky AG: Human Genetics: Problems and Approaches (Springer, Berlin, New York 1997).
9 Risch N, Reich EW, Wishnick MM, McCarthy JG: Spontaneous mutation and parental age in humans. Am J Hum Genet 1987;41:218–248.
10 Crow JF: The origins, patterns and implications of human spontaneous mutation. Nat Rev Genet 2000;1:40–47.
11 Penrose L: Paternal age and mutation. Lancet 1955;269:312–313.
12 Orioli IM, Castilla EE, Scarano G, Mastroiacovo P: Effect of paternal age in achondroplasia, thanatophoric dysplasia, and osteogenesis imperfecta. Am J Med Genet 1995;59:209–217.
13 Crow JF: How much do we know about spontaneous human mutation rates? [published erratum appears in Environ Mol Mutagen 1993;21:389]. Environ Mol Mutagen 1993;21:122–129.
14 Drost JB, Lee WR: Biological basis of germline mutation: comparisons of spontaneous germline mutation rates among drosophila, mouse, and human. Environ Mol Mutagen 1995;25:48–64.
15 Huttley GA, Jakobsen IB, Wilson SR, Easteal S: How important is DNA replication for mutagenesis? Mol Biol Evol 2000;17:929–937.
16 Hurst LD, Ellegren H: Sex biases in the mutation rate. Trends Genet 1998;14:446–452.
17 Nachman MW, Crowell SL: Estimate of the mutation rate per nucleotide in humans. Genetics 2000;156:297–304.
18 Kondrashov AS: Direct estimates of human per nucleotide mutation rates at 20 loci causing Mendelian diseases. Hum Mutat 2003;21:12–27.
19 Rousseau F, Bonaventure J, Legeai-Mallet L, Pelet A, Rozet JM, et al: Mutations in the gene encoding fibroblast growth factor receptor-3 in achondroplasia. Nature 1994;371:252–254.
20 Shiang R, Thompson LM, Zhu YZ, Church DM, Fielder TJ, et al: Mutations in the transmembrane domain of FGFR3 cause the most common genetic form of dwarfism, achondroplasia. Cell 1994;78:335–342.
21 Bellus GA, Hefferon TW, Ortiz de Luna RI, Hecht JT, Horton WA, et al: Achondroplasia is defined by recurrent G380R mutations of FGFR3. Am J Hum Genet 1995;56:368–373.
22 Tiemann-Boege I, Navidi W, Grewal R, Cohn D, Eskenazi B, Wyrobek AJ, Arnheim N: The observed human sperm mutation frequency cannot explain the achondroplasia paternal age effect. Proc Natl Acad Sci USA 2002;99:14952–14957.

23 Glaser RL, Broman KW, Schulman RL, Eskenazi B, Wyrobek AJ, Jabs EW: The paternal-age effect in Apert syndrome is due, in part, to the increased frequency of mutations in sperm. Am J Hum Genet 2003;73:939–947.
24 Goriely A, McVean GA, Rojmyr M, Ingemarsson B, Wilkie AO: Evidence for selective advantage of pathogenic *FGFR2* mutations in the male germ line. Science 2003;301:643–646.
25 Goriely A, McVean GA, van Pelt AM, O'Rourke AW, Wall SA, de Rooij DG, Wilkie AO: Gain-of-function amino acid substitutions drive positive selection of FGFR2 mutations in human spermatogonia. Proc Natl Acad Sci USA 2005;102:6051–6056.
26 Kan SH, Elanko N, Johnson D, Cornejo-Roldan L, Cook J, et al: Genomic screening of fibroblast growth-factor receptor 2 reveals a wide spectrum of mutations in patients with syndromic craniosynostosis. Am J Hum Genet 2002;70:472–486.
27 Hulten MA, Patel SD, Tankimanova M, Westgren M, Papadogiannakis N, Jonsson AM Iwarsson E: On the origin of trisomy 21 Down syndrome. Mol Cytogenet 2008;1:21.
28 Hulten M, Patel S, Jonasson J, Iwarsson E: On the origin of the maternal age effect in trisomy 21 Down syndrome: The Oocyte Mosaicism Selection (OMS) Model. Reproduction 2009;15:15.
29 Choi SK, Yoon SR, Calabrese P, Arnheim N: A germ-line-selective advantage rather than an increased mutation rate can explain some unexpectedly common human disease mutations. Proc Natl Acad Sci USA 2008;105:10143–10148.
30 Qin J, Calabrese P, Tiemann-Boege I, Shinde DN, Yoon SR, et al: The molecular anatomy of spontaneous germline mutations in human testes. PLoS Biol 2007;5:e224.
31 Liu Q, Sommer SS: Detection of extremely rare alleles by bidirectional pyrophosphorolysis-activated polymerization allele-specific amplification (Bi-PAP-A): measurement of mutation load in mammalian tissues. Biotechniques 2004;36:156–166.
32 Pollock PM, Gartside MG, Dejeza LC, Powell MA, Mallon MA, et al: Frequent activating *FGFR2* mutations in endometrial carcinomas parallel germline mutations associated with craniosynostosis and skeletal dysplasia syndromes. Oncogene 2007;26:7158–7162.
33 Crow JF: Age and sex effects on human mutation rates: an old problem with new complexities. J Radiat Res (Tokyo) 2006;47 (suppl B):B75–B82.
34 Yoon SR, Qin J, Glaser RL, Jabs EW, Wexler NS, et al: The ups and downs of mutation frequencies during aging can account for the Apert syndrome paternal age effect. PLoS Genet 2009;5:e1000558.
35 Dakouane Giudicelli M, Serazin V, Le Sciellour CR, Albert M, Selva J, Giudicelli Y: Increased achondroplasia mutation frequency with advanced age and evidence for G1138A mosaicism in human testis biopsies. Fertil Steril 2008;89:1651–1656.
36 Muenke M, Wilkie AO: The Online Metabolic and Molecular Bases of Inherited Disease, 2007 www.ommbid.com/OMMBID/the_online_metabolic_bases_of_inherited_disease/b/fulltext/part30/ch245/9.
37 Blank CE: Apert's syndrome (a type of acrocephalosyndactyly): observations on a British series of thirty-nine cases. Ann Hum Genet 1960;24:151–164.
38 Cohen MM Jr: An etiologic and nosologic overview of craniosynostosis syndromes. Birth Defects Orig Artic Ser 1975;11:137–189.
39 Herman-Giddens ME, Wang L, Koch G: Secondary sexual characteristics in boys: estimates from the national health and nutrition examination survey III, 1988–1994. Arch Pediatr Adolesc Med 2001;155:1022–1028.
40 Karpati AM, Rubin CH, Kieszak SM, Marcus M, Troiano RP: Stature and pubertal stage assessment in American boys: the 1988–1994 Third National Health and Nutrition Examination Survey. J Adolesc Health 2002;30:205–212.
41 Carlsen E, Giwercman A, Keiding N, Skakkebaek NE: Evidence for decreasing quality of semen during past 50 years. BMJ 1992;305:609–613.
42 Heller CG, Clermont Y: Spermatogenesis in man: an estimate of its duration. Science 1963;140:184–186.

Norman Arnheim, Peter Calabrese
Molecular and Computational Biology Program
University of Southern California
1050 Childs Way, Los Angeles, California, 90089-2910 (USA)
Tel. +1 213 740 7675, Fax +1 213 740 8631, E-Mail arnheim@usc.edu, petercal@usc.edu

Muenke M, Kress W, Collmann H, Solomon BD (eds): Craniosynostoses: Molecular Genetics, Principles of Diagnosis, and Treatment.
Monogr Hum Genet. Basel, Karger, 2011, vol 19, pp 67–88

Apert, Crouzon, and Pfeiffer Syndromes

M. Michael Cohen Jr.

Department of Pediatrics, Faculty of Medicine, Dalhousie University, Halifax, N.S., Canada

Abstract
This study is based on our research analysis of 136 cases of Apert syndrome, 61 cases of Crouzon syndrome, and a large number of patients with Pfeiffer syndrome. For Apert syndrome, the following topics are discussed: growth and development; visceral anomalies; central nervous system; performance; craniofacial findings; upper and lower respiratory compromise; anomalies of the hands, feet, shoulders, elbows, hips, knees, rib cage, and spine, including histologic, radiographic, and longitudinal data; cutaneous manifestations; prenatal diagnosis; and molecular genetics. For Crouzon syndrome, the following topics are discussed: central nervous system; upper and lower respiratory compromise; cervical anomalies; radiographic findings; craniofacial abnormalities; ophthalmologic, aural, and oral findings; and molecular genetics. For Pfeiffer syndrome, the following topics are discussed: subtypes of Pfeiffer syndrome; craniofacial features; central nervous system; hands and feet; vertebral abnormalities; other skeletal findings; miscellaneous abnormalities; and molecular genetics.

This chapter focuses on Apert [1], Crouzon [2], and Pfeiffer syndromes [3].

Apert Syndrome

This section is based on our analysis of 136 cases of Apert syndrome from 33 published articles covering all aspects of the disorder. Six of the novel subgroups addressed include (1) the neuropathology of the brain, (2) a study of cranial volume with a comparison to that of Crouzon syndrome, (3) a study of newborns, (4) a prenatal study of the limbs and trachea histologically, (5) a study of the shoulders, elbows, knees, and pelvis in 38 cases, and (6) a series of patients who never had any cranial, facial, or hand surgery, allowing us to follow the natural history of Apert syndrome [4].

Apert syndrome is characterized by craniosynostosis, midface deficiency, symmetric syndactyly of the hands and feet (fig. 1A–C), and many other abnormalities. Birth prevalence is approximately 15–16 per 1,000,000 newborns [5]. Inheritance is autosomal dominant with a male-to-female ratio of 1:1 with most cases representing new mutations. The rarity of familial cases can be explained by reduced genetic fitness of affected individuals, and the presence of mental deficiency, found in some cases, diminishes the likelihood of mating [6, 7]. Origin of new mutations is exclusively of paternal origin [8].

Growth and Development

Because megalencephaly and increased head height are characteristic of Apert syndrome (figs. 1L–N, 2C, 3A), the head is unusually heavy and the cranium is disproportionately high. Because these characteristics are present at birth, head circumference, length, and weight are above the normal 50th centile (table 1); 16% exceed 4,000 g in weight compared to about 5% in the general

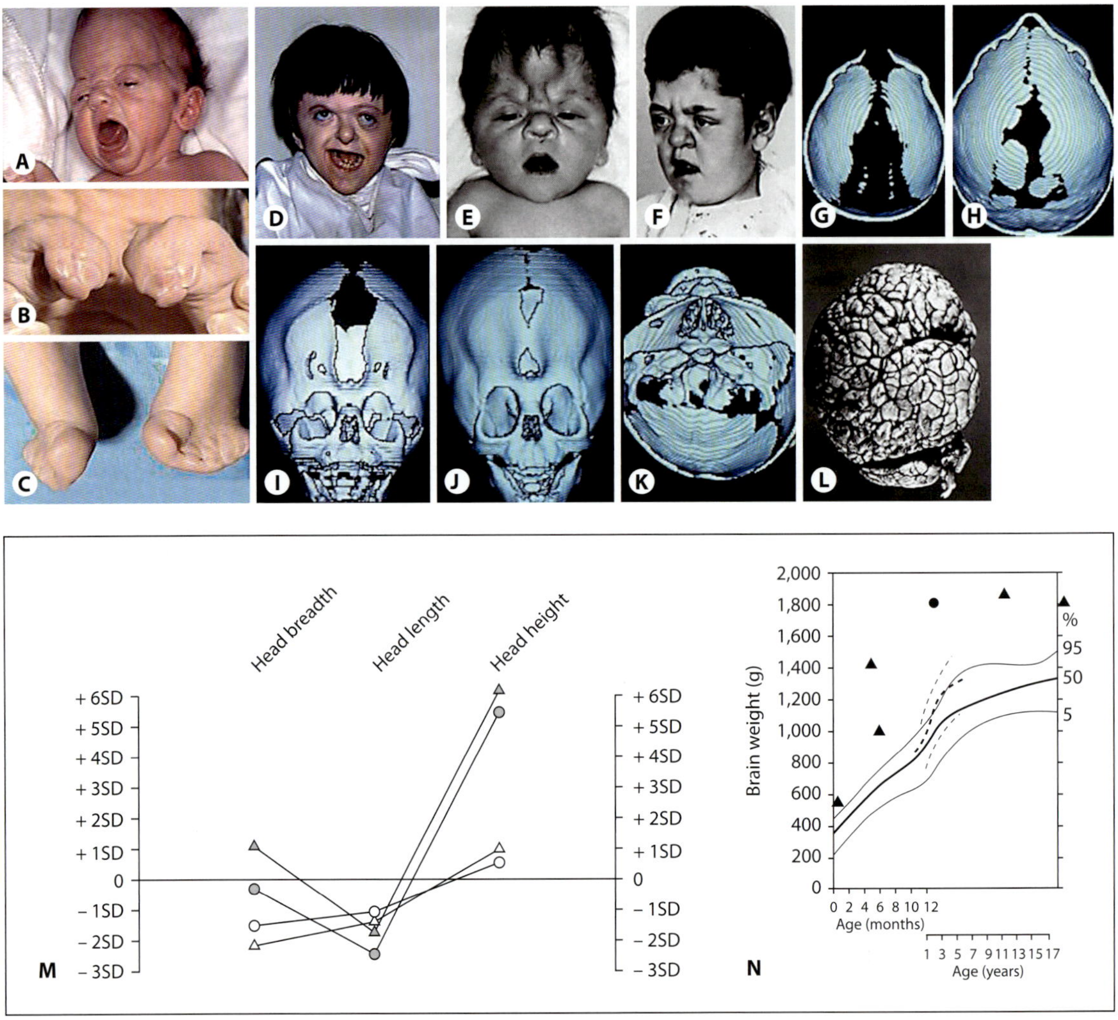

Fig. 1. Apert Syndrome. **A–C** Apert syndrome phenotype. **D** Facial asymmetry. **E, F** In **E**, note midline calvarial defect mimicking a 'frontal encephalocele' in an infant. In **F**, the same patient at 10 years of age with closure of the midline defect without any surgical intervention. **G–K** Three-dimensional radiographic views. **G, I** Note midline calvarial defect. In **I**, note abnormally large anterolateral fontanels extending into the orbits. **H, J** Note closure of midline calvarial defect with bony islands. **K** Asymmetry of the cranial base. **L** Megalencephaly and polymicrogyria at 34 weeks of gestation. **M** Average cranial profile pattern of 15 male and 12 female adults with Apert syndrome (solid circles, males; solid triangles, females). Pattern demonstrates that head breadth is either normal or slightly increased, head length is significantly short, and head height is dramatically increased. Open circles (males) and triangles (females) represent the profile pattern of adults with Crouzon syndrome for comparison; note dramatically different cranial configuration in the 2 syndromes. The Crouzon measurements demonstrate a much smaller skull. The horizontal 0 line represents the mean normal value. Vertical lines indicate standard deviations above and below mean normal values. **N** Megalencephaly is characteristic of Apert syndrome. Six brain weights from our own autopsy series at different ages (triangles, 5 females; circle, 1 male). Range of female brain weights is represented by the solid lines and the range of males brain weights is represented by the dotted lines (5th, 50th, and 95th centiles). All brain weights are dramatically above the 95th centile.

Table 1. Measurements of newborns with Apert syndrome [9]

Measurement		Sample size	Mean	Normal 50th centile
Birth length	males	26	53.0 cm	50.5 cm
	females	21	52.3 cm	49.9 cm
Birth weight	males	39	3.58 kg	3.27 kg
	females	37	3.54 kg	3.23 kg
Head circumference	males	15	35.4 cm	34.8 cm
	females	11	34.5 cm	34.3 cm

Table 2. Mean adult cranial volume in milliliters [17]

Group		Number of subjects	Estimated volume
Apert (using maximum head length)	males	15	1723
	females	12	1722
Apert (using regular OFC)	males	15	1632
	females	12	1589
Crouzon	males	18	1411
	females	17	1274
Normal	males	30	1548
	females	37	1425

population [9]. The growth pattern in childhood consists of a slowing of linear growth with most values falling between the 5th and 50th centiles. From adolescence to adulthood, slowing becomes more pronounced. This two-step deceleration results in large measure from rhizomelic shortness of the lower limbs (see below) [9, 10].

Visceral Anomalies

Cardiovascular and genitourinary anomalies occur in 10% and 9.6% of patients, respectively. Complex and multiple cardiac anomalies are frequently associated with an early death [1, 11]. Among genitourinary anomalies, hydronephrosis (3%) and cryptorchidism (4.5%, n = 66 males) occur most commonly. Both cardiovascular and genitourinary anomalies should be considered in the workup of all Apert syndrome newborns [11]. Anomalies of the respiratory system (1.5%) and gastrointestinal system (1.5%) occur with lower frequency [11]. Factors known to be associated with an early demise in Apert syndrome include prematurity, solid cartilaginous trachea (see below) [1, 11, 12], complex cardiovascular malformations, and frank cloverleaf skull (see below) [1, 13, 14].

Central Nervous Abnormalities

Benign distortion ventriculomegaly is characteristic of Apert syndrome infants (26/28 cases in our series [1, 9, 15]. Similarly, another group reported the same findings in 12 of 13 cases [16].

It is important to understand why benign distortion ventriculomegaly is characteristic of Apert syndrome: (1) our neuropathologic study of brains from 6 cases at different ages shows that brain weights are far in excess of the 95th centile [9] (fig. 1N), (2) our study demonstrates a cranial volume far in excess of normal [17] (table 2). In contrast, the cranial volume is much smaller than normal in Crouzon syndrome (fig. 1M, table 2); (3) the cranial shape in Apert syndrome is distorted (fig. 1L); (4) except for early closure of the coronal suture, a large midline calvarial defect is present during infancy (fig. 1I, G), the other sutures are patent, and the synchondroses are so widely patent that the abnormal anterolateral fontanels intrude into the orbits (fig. 1I). Thus, the Apert syndrome brain is megalencephalic, the skull is large and distorted, and sutures (except coronal) and synchondroses are widely patent. Thus, benign ventriculomegaly is the proper term [15]. Tokumaru et al. [18] also found distortion ventriculomegaly in their patients (n = 8). Noetzel et al. [19] spoke of 'nonprogressive ventriculomegaly'. We disagree with those who refer to this as 'arrested or compensated hydrocephalus' [20, 21] or those who feel that this issue is complex and not resolved [22].

With closure of the skull, however, there is a risk of increased intracranial pressure and even progressive hydrocephalus. Early surgical intervention is important in this regard, although continued monitoring for increased intracranial pressure is essential because progressive hydrocephalus may occur or recur. Combining our infant data [1] with that of the Australian group [16], progressive hydrocephalus occurred in 7.3% (n = 41). Renier and his coworkers [23, 24] reported a similar frequency in his patients (8%).

Comment. In one study [23, 24], 88% of all patients had surgery (n = 60), but only 61.6% had surgical intervention before 1 year of age. The others did not have surgery until later, and, further, 16.6% were institutionalized. Thus, the finding of raised intracranial pressure was related to closure of the skull. A second study [25] reported that 83% of patients (n = 24) developed increased intracranial pressure. The authors indicate that their rate was higher than ever reported earlier. In the protocol they adopted, Apert syndrome patients do not have any preemptive surgery. Rather, they waited until the intracranial pressure rose before they began treatment, so the high frequency of raised intracranial pressure was a function of their protocol.

In 1990 [15], we reported hypoplasia of the corpus callosum, agenesis of the corpus callosum and absent or defective septum pellucidum. In our neuropathologic study of 5 cases, we also noted polymicrogyria, dorsally displaced hippocampi and hippocampal gyri, hypoplastic white matter, and heterotopic gray matter. Renier et al. [23] confirmed some of our findings (no autopsies) in a large series (n = 60) with hypoplasia of the corpus callosum (27%), agenesis of the corpus callosum (3%), agenesis of the septum pellucidum (30%), and cavum septum pellucidum (25%). They [24] noted that anomalies of the septum pellucidum seemed to play a partial role in the mental prognosis of Apert syndrome: 50% of patients with a normal septum had an IQ > 70 compared to 18% in those with septal anomalies. Cinalli et al. [26] found tonsillar herniation in 1.7% (n = 44) compared to 72% in Crouzon syndrome.

Performance

Lefèbvre et al. [27] studied 25 children who underwent neurosurgery to correct craniosynostosis during infancy (average age: 3 months). The mean IQ was 73.6 with a range of 52–89 with 'only two patients functioning within the average range of intelligence'. In the series of Renier et al. (n = 60) [24], the main factor influencing the mental prognosis was the age at the time of surgery: IQ > 70 in 50% of the children operated on before one year of age compared to an IQ > 70 in only 8% of those who had surgery later. I have discussed other series elsewhere [1].

Five interesting outliers in our series of 136 patients include 4 college graduates: two without any cranial or craniofacial surgery whatsoever and two who had surgical procedures. Of the two who had surgery, one with minimal surgical

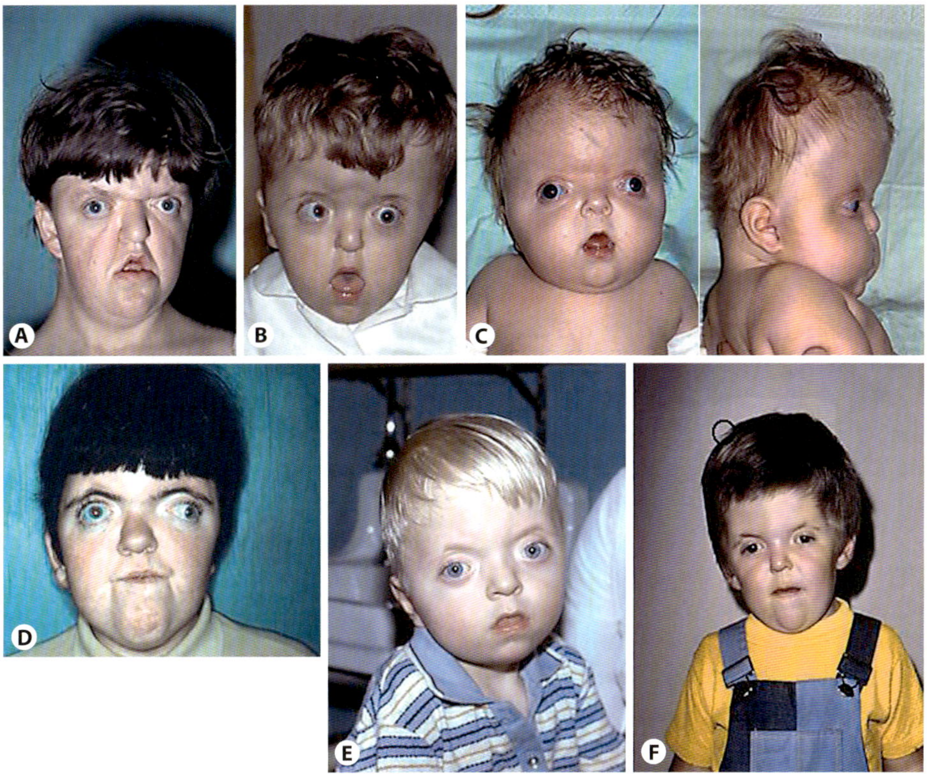

Fig. 2. Apert Syndrome. **A** Severe phenotype in a teenage girl. Note trapezoidal configuration of the lips at rest. **B** Severe phenotype with no cranial or craniofacial surgical procedure. Note esotropia. **C** Frontal and lateral view of a severely affected infant, who later had cranial surgical intervention followed by a craniofacial procedure at a much later date. Note strabismus, downslanting palpebral fissures, increased head height and decreased head length. **D** Asymmetric appearance. Note hypertelorism, asymmetrically downslanting palpebral fissures, and exotropia. Compare her degree of asymmetry to that of a younger patient with more severe asymmetry shown in figure 1D. **E** Crouzonoid appearance of a patient with classic syndactyly and other typical skeletal manifestations of Apert syndrome. **F** Mild facial phenotype.

intervention has two master's degrees. Another with cranial surgery, but with only a single surgical division of his middigital hand mass works at a television station and is the bicycling champion in his city. Another (separate) patient with a classic Apert syndrome appearance had open coronal sutures at 14.5 years of age.

Craniofacial Abnormalities

Craniofacial features may be severe, asymmetric, mild, or even Crouzonoid (fig. 2). In infancy, a wide midline calvarial defect is present extending from the glabella to the posterior fontanel. Bony islands, beginning anywhere within the defect, form and coalesce, resulting in complete obliteration during the first year or two of life (fig. 1H, J). No proper sagittal and metopic sutures ever form ab initio or later. The coronal suture is closed at birth, the anterolateral and posterolateral fontanels are abnormally large, the synchondroses are patent, and both lambdoid and squamosal sutures are patent. Thus, increased intracranial pressure is unlikely while all these are patent, but increases after closure without surgical intervention. Interestingly, sutural interdigitations fail to form ab initio in the midline defect, resulting in a suture default zone. Thus, the appropriate term is sutural agenesis, not craniosynostosis [28–30].

In frontal view during infancy, the midline calvarial defect may simulate an anterior encephalocele. Figure 1E shows such a patient at 2.5 weeks of age, but with closure of the midline calvarial defect, this disappears completely as can be seen in the same patient at 10 years (fig. 1F), who had no surgical intervention in this area. We do have one large (real) encephalocele in a single patient [13].

Variability in the facial phenotype is demonstrated in figure 2. Craniofacial asymmetry is common in Apert syndrome (figs. 1D, K, 2D) and is found in 42% (n = 62) of patients; it is related to megalencephaly combined with open sutures (except coronal), open fontanels, and open synchondroses. We recommend that during early infancy in Apert syndrome changing the head position on successive nights from back to left side to right side on a rotational basis [1, 28, 29].

Radiographic Findings in the Craniofacial Region
During infancy, thinning and hypoplasia are constant (100%, n = 16). Fused sutures (>4–30 years) include the coronal (100%, n = 67), sagittal (85%, n = 62), and lambdoid (81%, n = 67). Other craniofacial findings include frontal protrusion (63%, n = 70), marked craniofacial asymmetry (42%, n = 62), increased digital markings (81%, n = 58), enlargement of the sella turcica (66%, n = 70), absence of the frontal sinus (16+ years) (36%, n = 22), deviation of the nasal septum (73%, n = 63), obstruction of the nasopharynx (51%, n = 71), and calcification of the stylohyoid ligament (66%, n = 70) [31].

Respiratory Problems
The reduced nasopharyngeal dimensions and reduced patency of the posterior choanae pose a risk of respiratory embarrassment, obstructive sleep apnea, cor pulmonale and even sudden death. During infancy, the only option is tracheostomy with or without some air tubing at night. Apert syndrome patients should be monitored for snoring and/or an unusual amount of daytime somnolence and when apparent should be referred to a sleep center for proper diagnosis and treatment [12].

Cartilage Sleeve Abnormalities
Rarely, serious lower respiratory compromise in Apert syndrome is caused by failure of segmentation of the cartilaginous rings (n = 8), so that the trachea is solidly cartilaginous (fig. 4B, C). This results in the inability to handle respiratory secretions. MRI is recommended for any Apert syndrome infant with signs of lower respiratory compromise [12].

Ophthalmologic Abnormalities
Ocular findings include hypertelorism, proptosis (often asymmetric), and downslanting palpebral fissures (also often asymmetric). Most inner and outer canthal distances were increased above the 75th or 97th centiles (n = 30). Exotropia was characteristic. The V pattern was common with divergent upgaze and esotropic downgaze. Hyperopia, myopia, and astigmatism were found frequently. Strabismus and significant refractive errors sometimes caused amblyopia. Structural abnormalities of the extraocular muscles were found in some cases, particularly absence of the superior rectus muscle. The eyebrows sometimes have a break in continuity, which corresponds exactly to a specific defect of the supraorbital rims (fig. 3B) [31, 32].

Oral Manifestations
In the relaxed state, particularly during infancy, the lips assume a trapezoidal configuration (fig. 3F). The palate is highly arched and constricted with a median furrow in 94% (n = 68) (fig. 3C). Lateral palatal swellings increase in size with age and contain excess mucopolysaccharide, predominantly hyaluronic acid, and to a lesser extent, sulfated mucopolysaccharides (fig. 3D, E). The hard

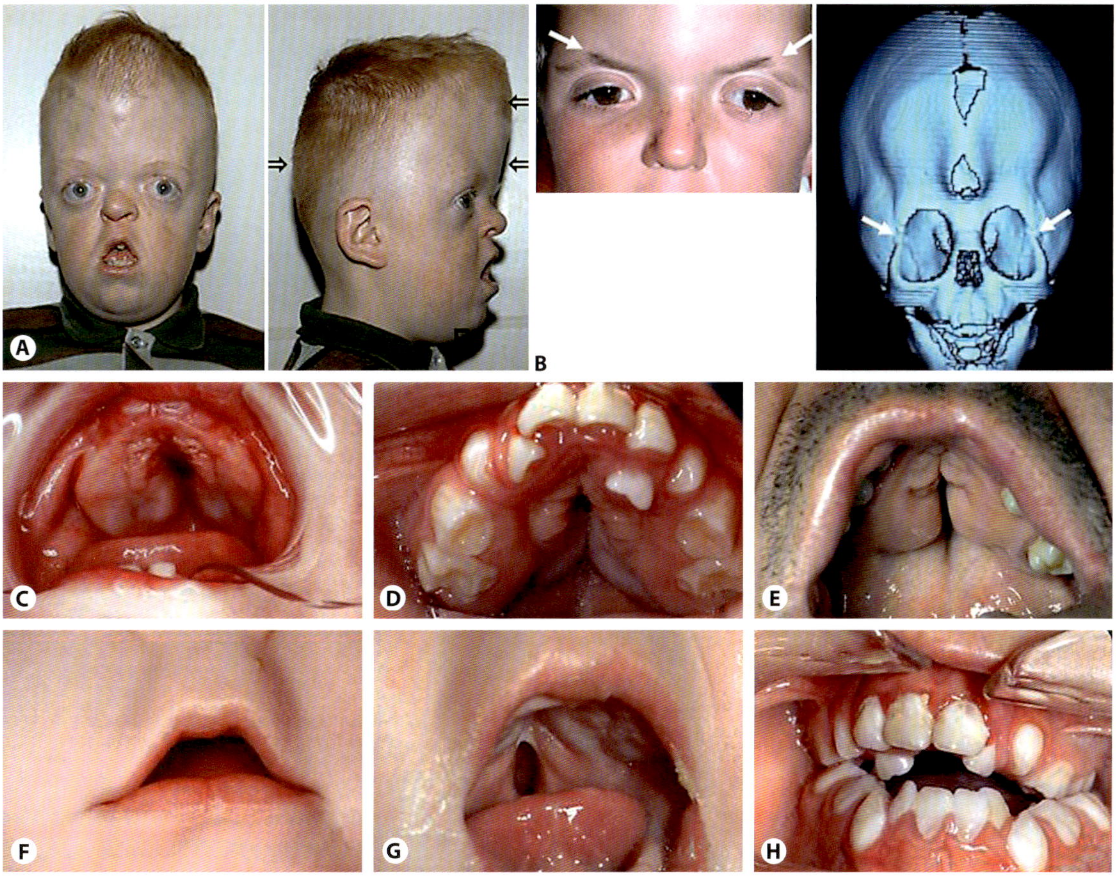

Fig. 3. Apert syndrome. **A** This boy has never had any cranial or craniofacial surgical procedures. Arrows show that the normal head circumference is not the maximum one possible. The top arrow shows that a head circumference measured at that point is dramatically higher. **B** Mild Apert syndrome phenotype. Arrows showing a break in the continuity of the eyebrows related to the corresponding defect in the supraorbital rims. **C** Highly arched and constricted palate. **D**, **E** Progressive increase of the size of the lateral palatal swellings with age. **F** Typical trapezoidal configuration of the lips at rest during infancy, but sometimes in adults as well. **G** Cleft palate. **H** Typical malocclusion with maxillary and mandibular crowding of teeth, more severe in the maxilla than in the mandible. Note the open bite, mandibular overjet, anterior crossbite, and posterior crossbite.

palate is shorter than normal and the soft palate is both longer and thicker than normal. Cleft soft palate (fig. 3G) occurs in 41% (n = 75) and bifid uvula in 35% (n = 75) of patients [33].

Dental anomalies include severely delayed eruption in 68% (n = 19), ectopic eruption in 50% (n = 54), and shovel-shaped incisors in 30% (n = 56). Crowding of teeth is more severe in the maxilla than the mandible (fig. 3H). Also found are anterior openbite in 73% (n = 73), posterior crossbite in 63% (n = 51), and mandibular overjet in 81% (n = 53) [33].

Ear, Temporal Area, and Aural Findings

Ear length measurements (n = 29) were above the 50th centile in 24% and of these 13% were between the 75th and 97th centiles [31]. The temporal muscle is shorter than normal in Apert

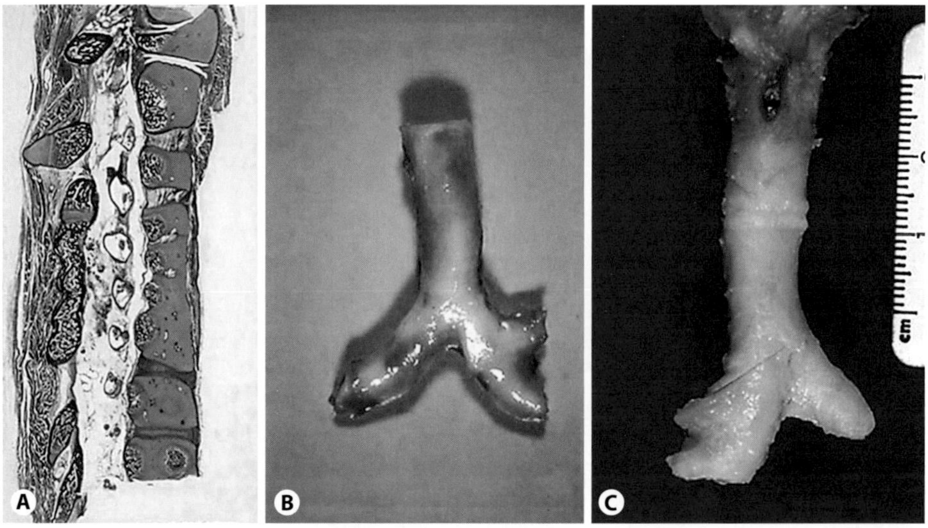

Fig. 4. Apert Syndrome. **A** Failure of cartilaginous segmentation of cervical vertebrae at 31 weeks of gestation. **B, C** Failure of cartilaginous segmentation of the trachea.

syndrome (mean = 89 mm, on the average) compared to 105 mm in control subjects. The superficial temporal fat pad is smaller in surface area than normal, but thicker than normal. The temporal bones are obliquely situated to various degrees. This determines whether the ear position is minimally oblique or whether mild, moderate, or severe cloverleafing will occur. Frank cloverleaf skull occurs in about 4% of Apert syndrome patients [13]. In a study of 20 patients with Apert syndrome, hearing loss occurred in 90% with 80% of them having conductive hearing loss. Inner ear anomalies were found in all of them with dilated vestibule, malformed semicircular canals, and cochlear dysplasia occuring most commonly [34].

Lack of Cervical Cartilaginous Segmentation

We studied 68 radiographs of the cervical spine, many longitudinal in nature. Histological study of failure of segmentation in a 31-week stillborn is shown in figure 4A involving the bodies of C4-C5-C6-C-7 and neural arches C3-C4-C5-C6-C7 and these are not visible radiographically. Specific cervical involvement was found in 46 of our 68 cases (68%): two vertebrae were unsegmented in 37% and multiple vertebrae were unsegmented in 31%. C5-C6 was most common alone or in combination with multiple vertebrae [35].

Hands and Feet

We studied 44 pairs of hands and 37 pairs of feet both clinically and radiographically [36]. Symmetric syndactyly of the hands and feet are of 3 types. Type 1 involves digits 2, 3, and 4 with 1 and 5 separate. Type 2 involves digits 2, 3, 4, and 5 with 1 separate. Type 3 involves all 5 digits. Types of hands and feet are congruent in 48.6% and noncongruent in the other 51.4%. Among congruent patterns, type 1 hands and feet are most common. Among noncongruent patterns, the most common are type 2 hands associated with type 3 feet [36].

It should be carefully noted that although most authors speak of various 'fusions' in the hands and feet in Apert syndrome, in all cases there is actually a lack of segmentation of cartilages. Figure 5A shows a histological section of a hand in a 31-week-old stillborn. The cartilage model shows lack of cartilaginous segmentation at the base of

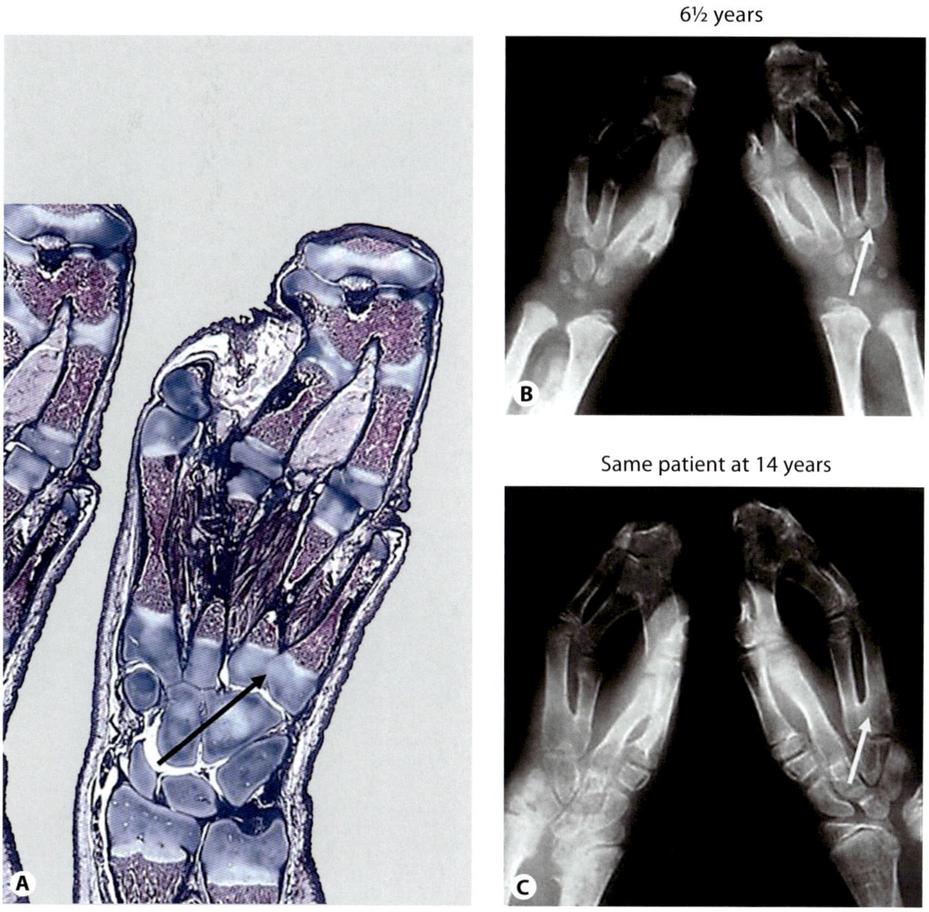

Fig. 5. Apert Syndrome. **A** Cross section of hand at 31 weeks showing lack of cartilaginous segmentation at the base of the 4th and 5th metacarpals. **B, C** Arrow points to base of 4th and 5th metacarpals in a radiograph at 6.5 years, but at 14 years, early failure of cartilaginous segmentation becomes evident.

the 4th and 5th metacarpals. Now compare figure 5B in a patient at 6.5 years in which the radiograph shows no 'coalition' at the base of the 4th and 5th metacarpals with same hand of this patient at 14 years (fig. 5C); it can be seen that they are now 'coalesced', but this is not 'fusion' because they were like this ab initio because of lack of cartilaginous segmentation during embryonic life, and calcification has now made that evident [36].

Lack of cartilaginous segmentation of the proximal and middle phalanges becomes evident with calcification, so that it looks like those fingers have only one bone. Lack of cartilaginous segmentation also involves the carpals, particularly the capitate and hamate. We also noted postaxial polydactyly in 3 patients (n = 44) [36]. We have dealt with abnormalities of the palmar aponeurosis, flexor retinaculum, extrinsic flexor tendons, extrinsic extensor tendons, and the intrinsic musculature elsewhere [36].

Some feet have 5 metatarsals (fig. 6A) and some have 6 (fig. 6B). It is important to assess this early

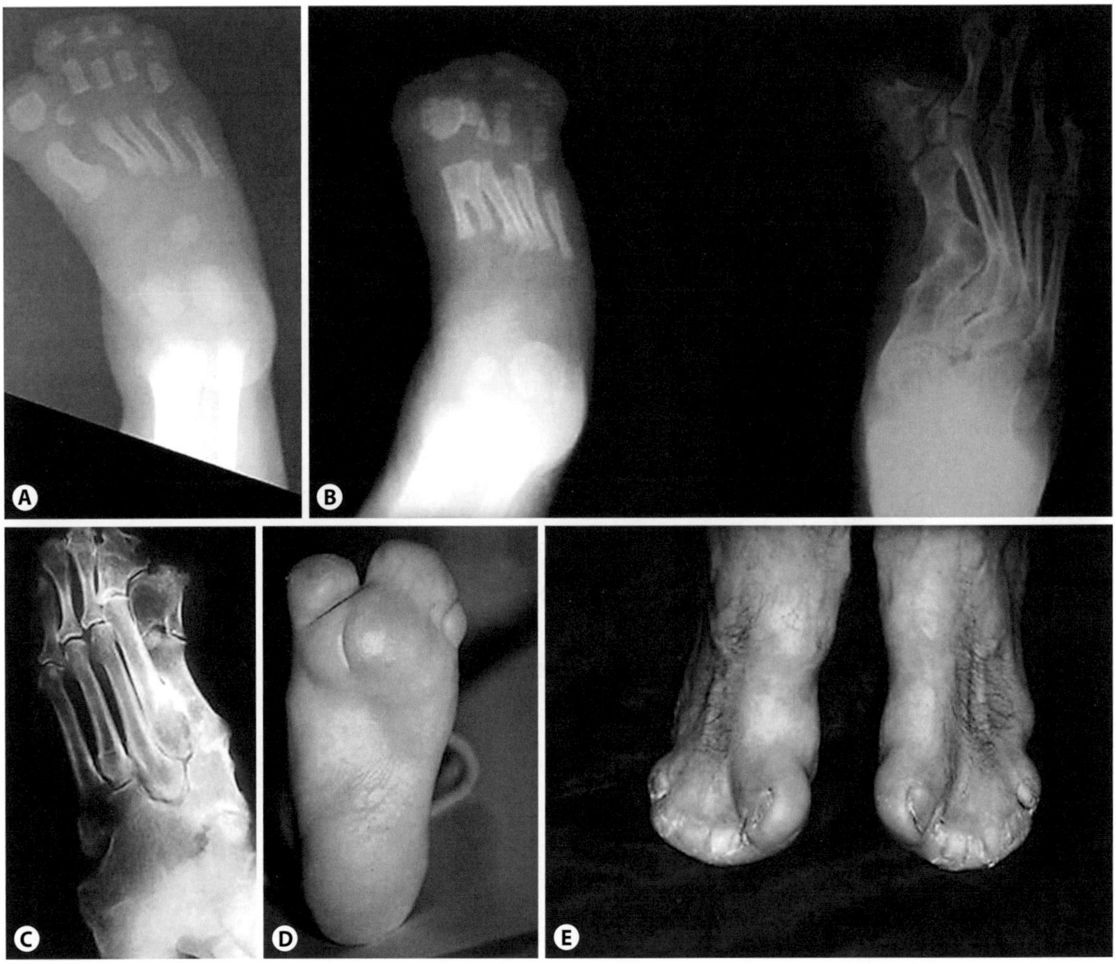

Fig. 6. Apert Syndrome. **A** Radiograph showing 5 metatarsals. **B** Radiograph showing 6 metatarsals (left), predicting a more severe defect in the foot (right). **C** Radiograph showing severe defect in the foot. **D** Callosities on the ball of the foot with 5 metatarsals. **E** Callosities on the sides of the foot with 6 metatarsals. Patient walks bearing weight on the lateral surfaces of the feet.

because patients with 6 metatarsals will eventually have more severe distortion of the foot with age (fig. 6B (right), C). Lack of cartilaginous segmentation in the foot includes all tarsals and metatarsals, commonly sparing only the talonavicular joint. Foot abnormalities frequently include valgus position of the ankle, metatarsus adductus, dorsiflexion of the hallux, and gradual supination of the foot. The callosities on the feet are of two patterns: those with 5 metatarsals develop callosities on the balls of the feet (fig. 6D), whereas those with 6 metatarsals develop callosities of the lateral surfaces of the feet (fig. 6E) [36].

Skeletal Abnormalities

We studied the shoulders, humeri, elbows, hips, knees, rib cage, and spine at different ages both clinically and radiographically in 38 patients. Mobility at the glenohumeral joint is limited. Progressive limitation in abduction, forward

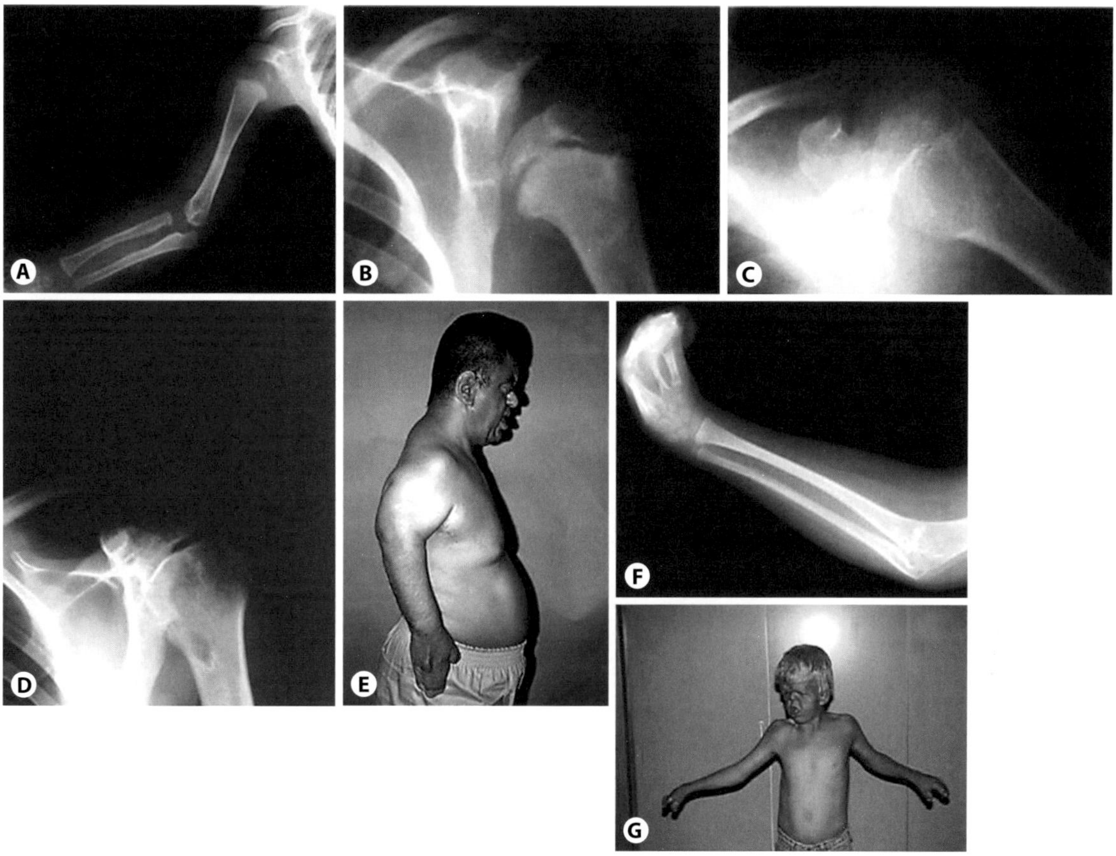

Fig. 7. Apert Syndrome. **A–D** Radiographs showing alterations at the shoulder with age. **A** Delayed appearance of the ossification center of the humeral head. **B** Irregular flattening of the humeral head, beaking of the metaphysis, small irregular glenoid fossa, small scapula, extreme hypoplasia of the coracoid process, and a prominent acromion are evident by age 6. **C** By age 12, the humeral head becomes more flattened, more irregular with age and a radiolucency develops at the end of the humeral head together with a small irregular glenoid fossa, and a short irregular coracoid process. **D** By age 18, the humeral head is oblong-shaped with a small irregular glenoid fossa and a proximal humeral radiolucency. **E** Dramatically short humerus. **F** Lack of cartilaginous segmentation at the elbow, which appears 'fused' in the radiograph. **G** Limited shoulder mobility and limited elbow mobility.

flexion, and external rotation with growth was virtually a constant finding. The acromioclavicular joint was prominent and sometimes had an angular, pointed appearance clinically. This was often associated with atrophic musculature and winging of the scapula. Limited elbow mobility was common and usually mild in degree. Decreased elbow extension was most often found with decreased flexion, pronation, and supination occurring less frequently. Limited elbow mobility did not change significantly with growth in contrast to the increasing severity observed in the shoulder joint. Short humeri were a constant finding [10].

The appearance of the ossification center of the humeral head is always delayed (fig. 7A). Irregular flattening of the humeral head, beaking of the metaphysis, small irregular glenoid fossa, small scapula, extreme hypoplasia of the coracoid process, and a prominent acromion are evident by age 6 (fig. 7B). By age 12, the humeral head

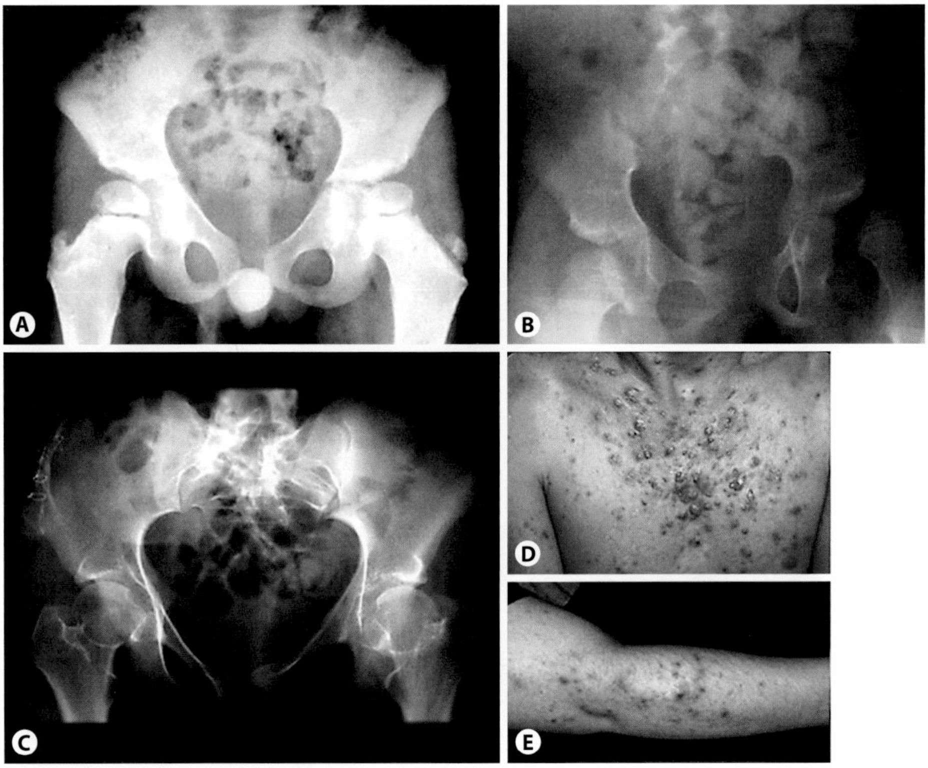

Fig. 8. Apert Syndrome. **A** Stippling of the ossification centers of the greater trochanters. **B** Unilateral acetabular dysplasia and hip dislocation. **C** Short broad femoral necks, prominent greater trochanters, wide interpubic distance, and spina bifida of L5 and S1. Note wiring on the iliac crest, which was where bone was harvested for a craniofacial procedure. **D** Severe conglobate acne vulgaris of the chest. **E** Acneiform lesions of the forearms.

becomes more flattened and more irregular with age and a radiolucency develops at the humeral head together with a small irregular glenoid fossa, and a short irregular coracoid process (fig. 7C). By age 18, the humeral head is oblong-shaped with a small irregular glenoid fossa and a proximal humeral radiolucency (fig. 7D) [10].

The humerus was short by measurement in 36 of 38 patients and was dramatically short in 6 of our 136 patients (fig. 7E). Limited elbow mobility was found in 26 of 38 patients and 3 of 38 had radiohumeral synostosis (fig. 7F). A boy with both limited shoulder mobility and limited elbow mobility is shown in figure 7G. Genua valga was found in 6 of 38 patients; one patient had osseous 'ankylosis' of the knee (lack of segmentation) [10].

Findings in the spine and chest included spina bifida (3/38), hemivertebrae (L2, L3, and L4; 1/38), lack of lumbar cartilage segmentation (T3-T4, T7-T8; 1/38), thoracic or thoracolumbar scoliosis (9/38), and lumbar or thoracolumbar lordosis (7/38). Other findings included pectus excavatum (13/38), flattening of the chest wall (5/38), and asymmetric chest wall (2/38). [10].

Pelvic findings (11 cases) included abnormalities of the acetabulum, femoral head, and femoral neck. Figure 8A shows stippling of the ossification centers of the greater trochanters. Figure 8B shows unilateral acetabular dysplasia and hip

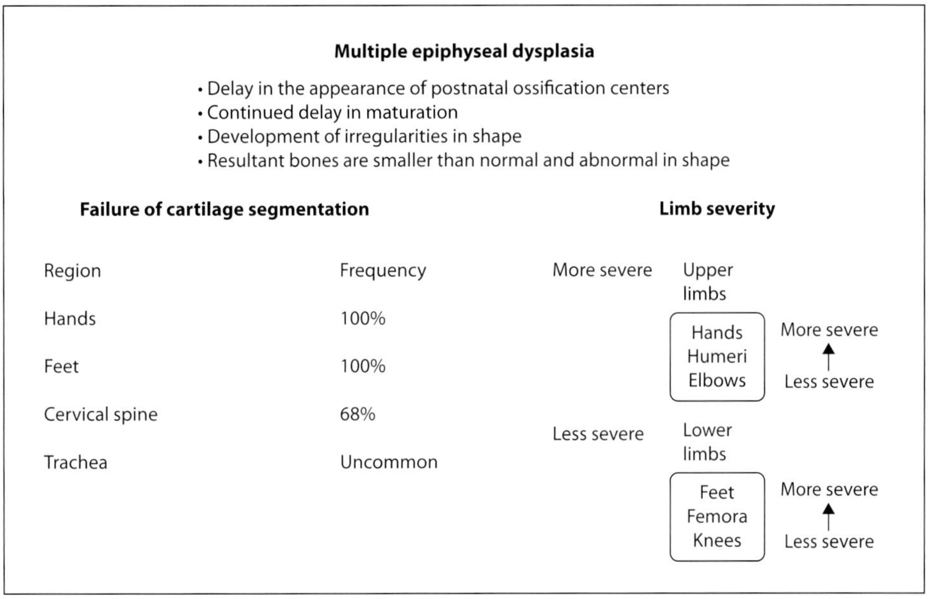

Fig. 9. Apert Syndrome. See text.

dislocation. Figure 8C shows short broad femoral necks, prominent greater trochanters, wide interpubic distance, and spina bifida of L5 and S1 [10].

Skeletal Biology of Apert Syndrome

Figure 9 summarizes (1) the multiple epiphyseal dysplasia that characterizes Apert syndrome, (2) some of the main regions subject to failure of cartilaginous segmentation, and (3) differences in severity of various limb parts [1, 10].

Cutaneous Manifestations

During infancy, skin dimples are usually observed at the shoulders, elbows, and knuckles. Excessive sweating is common, particularly during sleep when the head becomes soaked. Sweating may also occur during breast feeding, crying, exertion, and sympathomimetic activity. Temperature elevations may occur. Palmar hyperhidrosis is common and severe. During adolescence, profuse sweating is common. At adolescence and thereafter, the skin becomes oily. Acneiform lesions are particularly prevalent on the face, chest (fig. 8D), and back. The forearms are affected in some (14/19) (fig. 8E) and the eruption may extend to the buttocks and thighs (4/19) [37].

Biopsies of the skin have established an increased number of sweat glands and sebaceous glands in Apert syndrome patients compared with those in the general population. The unusual extension of severe acne vulgaris to the forearms and elsewhere in Apert syndrome suggests an exquisite end-organ responsiveness to steroid hormones that might be a fruitful area for further investigation [37].

Prenatal Diagnosis

I have discussed prenatal diagnosis in FGFR syndromes [7] and also Apert syndrome in particular [1]. At least 16 familial cases have been reported and in such instances, prenatal molecular diagnosis is faciliated by the two possible mutations (Ser252Trp and Pro253Arg) that account for 98% of all cases. However, the overwhelming majority of cases are sporadic. Many ultrasonic studies are carried out during the third trimester and when a diagnosis of

Table 3. Differences in FGFR2 molecular biology in Apert and Crouzon syndromes [7]

Syndrome	Apert syndrome	Crouzon syndrome
Mutation sites	two specific mutations in the IgII-IgIII linker region	more than 30 mutations in IgIII and sometimes elsewhere
Types of mutations	bulky amino acid substitutions (Ser252Trp, Pro253Arg)	frequently involve cysteine residues
Consequences of mutations	gain-of-function mechanism with specific effects on skeletogenesis	gain-of-function mechanism with specific effects on skeletogenesis
Mechanisms	enhanced ligand-binding specificity	ligand-independent expression
Phenotypic/molecular correlations	Yes	No

Apert syndrome is made, it is by coincidence. Mid-second trimester ultrasonic screening for congenital malformations usually fails to detect the anomalies of Apert syndrome, including syndactyly. In a retrospective study of the ultrasonic studies of 30 patients with Apert syndrome, it has been shown that prenatal ultrasonic identification of mild ventriculomegaly or agenesis of the corpus callosum should stimulate a careful search for features of Apert syndrome with prompt follow-up imaging for bony abnormalities that have a later onset, but the possibility of molecular testing should be considered with these 2 findings together [38].

Molecular Genetics

Apert syndrome results from 2 mutations in the linker region between the second and third immunoglobulin-like loops (IgII and IgIII): c.755C>G, resulting in p.Ser252Trp, and c.758C>G, resulting in p.Pro253Arg. The frequency estimates of various mutations for Apert syndrome are as follows: p.Ser252Trp (~66%), p.Pro253Arg (~33%), and rare mutations (~1%). Such rare mutations include 2 *Alu* insertions, an acceptor splice site mutation, and a double nucleotide substitution, c.755_756CG>TT, resulting in p.Pro252Phe [7, 39, 40].

Other unusual findings include a somatic p.Ser252Trp mutation in an upper limb with acne vulgaris in an otherwise normal person and isolated Apert-type syndactyly with a normal craniofacial appearance and 2 heterozygous mutations (c.755C>T, resulting in p.Ser252Lys, and c.934G>T, resulting in p.Ala315Ser) [41].

Genotype-phenotype correlations indicate that p.Ser252Trp is more frequently found with cleft palate and more severe facial anomalies, whereas p.Pro253Arg is more frequently associated with severe syndactyly [42].

p.Ser252Trp and p.Pro253Arg are both bulky mutations that alter the tertiary structure of FGFR2, resulting in enhanced ligand-binding affinity, which is the pathogenetic mechanism that produces Apert syndrome (see table 3 for a comparison of the mechanisms in Apert and Crouzon syndromes). By analyzing FGFR2 expression in keratinocytes and fibroblast cell lines from an Apert *Alu* patient, ectopic expression of alternative spliceform IgIIIb suggests that signaling through IgIIIb causes the syndactyly in Apert syndrome [40].

Evidence has been found [43] that clonal expansion of testicular spermatogonial stem cells is driven by positive selection of pathogenetic *FGFR2* mutations, which confers gain-of-function to the mutant cell, explaining the high levels of specific mutations in the spermatogonia as well as the paternal age effect.

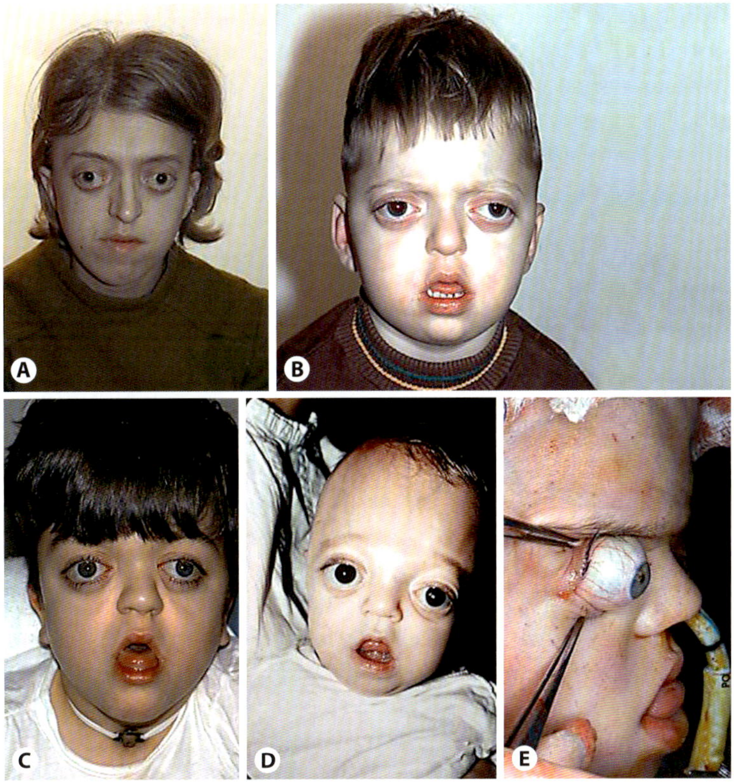

Fig. 10. Crouzon Syndrome. **A, B** Crouzon syndrome in a mother and child. **C** Compromised airway requiring tracheostomy. **D** Pronounced ocular proptosis and hypertelorism. **E** Subluxation of the eyeglobe.

Crouzon Syndrome

Our study of Crouzon syndrome comprises 61 cases in over 16 published articles [2, 44]. The syndrome is characterized by craniosynostosis, maxillary hypoplasia, shallow orbits, and ocular proptosis [2, 44] (fig. 10). Inheritance is autosomal dominant (fig. 10A, B). The birth prevalence is 5–16 per one million newborns by both direct and indirect methods [2]. The syndrome accounts for 4.5% of all cases of craniosynostosis [2]. In one large study [45], 67% were familial and 33% were sporadic; in the other large study [44], 44% were familial and 56% were sporadic. We reported germinal mosaicism for Crouzon syndrome in two siblings [2]. New mutations are of paternal origin [44]. Most cases are associated with brachycephaly, but trigonocephaly, scaphocephaly, and even cloverleaf skull have also been noted [2, 44].

Nowhere is this more apparent than in the large pedigree reported by Shiller [46]. The proband had cloverleaf skull. Several family members had classic Crouzon syndrome and others had ocular proptosis and midface deficiency without craniosynostosis. We have observed a family in which some members had brachycephaly and others had scaphocephaly [2, 44].

Central Nervous System

In our study of head size in Crouzon syndrome, we found that head length, head width, and head height are much smaller in Crouzon syndrome than in Apert syndrome (fig. 1M) [9]. The cranial volume is also much smaller than the volume in Apert syndrome. Furthermore, it is smaller than the average volume in the general population (table 2) [17]. Abnormalities of the central nervous system include shunted hydrocephalus (25.5%, n = 86) [44], chronic tonsillar herniation (72%, n = 44) [26], jugular foramen stenosis with venous obstruction (3/10) [47], seizures (~10%, n = 52), frequent headaches (29%, n = 52), mental deficiency (3%, n = 61), and agenesis of the corpus callosum in one documented case [44].

Respiratory Problems
Because of the severe maxillary deficiency, patients should be monitored for snoring and daytime somnolence. If severe in infancy, tracheostomy is the only option with or without some air tubing at night, and if severity persists, tracheostomy is sometimes used longer (fig. 10C). In older children and during adolescence, referral is necessary for polysomnographic study. A number of options are available, including various types of CPAP. Sequelae from obstructive sleep apnea may include failure to thrive or growth deficiency, hypertension, cardiorespiratory failure, and neurological damage [2].

Lower Respiratory Compromise
Solid cartilaginous trachea, from lack of segmentation of cartilage rings (erroneously referred to as 'fusion') results in the inability to clear secretions and most often leads to an early demise. MRI is mandatory for any Crouzon syndrome patient with lower respiratory compromise [2].

Cervical Anomalies
Failure of cervical vertebral cartilage modeling (erroneously referred to as 'progressive fusion of vertebrae') is found in 25% of Crouzon syndrome patients. All involve C2-C3. Any anomalies should be assessed before undergoing anesthesia for any cranial procedure because cervical anomalies may compound an already problematic airway, resulting from a relatively inflexible neck [see 35].

Radiographic Findings
Common radiographic findings include increased digital marking and maxillary deficiency. The cervical spine should always be assessed. If no skeletal anomalies appear, it is important to remember that any asymmetry of the vertebral column presages lack of segmentation of cartilaginous modeling before the appearance of what radiologists call 'progressive fusion.' Calcification of the stylohyoid ligament is found in 88% of older children, teenagers, and adults with Crouzon syndrome (n = 61) [44]. Stiffness of the elbows has been reported in 16% of patients (n = 61), and in 2 cases, subluxation of the radial head was evident [2, 44].

Craniofacial Abnormalities
Cranial malformation in Crouzon syndrome depends on the order and rate of progression of sutural synostosis. Craniostenosis may be evident at birth or develop during the first year of life. An important diagnostic feature is shallow orbits with ocular proptosis [32]. Craniosynostosis is eventually found in 100% of cases (n = 47), with synostosis of the coronal in 2% (n = 47); coronal and sagittal in 19% (n = 47); coronal, sagittal, and lambdoid in 75% (n = 47); and sagittal and lambdoid sutures in 4% (n = 47) [44, 48]. Note above that some classical cases in the family reported by Shiller [46] had no craniosynostosis.

Ophthalmologic Findings
These include hypertelorism, ocular proptosis (fig. 10D) in 100% (n = 61), exotropia in 76.6% (n = 60), exposure conjunctivitis in 51.9% (n = 52), poor vision in one or both eyes in 46.3% (n = 54), optic atrophy in one or both eyes in 22.2% (n = 45), exposure keratitis in 11.5% (n = 52), nystagmus in 11.5% (n = 52), blindness in 6.6% (n = 61), and iris coloboma in 1.7% (n = 60) [32, 44]. Luxation of the eyeglobes is observed in some instances (fig. 10E) [32]. Low frequency findings include aniridia, correctopia, microcornea, megalocornea, keratoconus, cataract, ectopia lentis, blue sclera, and glaucoma [2, 32].

Aural Findings
Mild-to-moderate conductive hearing deficit occurs in 55% (n = 49) and atresia of the external auditory canal is found in 13% of patients (n = 53). Deviation of the nasal septum is found in 33% of patients (n = 60) [44].

Oral Findings
These include lateral palatal swellings in 50% (n = 54). Other findings include obligatory mouth breathing in 32% (n = 53), bifid uvula in 9% (n = 53), cleft palate in 9% (n = 61), and cleft lip in 2% (n = 61). The maxillary dental arch is shortened with posterior crossbite, crowding of teeth, and ectopic eruption of maxillary first molars in 47% (n = 17). Anterior open bite, mandibular overjet, and crowding of mandibular anterior teeth are common [44].

Molecular Genetics
Well over 30 *FGFR2* mutations for Crouzon syndrome are known. All show ligand independent dimerization. Most are located on IgIII. At least half a dozen mutations are identical to those that cause Pfeiffer syndrome, and one 9-bp deletion overlaps with an 18-bp deletion in Pfeiffer syndrome. One common mutation, c.1032G>A, does not result in an amino acid substitution (p.Ala344Ala), but produces a cryptic donor splice site, causing a deletion of 17 amino acids and shortening the distance from the disulfide bond of IgIIIc to the transmembrane domain [7]. Two rare mutations are found, respectively, on IgI, c.314A>G, resulting in p.Tyr105Cys, and in the linker region between IgII and IgIII, c.755C>T, resulting in p.Ser252Leu [49]. In the latter mutation, the Crouzon phenotype was very mild. Other family members with this mutation were normal [49]. Mutations have also been reported in the split kinase domain [50]. One mutation was found in the first kinase domain: c.1645A>C, resulting in p.Asn549His, which occurs at the equivalent residue to the FGFR3 540 residue, a mutational hot spot for hypochondroplasia. Another mutation was found in the second kinase domain: c.2032A>G, resulting in p.Arg678Gly.

Unfortunately, a mutation on *FGFR3* has been said to cause Crouzon syndrome with acanthosis nigricans, suggesting that Crouzon syndrome is genetically heterogeneous. However, radiographic evidence has demonstrated cementomas of the jaws on occasion and, more often, mild alterations of the interpediculate distances of the distal vertebral column (the frequency is not known), which are clinically silent. I have named this condition Crouzonodermoskeletal syndrome and it is caused by a highly specific mutation 11 amino acids away from the common mutation for achondroplasia, which has more severe alterations in the interpediculate distances of the distal vertebral column [51]. It should also be noted that in most reported series of patients, the CNS findings in Crouzon syndrome have a high frequency of jugular foramen stenosis with venous obstruction. Since 100% of patients with FGFR3 Crouzonodermoskeletal syndrome have this feature, such estimates for Crouzon syndrome for this feature cannot be trusted because this distinction is not made. Robson and Mulliken [47] who did make the distinction found only 3 of 10 patients with Crouzon syndrome had this finding.

Pfeiffer Syndrome

Our studies of Pfeiffer syndrome include a number of cases based on 9 published studies. The syndrome is characterized by craniosynostosis, midface deficiency, broad thumbs, broad great toes, brachydactyly, variable soft tissue syndactyly, and other anomalies (fig. 11). Inheritance is autosomal dominant with many sporadic cases. Three clinical subtypes have been proposed (fig. 11, table 4). Type 1 consists of Pfeiffer syndrome as just described. Type 2 is characterized, in addition, by cloverleaf skull and often elbow ankylosis/synostosis and by a cluster of unusual anomalies. Type 3 comprises a very short anterior cranial base, severe

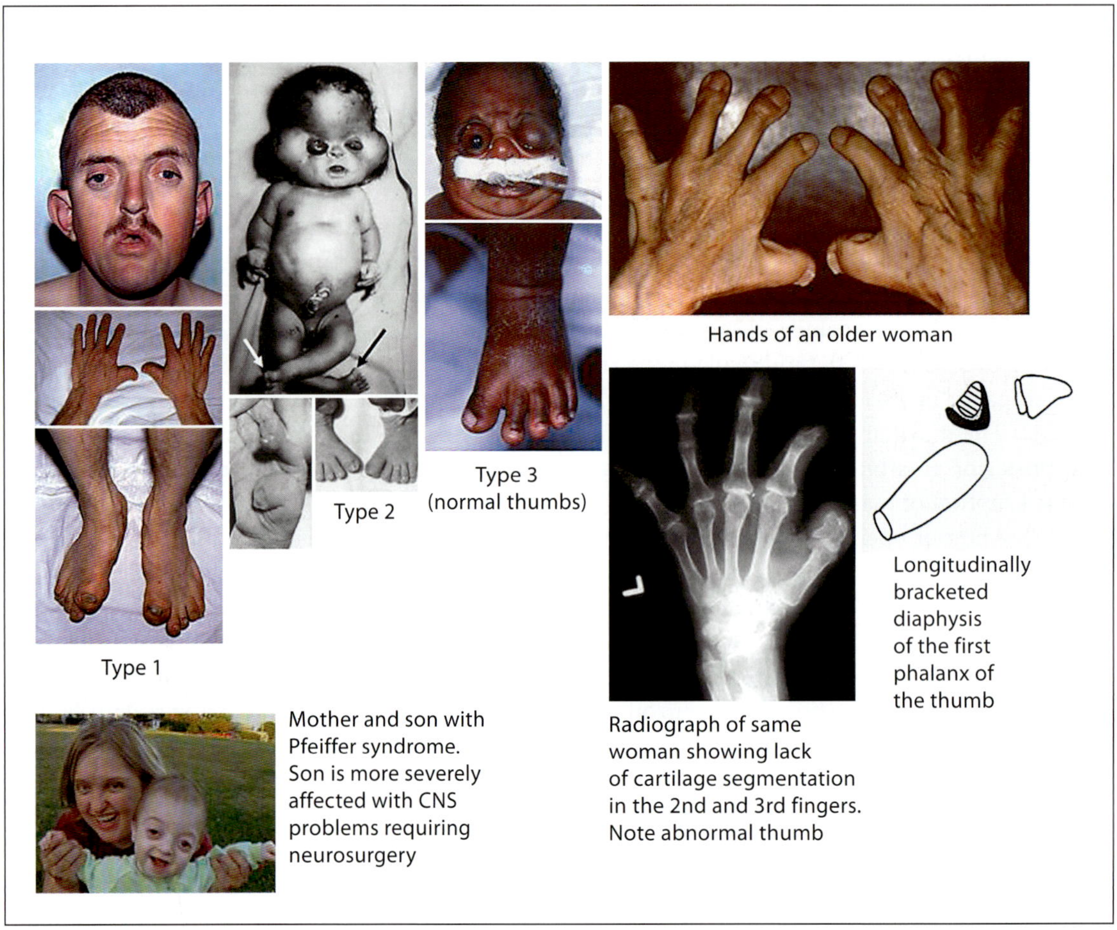

Fig. 11. Pfeiffer Syndrome. Pfeiffer syndrome, types 1, 2, and 3. Stillborn type 2 Pfeiffer syndrome with severe cloverleaf skull (arrows point to broad great toes). The close-up of the hands and feet below are from another type 2 case. Mother and son with Pfeiffer syndrome. Son is more severely affected with CNS problems requiring neurosurgery. Hands of an older woman showing brachydactyly and broad thumbs. Radiograph shows lack of cartilaginous segmentation in the 2nd and 3rd fingers. The 2nd finger deviates to the radial side. Note the abnormal thumb. Diagram shows a longitudinally bracketed diaphysis of the first phalanx of the thumb. Note the triangular shape and position on the ulnar side of the first metacarpal. As growth takes place, deviation of the thumb becomes more pronounced. Black = osseous part of bracket. Dotted = cartilaginous part of bracket.

ocular proptosis, elbow ankylosis/synostosis, and a cluster of unusual anomalies. Although these subtypes are useful they have limited nosologic status and some clinical overlap does occur [3, 52].

Craniofacial Features
These include brachycephaly, particularly involving the coronal suture, hypertelorism, ocular proptosis, and midface deficiency. Type 2 Pfeiffer syndrome has cloverleaf skull and type 3 has severe ocular proptosis associated with a very short cranial base (table 4) [3, 52].

Central Nervous System
Distortion ventriculomegaly, midline calvarial defect, progressive hydrocephalus, and cerebellar

Table 4. Clinical trends[a] in subtypes of Pfeiffer syndrome

Major characteristics		Other anomalies	Prognosis
Type 1	craniosynostosis, broad thumbs and great toes, brachydactyly, variable syndactyly	variable low frequency anomalies (e.g., vertebral anomalies)	usually normal development
Type 2	cloverleaf skull, severe ocular proptosis, broad thumbs and great toes, brachydactyly, variable syndactyly	elbow 'ankylosis' (lack of cartilage segmentation at the elbows), unusual cluster of anomalies	increased risk for neurodevelopmental abnormalities
Type 3	craniosynostosis, very short anterior cranial fossa, severe ocular proptosis, broad thumbs and great toes, brachydactyly, variable syndactyly	elbow 'ankylosis' (lack of cartilage segmentation at the elbows), unusual cluster of anomalies	increased risk for neurodevelopmental abnormalities

[a]The term 'trends' is used to indicate that there are some cases with overlapping features. Also, some patients have broad great toes with normal thumbs.

herniation are common. Progressive hydrocephalus is much more common in Pfeiffer and Crouzon syndromes than in Apert syndrome. Gyral abnormalities and cerebellar herniation have been recorded in some patients. CNS involvement occurs with much higher frequency in type 2 and type 3 patients than in type 1 patients [3].

Relative to all cases of cloverleaf skull, type 2 Pfeiffer syndrome with cloverleaf skull (fig. 11) accounts for 15% of the cases. While this may appear to be high, type 2 thanatophoric dysplasia accounts for 40% of these and isolated cloverleaf skull accounts for 20% of the cases [14]. Types 2 and 3 have been reviewed extensively. Plomb et al. [53] reported 5 patients with type 2. They all had cloverleaf skull, severe proptosis, 'ankylosis' of the elbows, broad thumbs and/or broad halluces, and varying other anomalies. In their literature review, most patients died shortly after birth. Causes of death included pulmonary problems, brain abnormalities, prematurity, and postoperative complications. Robin et al. [54] reported the prognosis with Pfeiffer syndrome types 2 and 3. Although of increased risk for neurodevelopmental difficulties, a favorable outcome can be achieved in some cases with aggressive medical and surgical management. However, normal outcome is not the rule and neurodevelopmental outcome and life expectancy remain guarded in most cases.

Hands and Feet

The thumbs are broad and may deviate medially. In some cases, the thumbs are normal. Brachydactyly is very common and mild soft tissue syndactyly may accompany some cases. The great toes are broad and partial soft tissue syndactyly between the toes may be found in some cases, particularly involving the second and third toes [3]. Some of the same types of lack of cartilaginous segmentation found in Apert syndrome may also be found in Pfeiffer syndrome. Findings may include absence of the middle phalangeal joints, particularly in the second finger; lack of segmentation of the 4th and 5th metacarpals at their proximal ends; brachymesophalangy; radial deviation of the thumb; progressive varus deformity of the hallux; accessory epiphyses of the 1st and 2nd metatarsals; and double ossification centers of the proximal phalanx of the hallux and, in some cases, with duplication. The 1st metatarsal is broad, may be short, and may exhibit partial duplication. In some cases, lack of segmentation may occur in the carpal, metacarpal, tarsal, and metatarsal bones [3].

Figure 11 shows the hands of an older woman illustrating broad thumbs, brachydactyly, and radial deviation of the second fingers. The radiograph shows lack of cartilaginous segmentation of the 2nd and 3rd fingers. The thumb is very abnormal and its explanation lies in a longitudinally bracketed diaphysis of the 1st phalanx of the thumb.

Vertebral Abnormalities

Failure of cartilaginous segmentation of the vertebrae occurs in about 70% of patients. Findings have included lack of segmentation of two vertebrae and sometimes involve multiple vertebrae. C2-C3 is most common, but lack of segmentation may involve C3-C4, C4-C5; C5-C6; and lumbar vertebrae in some cases [3].

Other Skeletal Findings

These include many cases of elbow 'ankylosis/synostosis', short humerus, and scapulohumeral joint limitation. Other reported findings have included short femoral neck, coxa valga, limited knee extension, kyphoscoliosis and sacrococcygeal eversion [3].

Miscellaneous Abnormalities

Many have been noted. Cardiovascular findings have included ventricular septal defect, patent ductus arteriosus, bicuspid aortic valve, and single umbilical artery. Gastrointestinal findings have included pyloric stenosis, common mesentery, absent lesser omentum, hypoplastic gallbladder, imperforate anus, malposed anus, intestinal malrotation, and prune belly. Genitourinary findings have included urogenital septum defect, hydronephrosis, pelvic kidney, ovarian cyst, hypospadias, bifid scrotum, and cryptorchidism [3].

Molecular Genetics

Pfeiffer syndrome is genetically heterogeneous with one *FGFR1* mutation in the linker region between IgII and IgIII (c.755C>G, resulting in p.Pro252Arg) and many *FGFR2* mutations. The mutation in the linker region on *FGFR1* shows enhanced ligand-binding affinity [7]. All mutations on *FGFR2* show ligand-independent dimerization. Most *FGFR2* mutations cluster in the third IgIII loop, but others have been found, including one near the transmembrane domain and several in the split kinase domain. Well over 30 mutations are known and about half a dozen have also been found with Crouzon syndrome. One 18-bp deletion overlaps with a 9-bp deletion in Crouzon syndrome. Many mutations involve p.Cys278 and particularly p.Cys342. Splice site mutations occur less commonly. A severe Pfeiffer syndrome phenotype occurs with c.1052C>G, resulting in p.Ser351Cys; c.870G>T, resulting in p.Trp290Cys; and c.1124A>G, resulting in p.Tyr375Cys. This later mutation is associated with several cases of Beare-Stevenson cutis gyrata syndrome. The c.940–2A>G substitution of the 3′-splice site upstream of exon 9 is associated with a relatively severe phenotype, particularly with respect to the hands and feet [55–57]. Passos-Bueno et al. [58] reported a Pfeiffer splice site mutation with an Apert-like phenotype. A Pfeiffer-like phenotype with a nucleotide change of c.755C>G, resulting in p.Ser252Trp, was noted with the most common mutation for Apert syndrome [59]. The mutation p.Ser252Trp/p.Pro253Arg, resulting in Pfeiffer syndrome, is extremely rare because it requires 3 nucleotide substitutions (c.755_757CGC>TCT) [17]. One unusual Pfeiffer syndrome mutation is an insertion (c.1084_1085insTCAACA), which activates a cryptic splice site (p.Gly345_Pro361del) [60].

Type 1 Pfeiffer syndrome is often associated with the *FGFR1* mutation and tends to result in a milder phenotype than those on *FGFR2*. Although type 2 and type 3 cases tend to be associated with *FGFR2* mutations, some type 1 cases have also been noted [4]. Abnormalities of the hands and feet tend to be more severe with *FGFR2* splice-site mutations. A severe limb phenotype with very broad thumbs and great toes together with cutaneous syndactyly of digits 2 to 5 occurs with a 2-nucleotide *FGFR2* IgII mutation, c.514_515GC>TT, resulting in p.Ala172Phe. Mutations in the split kinase domain tend to exhibit mild broadening of the thumbs and great toes [41, 50].

Acknowledgement

This chapter 'Apert, Crouzon, and Pfeiffer Syndromes' is dedicated to my friend, Jaime L. Frías, MD, Professor Emeritus of Pediatrics, University of South Florida, for his excellent work in pediatrics and dysmorphology and to my friend Bernarda Strauss, MD, Children's Mercy Hospital, University of Missouri at Kansas City, for her excellent work in art history, pediatrics, and medical genetics.

References

1 Cohen MM Jr: Apert syndrome; in Cohen MM Jr, MacLean RE (eds): Craniosynostosis: Diagnosis, Evaluation, and Management, ch 24, pp 316–353 (Oxford University Press, New York, 2000).
2 Cohen MM Jr: Crouzon syndrome; in Cohen MM Jr, MacLean RE (eds): Craniosynostosis: Diagnosis, Evaluation, and Management, ch 26, pp 361–365 (Oxford University Press, New York, 2000).
3 Cohen MM Jr: Pfeiffer syndrome; in Cohen MM Jr, MacLean RE (eds): Craniosynostosis: Diagnosis, Evaluation, and Management, ch 25, pp 354–360 (Oxford University Press, New York, 2000).
4 Cohen MM Jr: An updated pediatric perspective on the Apert syndrome. Am J Dis Child 1993;147:989–993.
5 Cohen MM Jr, Kreiborg S, Lammer EJ, Cordero JF, Mastroiacovo P, et al: Birth prevalence study of the Apert syndrome. Am J Med Genet 1992;42:655–659.
6 Cohen MM Jr, Kreiborg S: Genetic and family study of Apert syndrome. J Craniofac Genet Dev Biol 1991;11:7–17.
7 Cohen MM Jr: FGFs/FGFRs and associated disorders; in Epstein CJ, Erickson RP, Wynshaw-Boris A (eds): Inborn Errors of Development, ch 33, pp 380–400 (Oxford University Press, New York, 2004).
8 Moloney DM, Slaney SF, Oldridge M, Sahlin P, Stenman G, Wilkie AOM: Exclusive paternal origin of new mutations in Apert syndrome. Nat Genet 1996;13:48–53.
9 Cohen MM Jr, Kreiborg S: Growth and development in the Apert syndrome. Am J Med Genet 1993;47:617–623.
10 Cohen MM Jr, Kreiborg S: Skeletal abnormalities in the Apert syndrome. Am J Med Genet 1993;47:624–632.
11 Cohen MM Jr, Kreiborg S: Visceral anomalies in the Apert syndrome. Am J Med Genet 1993;45:758–760.
12 Cohen MM Jr, Kreiborg S: Upper and lower airway compromise in the Apert syndrome. Am J Med Genet 1992;44:90–93.
13 Cohen MM Jr, Kreiborg S: Unusual cranial aspects of the Apert syndrome. J Craniofac Genet Dev Biol 1994;14:48–56.
14 Cohen MM Jr: Cloverleaf skulls: Etiologic heterogeneity and pathogenetic variability. J Craniofac Surg 2009;20: 652–656.
15 Cohen MM Jr, Kreiborg S: The central nervous system in the Apert syndrome. Am J Med Genet 1990;35:36–45.
16 Hanieh A, David DJ: Apert's syndrome. Childs Ner Syst 1993;9:289–291.
17 Cohen MM Jr, Kreiborg S: Cranial size and configuration in the Apert syndrome. J Craniofac Genet Dev Biol 1994; 14:153–162.
18 Tokumara AM, Barkovich J, Ciricillo SF, Edwards MSB: Skull base and calvarial deformities: Association with intracranial changes in craniofacial syndromes. Am J Neuroradiol 1966;17:619–630.
19 Noetzel MJ, Marsh JL, Palkes H, Gado M: Hydrocephalus and mental retardation in craniosynostosis. 1985;107:885–892.
20 Fishman MA, Hogan GR, Dodge PR: The concurrence of hydrocephalus and craniosynostosis. J Neurosurg 1971;34:621–629.
21 Hogan GR, Bauman ML: Hydrocephalus in Apert's syndrome. J Pediatr 1971;79: 782–787.
22 Collmann H, Sörensen N, Krauss J: Hydrocephalus in craniosynostosis: A review. Childs Nerv Syst 2005;21:902–912.
23 Renier D, Arnaud E, Cinalli G, Sebag G, Zerah M, Marchac D: Prognosis for mental function in Apert's syndrome. J Neurosurg 1966;85:66–72.
24 Renier D, Arnaud E, Cinalli G, Marchac D, Brunet L, et al: Mental prognosis of Apert syndrome. Arch Pédiatr 1996;3: 752–760.
25 Marucci DD, Dunaway DJ, Jones BM, Hayward RD: Raised intracranial pressure in Apert syndrome. Plast Reconstr Surg 2008;122:1162–1168.
26 Cinalli G, Renier D, Sebag G, Sainte-Rose C, Arnaud E, Pierre-Kahn A: Chronic tonsillar herniation in Crouzon's and Apert's syndrome: The role of premature synostosis of the lambdoid suture. J Neurosurg 1995;83:575–582.
27 Lefèbvre A, Travis F, Arndt EM, Munro IR: A psychiatric profile before and after reconstructive surgery in children with Apert's syndrome. Br J Plast Surg 1986; 39:510–513.
28 Cohen MM Jr, Kreiborg S: Suture formation, premature sutural fusion, and suture default zones in Apert syndrome. Am J Med Genet 1996;62:339–344.
29 Kreiborg S, Cohen MM Jr: Characteristics of the infant Apert skull and its subsequent development. J Craniofac J Dev Biol 1990;10:399–410.
30 Kreiborg S, Marsh JL, Cohen MM Jr, Liversage M, Pedersen H, et al: Comparative three-dimensional analysis of CT-scans of the calvaria and cranial base in Apert and Crouzon syndromes. J Craniomaxillofac Surg 1993;21:181–188.

31 Cohen MM Jr, Kreiborg S: A clinical study of the craniofacial features in Apert syndrome. Int J Oral Maxillofac Surg 1996;25:45–53.
32 Kreiborg S, Cohen MM Jr: Ocular manifestations of Apert and Crouzon syndromes: Qualitative and quantitative findings. J Craniofac Surg 2010;21:1354–1357.
33 Kreiborg S, Cohen MM Jr: The oral manifestations of Apert syndrome. J Craniofac Genet Dev Biol 1992;12:41–48.
34 Zhou G, Schwartz LT, Gopen Q: Inner ear anomalies and conductive hearing loss in children with Apert syndrome: An overlooked otologic aspect. Otol Neurotol 2009;30: 184–189.
35 Kreiborg S, Barr M Jr, Cohen MM Jr: Cervical spine in the Apert syndrome. Am J Med Genet 1992;43:704–708.
36 Cohen MM Jr, Kreiborg S: Hands and feet in the Apert syndrome. Am J Med Genet 1995;57:82–96.
37 Cohen MM Jr, Kreiborg S: Cutaneous manifestations of the Apert syndrome. Am J Med Genet 1995;58:94–96.
38 Quintero-Rivera F, Robson CD, Reiss RE, Levine D, Benon C, Mulliken JB, Kimonis E: Apert syndrome: what prenatal radiographic findings should prompt its consideration? Prenat Diagn 2006;26: 966–972.
39 Wilkie AOM, Slaney SF, Oldridge M, Poole MD, Ashworth GJ, et al: Apert syndrome results from localized mutations of *FGFR2* and is allelic with Crouzon syndrome. Nat Genet 1995;9:165–172.
40 Oldridge M, Zackai EH, McDonald-McGinn DM, Iseki S, Moriss-Kay GM, et al: De novo Alu element insertions in *FGFR2* identify a distinct pathological basis for Apert syndrome. Am J Hum Genet 1999;64:446–461.
41 Wilkie AOM: Abnormal spliceform expression associated with splice acceptor mutations in exon IIIc of *FGFR2*. Am J Med Genet 2002;111:105.
42 Slaney SF, Oldridge M, Hurst JA, Moriss-Kay GM, Hall CM, Poole MD, Wilkie AOM: Differential effects of FGFR2 mutations on syndactyly and cleft palate in Apert syndrome. Am J Hum Genet 1996;58:923–932.
43 Goriely A, McVean GAT, Röjmyr M, Ingemarsson B, Wilkie AOM: Evidence for selective advantage of pathogenic FGFR2 mutations in the male germ line. Science 2003;301:643–646.
44 Kreiborg S: Crouzon syndrome. A clinical and roentgencephalometric study. Scand J Plast Reconstr Surg Hand Surg 1981;(suppl 18):1–198.
45 Atkinson FRB: Heredity, craniofacial dysostosis, or Crouzon disease. Méd Press Circular 1937;195:118–124.
46 Shiller G: Craniofacial dysostosis of Crouzon: A case report and pedigree with emphasis on heredity. Pediatrics 1959;23:107–112.
47 Robson CD, Mulliken JB: Prominent basal emissary foramina in craniosynostosis. Am J Neuroradiology 2000;21: 1707–1717.
48 Kreiborg S: Postnatal growth and development of the craniofacial complex in premature craniosynostosis, in Cohen MM Jr, MacLean RE (eds): Craniosynostosis: Diagnosis, Evaluation, and Management, ch 13, pp 158–174 (Oxford University Press, New York, 2000).
49 Oldridge M, Lunt PW, Zackai EH, McDonald-McGinn DM, Muenke M, et al: Genotype-phenotype correlations for nucleotide substitutions in the IgII-IgIII linker of FGFR2. Hum Mol Genet 1997; 6:137–143.
50 Kan S-H, Elanko N, Johnson D, Cornejo-Roldan L, Cook J, et al: Genomic screening of fibroblast growth factor receptor 2 reveals a wide spectrum of mutations in patients with syndromic craniosynostosis. Am J Med Genet 2002;70:472–486.
51 Cohen MM Jr: Let's call it 'Crouzondermoskeletal syndrome' so we won't be prisoners of our own conventional terminology. Am J Med Genet 1999;84:74.
52 Cohen MM Jr: Pfeiffer syndrome update, clinical subtypes, and guidelines for differential diagnosis. Am J Med Genet 1993;45:300–307.
53 Plomp AS, Hamel BCJ, Cobben JM, Verloes A, Offermans JPM, et al: Pfeiffer syndrome type 2: Further delineation and review of the literature. Am J Med Genet 1998;75:245–251.
54 Robin NH, Scott JA, Arnold JF, Goldstein JA, Shilling BB, Marion RW, Cohen MM Jr: Favorable prognosis for children with Pfeiffer syndrome types 2 and 3: Implications for classification. Am J Med Genet 1998;75:240–244.
55 Muenke M, Schell T, Hehr A, Robin NH, Losken HW, et al: A common mutation in the fibroblast growth factor 1 gene in Pfeiffer syndrome. Nat Genet 1994;8: 269–273.
56 Gripp KW, Stolle CA, McDonald-McGinn DM, Markowitz RI, Bartlett SP, et al: Phenotype of fibroblast growth factor receptor 2 Ser351Cys mutation: Pfeiffer syndrome III. Am J Med Genet 1998;78:356–360.
57 Cornejo-Roldan LR, Roessler E, Muenke M: Analysis of the mutational spectrum of the *FGFR2* gene in Pfeiffer syndrome. Hum Genet 1999;104:425–431.
58 Passos-Bueno MR, Sertié AL, Zatz M, Richieri-Costa A: Pfeiffer syndrome in an Apert patient: How wide is the spectrum of variability due to mutations in the FGFR2 gene? Am J Med Genet 1997; 71:243–245.
59 Passos-Bueno MR, Richieri-Costa A, Sertié AL, Kneppers A: Presence of the Apert canonical S252W *FGFR2* mutation in a patient without severe syndactyly. J Med Genet 1998;35:677–679.
60 Meyers GA, Day D, Goldberg R, Daentl DL, Przylepa KA, et al: *FGFR2* exon IIIa and IIIc mutations in Crouzon syndrome, Jackson-Weiss, and Pfeiffer syndromes: Evidence for missense changes, insertions, and a deletion due to alternative RNA splicing. Am J Hum Genet 1996;58:491–498.

M. Michael Cohen Jr.
Department of Pediatrics, Faculty of Medicine
Dalhousie University
5981 University Avenue, Halifax (NS) B3H 1W2 (Canada)
Tel. +1 902 477 8589, Fax +1 902 477 8589, E-Mail mmichael.cohenjr@gmail.com

Muenke M, Kress W, Collmann H, Solomon BD (eds): Craniosynostoses: Molecular Genetics, Principles of Diagnosis, and Treatment.
Monogr Hum Genet. Basel, Karger, 2011, vol 19, pp 89–97

Muenke Syndrome

B.D. Solomon · M. Muenke

Medical Genetics Branch, National Human Genome Research Institute, National Institutes of Health, Bethesda, Md., USA

Abstract

Muenke syndrome is defined by the presence of the p.P250R mutation in *FGFR3*, and is an autosomal dominant disorder with incomplete penetrance and variable expressivity. Typical manifestations of Muenke syndrome include coronal craniosynostosis, hearing loss, developmental delay/cognitive impairment, and relatively minor hand and foot anomalies. Clinical diagnosis is difficult because of phenotypic overlap and diagnosis is always made by molecular testing. Optimal management of patients involves a coordinated, multidisciplinary team familiar with the condition.

Craniosynostosis occurs in approximately 1 in 3,000 live births, and is a component feature in over 150 described syndromes [1]; see Chapter 11 in this volume. Relatively common craniosynostosis syndromes include Apert syndrome, Crouzon syndrome, Pfeiffer syndrome, Saethre-Chotzen syndrome, and Muenke syndrome (see Chapters 7 and 9 in this volume for specific discussions of the syndromes other than Muenke syndrome). Among these common syndromes, Muenke syndrome is the most common condition, accounting for approximately 8% of patients with craniosynostosis and over 25% of cases with an identified genetic cause; the condition is diagnosed in approximately 1 in 30,000 infants [2–4]. Additionally, as many patients with Muenke syndrome may be diagnosed with nonsyndromic craniosynostosis and may never undergo molecular genetic testing, the prevalence is likely to be underestimated [2, 5, 6].

Muenke syndrome was first defined in 1996 as a syndrome including craniosynostosis secondary to a recurrent p.P250R mutation in the gene *FGFR3* [7]. Since the discovery of the genetic basis of Muenke syndrome, advances on many fronts have contributed to an understanding of the disease. These areas of increased knowledge include a delineation of the molecular pathogenesis, patterns of inheritance, a more precise description of clinical features, and specifics of diagnosis, management, and genetic counseling. Muenke syndrome thus offers a clear example of how research in diverse areas contributes to the overall advancement of human clinical genetics. Most importantly, this improved understanding of many facets of Muenke syndrome has led to better outcomes for affected patients and families, and should serve as an inspiration to all who study and care for patients with rare diseases.

Gene Discovery

In 2 families clinically diagnosed with Pfeiffer syndrome, linkage analysis excluded the chromosomes known to be associated with Pfeiffer syndrome, and showed evidence instead of linkage to chromosome 4p16.3. *FGFR3* was located within the linked region on chromosome 4, and sequencing revealed segregation of the disease phenotype with the presence of a recurrent c.749C>G mutation, resulting in p.P250R [5, 7]. Strikingly, this was the paralogous mutation to that observed in Pfeiffer syndrome type I (p.P252R in FGFR1) and Apert syndrome (p.P253R in FGFR2) [8, 9].

Subsequent analysis of members of 8 additional families with various forms of craniosynostosis, who had been previously clinically diagnosed as having Pfeiffer syndrome (later, patient findings suggestive of Crouzon syndrome, Saethre-Chotzen, Jackson-Weiss syndrome, and even non-syndromic craniosynostosis were studied) revealed multiple additional patients with the same mutation [5, 7]. Furthermore, craniosynostosis in a large Australian kindred with 'Adelaide type' craniosynostosis was separately linked to chromosome 4p and identified to have the characteristic mutation [5]. Since this initial discovery of the cause of Muenke syndrome, the condition has been recognized as relatively common, with well over 300 affected patients reported in the literature [10]. The breadth of clinical diagnoses initially assigned to these early patients emphasizes the challenge of assigning a diagnosis based on clinical findings alone.

Muenke syndrome stands out as a classic example of the transition in the diagnosis of genetic conditions. Before the current era of rapid gene discovery, conditions were defined on purely clinical grounds, and diagnosis was often quite challenging and remains controversial to the present day; a classic example of this is the craniosynostosis-associated condition called Antley-Bixler syndrome (see Chapter 11 in this volume). With the advent of new genetic technologies, the etiologies of many Mendelian conditions have been elucidated, and a shift is taking place, in which definitions based on phenotype alone have transitioned to molecularly-based diagnostic criteria in conjunction with careful clinical assessment. Recent advances in genomic research will undoubtedly accelerate this process.

Inheritance and Genetic Counseling

Muenke syndrome is a classic autosomal dominant disorder with incomplete penetrance and highly variable expressivity [5, 11]. Despite examination by highly experienced clinicians with great familiarity with craniosynostosis in general and Muenke syndrome in particular, mutation carriers may be found to lack even subtle characteristics of disease [5, 12]. Penetrance is higher in females (87%) than males (76%), and there are additional gender-specific differences in manifestations, such as the suture involved in craniosynostosis [10, 13]. In 1 comprehensive review of patients, 58% of females had bilateral craniosynostosis, compared to only 37% of males [10].

As in many Mendelian disorders, the incomplete penetrance and variable expressivity provide evidence for multiple interacting genetic and environmental factors. These factors likely affect the degree of severity as well as the presence or absence of specific findings [14]. For example, monozygotic twins, both with Muenke syndrome but with significant phenotypic variability, have been reported, and animal models show variable phenotypes depending on the breed's genetic background [15, 16].

De novo mutations in *FGFR3* are of paternal origin, and are associated with increased paternal age [3]. The majority of mutations are de novo, though the exact proportion of de novo mutations is not known in probands with Muenke syndrome [2]. The mutation rate at the disease-causing nucleotide, the highest of any transversion in the human genome, is estimated to occur at up to 8×10^{-6}

per haploid genome (compared with the highest rate in the human genome, the c.1138G>A transition resulting in the common achondroplasia mutation, which occurs at a rate of $5–28 \times 10^{-6}$) [17].

Given the range of possibilities of phenotypic manifestations, and complexities regarding the inheritance of mutations, genetic counseling for affected patients and families can be intricate, and is therefore best handled by clinicians familiar with nuances of Muenke syndrome and other craniosynostosis syndromes. As some patients may have a degree of neurocognitive impairment, and because hearing loss is common (see below), counseling must additionally take into account challenges involving communication with patients and families.

Clinical Findings and Diagnosis

Patients with the defining FGFR3 p.P250R mutation demonstrate a wide range of findings, even within a single family [5, 11]. The majority of patients have coronal craniosynostosis, which can be unilateral or bilateral. A substantial proportion of mutation-positive patients (up to 17%) do not appear to have frank sutural abnormalities, and sutures in addition to the coronal sutures may be craniosynostotic [10, 12, 18]. Most patients with Muenke syndrome exhibit craniofacial findings typical of patients with craniosynostosis in general. These facial features, the severity of which is related to the degree of craniosynostosis, include brachycephaly, plagiocephaly, or trigonocephaly (the latter finding was described in one striking case report, though the connection between the defining mutation and metopic synostosis in this case is not clear), very mild midface hypoplasia, hypertelorism, ptosis, and a high palate [5, 10, 19] (fig. 1). Turricephaly, a depressed nasal bridge, and temporal bulging may be especially apparent [13], in contrast to isolated coronal synostosis. Early surgical correction can improve craniofacial anomalies and the overall cosmetic appearance [20]. However, compared to patients with non-syndromic coronal craniosynostosis, patients with Muenke syndrome are more likely to require multiple surgeries for craniosynostosis, and cosmesis may be less satisfactory [20–22] (see Chapter 18 in this volume).

In addition to craniosynostosis (though these manifestations may be present in mutation-positive patients who do not have craniosynostosis), common phenotypic findings in affected patients can include macrocephaly, low-frequency sensorineural hearing loss, and developmental delay/mental retardation. Hydrocephalus may also be present (table 1) [5, 10, 23]. It is unclear if cognitive dysfunction in patients is a primary part of the disease or if there is an additional contribution by deformational forces (and may in fact, be a combination of the two), but there are some authors who have reported that early neurosurgical intervention is associated with a more positive neurological outcome) [24, 25]. Patients with Muenke syndrome may be more likely to have intellectual impairment than patients with other *FGFR*-related syndromic craniosynostoses [10, 26].

Although craniosynostosis is the primary skeletal anomaly, brachydactyly and clinodactyly occur in approximately one-third of patients, and additional, relatively mild and easily overlooked skeletal anomalies are frequent, including coned epiphyses, carpal fusion, thimble-like or absent/fused middle phalanges, calcaneo-cuboidal fusion, and short and broad middle phalanges [5] (fig. 2). Patients with Muenke syndrome do not tend to have long-bone or other severe skeletal anomalies associated with other mutations in *FGFR3* [28]. In addition to the classic features associated with Muenke syndrome, unusual reported findings (which may be coincident) include Sprengel anomaly of the shoulder, cervical spine anomalies, bilateral medial temporal lobe dysgenesis, and (likely) upper airway obstruction leading to sudden infant death [29–31].

As described, clinical features of Muenke syndrome overlap that of other craniosynostosis

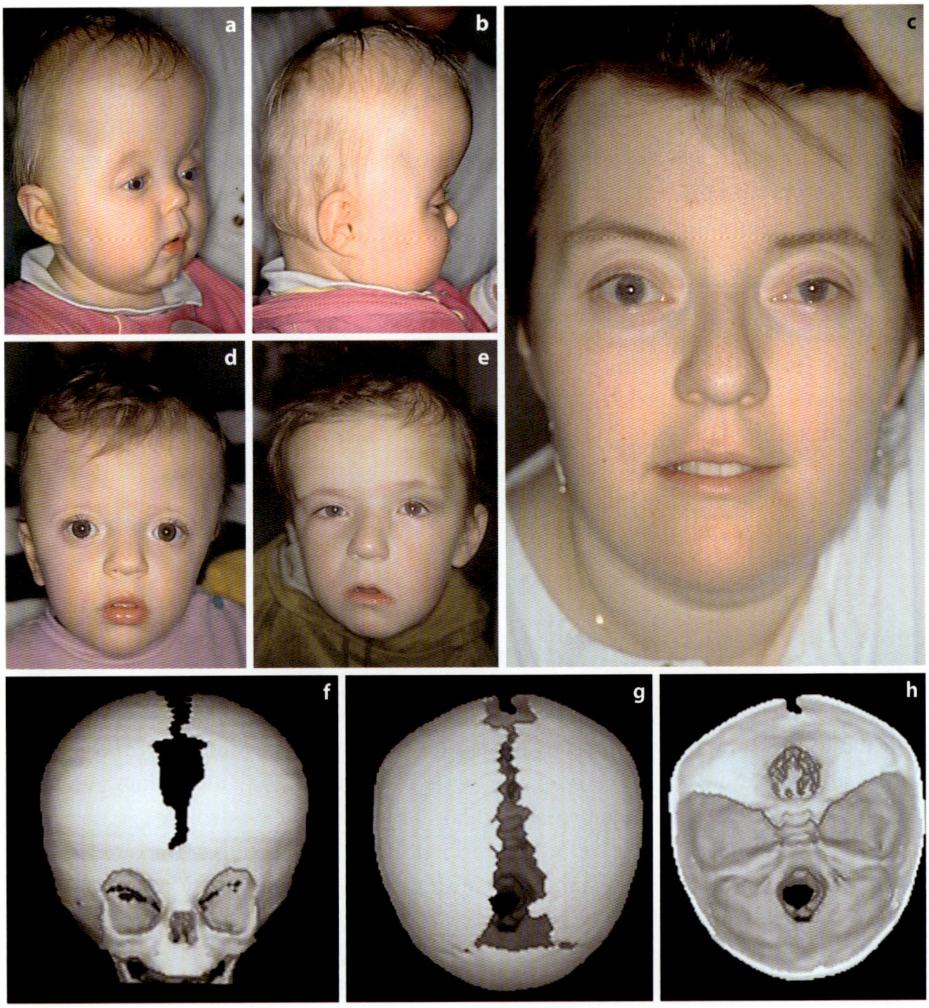

Fig. 1. a–e Patients with Muenke syndrome demonstrate a wide range of severity (dependent upon the degree of craniosynostosis) in terms of facial findings. Patients are shown pre-operatively at: **a**, **b** 11 months, demonstrating typical brachy-turricephaly, with a bulging forehead; **c** adulthood, showing brachycephaly and slight left ptosis; **d** 16 months, showing brachycephaly, with a high forehead, bulging temporal squama, and mild hypertelorism; **e** 45 months, showing anterior plagiocephaly due to left unilateral coronal synostosis. **f–h** Three-dimensional reformatted computed tomography of a 4-month-old (same patient as **d**), demonstrating brachycephaly and incomplete midline ossification, as well as a shortened anterior cranial base. Photos courtesy of H. Collmann, and published with consent from participating patients and families.

syndromes as well as non-syndromic craniosynostosis, and definitive diagnosis of Muenke syndrome depends on molecular testing (see Chapter 9 in this volume). Testing is available both on a commercial and on a research basis. As it is impossible for even the most experienced clinician to diagnose the condition on purely clinical grounds, testing may be performed as part of a multi-gene

Table 1. Prevalence of clinical features in patients with Muenke syndrome

Finding	Estimated prevalence (%)	Reference
Craniosynostosis	83	[10]
Bilateral coronal craniosynostosis	55	[10]
Unilateral coronal craniosynostosis	26	[10]
Other craniosynostosis type	5	[10]
Macrocephaly	3	[10]
Hearing loss[a]	40	[10, 27]
Cognitive impairment	35	[27]
Hand anomalies	65	[5]
Foot anomalies	55	[5]

[a] The prevalence of hearing loss may be shown to be much more common when sophisticated testing techniques are available.

panel looking for common mutations in genes associated with craniosynostosis (see Chapter 15 in this volume).

Management

Patients with Muenke syndrome may require treatment for a number of medical issues, but 3 areas are especially important: neurological development, management of hearing loss, and surgical treatment of craniosynostosis. As in many genetic conditions that affect multiple organ systems, optimal management of affected patients and families involves a multidisciplinary approach through a team experienced with the disorder [26, 32]. Many large pediatric centers have a dedicated craniofacial team to allow streamlining of care, which can be enormously beneficial both for patients and caregivers. In addition to a dedicated primary care doctor or medical home, required specialists may include experts in audiology, clinical genetics, dentistry, development, neurology and neuroradiology, ophthalmology, and surgery (neurosurgery, craniofacial surgery, and plastic surgery).

Diagnosed patients should be tested for hearing loss, and monitoring should continue even if the initial evaluation (including on neonatal screening) is normal. Similarly, patients should have initial and subsequent regular developmental evaluations in childhood, with implementation of treatment as necessary [10]. Surgical management algorithms for patients with Muenke syndrome, as well as other syndromic craniosynostoses, have been proposed. These algorithms include initial surgery in the first year of life and at least annual multidisciplinary evaluations [20, 26]. Fronto-orbital advancement and reshaping is typically the initial surgery. Patients may require a secondary additional revision, and most patients require secondary (and sometimes tertiary) extracranial contouring procedures, though the timing for these latter procedures is variable [20].

Molecular Pathogenesis

FGFR3 negatively regulates bone growth, and a number of chondrodysplasias (including hypochondroplasia, achondroplasia, and thanatophoric dysplasia) with varying severity result

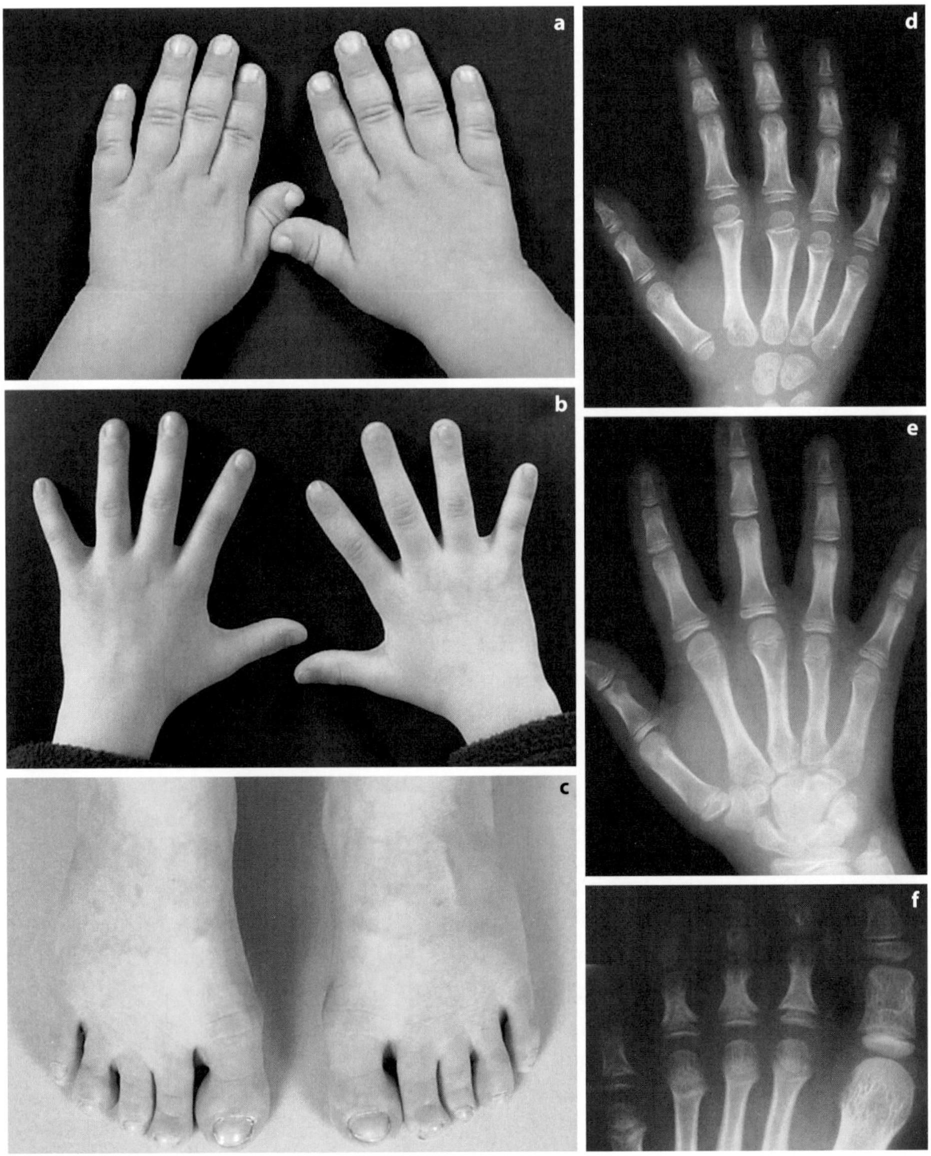

Fig. 2. The extremities of patients (5 different patients are shown) with Muenke syndrome show subtle but distinct anomalies. **a**, **b** Fifth finger brachydactyly in patients at 6 years (**a**) and 10 years (**b**) of age; **c** lower extremity brachydactyly (same patient as **b**); **d** thimble-like intermediate second phalanx with cone-shaped epiphysis and an abnormally short intermediate fifth phalanx (female, 7 years); **e** short intermediate fifth phalanx and fusion of the hamatum and capitatum (female, 11 years); **f** cone-shaped epiphyses of proximal phalanges I-V (same patient as **b**). Photos courtesy of H. Collmann.

from constitutively activating mutations in *FGFR3* [28, 33, 34]. While the mechanism has not been precisely defined, the current model as related to these conditions involves at least partial ligand-independent FGFR3 activation leading to reduced chondrocyte proliferation and differentiation and resultant decreased bone growth, due to the inhibitory effect of increased FGFR3 signaling in chondrocytes [16, 28]. In Muenke syndrome, on the other hand, long bones are not affected, suggesting a different, but still poorly understood pathogenetic mechanism. Animal models do not recapitulate the human spectrum well, but suggest a different mechanism than that underlying the allelic chondrodysplasias [16].

The defining proline to arginine mutation in amino acid 250 of FGFR3, located between second and third extracellular immunoglobulin-like FGF binding domains, results in enhanced ligand binding through the presence of additional hydrogen bonds [35]. A similar process underlies the pathogenesis of the analogous mutations in *FGFR1* and *FGFR2* [35]. Unlike the allelic chondrodysplasias, this enhanced ligand binding appears to remain ligand-dependent [16]. Further, the effect of very specific FGF ligand binding activity to mutant FGFR3 may explain differences in limb phenotypes in Muenke syndrome as opposed to other *FGFR*-related craniosynostoses [35].

Knowledge of FGFR3's role in sutural development is less robust than that of other craniosynostosis-related genes. Additionally, the interplay between FGFR3 and other molecules involved in craniosynostosis is not well-understood, but there is some evidence that TWIST1 may be a negative regulator of *FGFR3* transcriptional activation by E2A (see Chapter 4 in this volume). Clinically, Muenke syndrome has some similarities with Saethre-Chotzen syndrome (which is due to mutations in *TWIST1*), as well as to nonsyndromic craniosynostosis, and scalp fibroblasts in patients with the 3 disorders have been reported to have shared expression profiles [36, 37].

As mentioned, mouse models of Muenke syndrome have revealed some insights, but the animal systems do not recapitulate all aspects of the human disease. Twigg et al. showed that coronal craniosynostosis is not reliably reproduced in the mouse, though the mouse model may be nonetheless informative with regards to more general bone development [16]. The mouse model does provide a good system for the study of hearing loss in Muenke syndrome, which could be important in the development of molecular therapies [29].

Conclusions

Patients with Muenke syndrome present a complex picture to both the research scientist and the managing clinician. While impressive progress has been made in the laboratory, the clinic, and the operating theater, much work remains. Future questions that demand more complete answers include improved understanding of the molecular pathogenesis, unraveling gender-specific differences observed in patients, both in terms of inheritance and clinical manifestations, and optimization of management algorithms for affected patients and families.

Acknowledgements

This work was supported by the Division of Intramural Research, National Human Genome Research Institute, National Institutes of Health, Department of Health and Human Services, United States of America.

References

1 Boulet SL, Rasmussen SA, Honein MA: A population-based study of craniosynostosis in metropolitan Atlanta, 1989–2003. Am J Med Genet A 2008; 146A:984–991.
2 Moloney DM, Wall SA, Ashworth GJ, Oldridge M, Glass IA, et al: Prevalence of Pro250Arg mutation of fibroblast growth factor receptor 3 in coronal craniosynostosis. Lancet 1997;349:1059–1062.
3 Rannan-Eliya SV, Taylor IB, De Heer IM, Van Den Ouweland AM, Wall SA, Wilkie AO: Paternal origin of *FGFR3* mutations in Muenke-type craniosynostosis. Hum Genet 2004;115:200–207.
4 Wilkie AO, Byren JC, Hurst JA, Jayamohan J, Johnson D, et al: Prevalence and complications of single-gene and chromosomal disorders in craniosynostosis. Pediatrics 2010;126:e391–e400.
5 Muenke M, Gripp KW, McDonald-McGinn DM, Gaudenz K, Whitaker LA, et al: A unique point mutation in the fibroblast growth factor receptor 3 gene (*FGFR3*) defines a new craniosynostosis syndrome. Am J Hum Genet 1997;60: 555–564.
6 Gripp KW, McDonald-McGinn DM, Gaudenz K, Whitaker LA, Bartlett SP, et al: Identification of a genetic cause for isolated unilateral coronal synostosis: a unique mutation in the fibroblast growth factor receptor 3. J Pediatr 1998;132: 714–716.
7 Bellus GA, Gaudenz K, Zackai EH, Clarke LA, Szabo J, Francomano CA, Muenke M: Identical mutations in three different fibroblast growth factor receptor genes in autosomal dominant craniosynostosis syndromes. Nat Genet 1996; 14:174–176.
8 Muenke M, Schell U, Hehr A, Robin NH, Losken HW, et al: A common mutation in the fibroblast growth factor receptor 1 gene in Pfeiffer syndrome. Nat Genet 1994;8:269–274.
9 Wilkie AO, Slaney SF, Oldridge M, Poole MD, Ashworth GJ, et al: Apert syndrome results from localized mutations of *FGFR2* and is allelic with Crouzon syndrome. Nat Genet 1995;9:165–172.
10 Doherty ES, Lacbawan F, Hadley DW, Brewer C, Zalewski C, et al: Muenke syndrome (*FGFR3*-related craniosynostosis): expansion of the phenotype and review of the literature. Am J Med Genet A 2007;143A:3204–3215.
11 Golla A, Lichmer P, von Gernet S, Winterpacht A, Fairley J, Murken J, Schuffenhauer S: Phenotypic expression of the fibroblast growth factor receptor 3 *(FGFR3)* mutation P250R in a large craniosynostosis family. J Med Genet 1997;34:683–684.
12 Robin NH, Scott JA, Cohen AR, Goldstein JA: Nonpenetrance in *FGFR3*-associated coronal synostosis syndrome. Am J Med Genet 1998;80:296–297.
13 Lajeunie E, El Ghouzzi V, Le Merrer M, Munnich A, Bonaventure J, Renier D: Sex related expressivity of the phenotype in coronal craniosynostosis caused by the recurrent P250R *FGFR3* mutation. J Med Genet 1999;36:9–13.
14 Ming JE, Muenke M: Multiple hits during early embryonic development: digenic diseases and holoprosencephaly. Am J Hum Genet 2002;71:1017–1032.
15 Escobar LF, Hiett AK, Marnocha A: Significant phenotypic variability of Muenke syndrome in identical twins. Am J Med Genet A 2009;149A:1273–1276.
16 Twigg SR, Healy C, Babbs C, Sharpe JA, Wood WG, et al: Skeletal analysis of the Fgfr3(P244R) mouse, a genetic model for the Muenke craniosynostosis syndrome. Dev Dyn 2009;238:331–342.
17 Bellus GA, Hefferon TW, Ortiz de Luna RI, Hecht JT, Horton WA, et al: Achondroplasia is defined by recurrent G380R mutations of FGFR3. Am J Hum Genet 1995;56:368–373.
18 Renier D, El-Ghouzzi V, Bonaventure J, Le Merrer M, Lajeunie E: Fibroblast growth factor receptor 3 mutation in nonsyndromic coronal synostosis: clinical spectrum, prevalence, and surgical outcome. J Neurosurg 2000;92:631–636.
19 van der Meulen J, van den Ouweland A, Hoogeboom J: Trigonocephaly in Muenke syndrome. Am J Med Genet A 2006;140:2493–2494.
20 Honnebier MB, Cabiling DS, Hetlinger M, McDonald-McGinn DM, Zackai EH, Bartlett SP: The natural history of patients treated for *FGFR3*-associated (Muenke-type) craniosynostosis. Plast Reconstr Surg 2008;121:919–931.
21 Arnaud E, Meneses P, Lajeunie E, Thorne JA, Marchac D, Renier D: Postoperative mental and morphological outcome for nonsyndromic brachycephaly. Plast Reconstr Surg 2002;110:6–12.
22 Thomas GP, Wilkie AO, Richards PG, Wall SA: *FGFR3* P250R mutation increases the risk of reoperation in apparent 'nonsyndromic' coronal craniosynostosis. J Craniofac Surg 2005;16: 347–352.
23 Mansour SL, Twigg SR, Freeland RM, Wall SA, Li C, Wilkie AO: Hearing loss in a mouse model of Muenke syndrome. Hum Mol Genet 2009;18:43–50.
24 Lekovic GP, Bristol RE, Rekate HL: Cognitive impact of craniosynostosis. Semin Pediatr Neurol 2004;11:305–310.
25 Mathijssen I, Arnaud E, Lajeunie E, Marchac D, Renier D: Postoperative cognitive outcome for synostotic frontal plagiocephaly. J Neurosurg 2006;105:16–20.
26 Flapper WJ, Anderson PJ, Roberts RM, David DJ: Intellectual outcomes following protocol management in Crouzon, Pfeiffer, and Muenke syndromes. J Craniofac Surg 2009;20:1252–1255.
27 Kress W, Schropp C, Lieb G, Petersen B, Büsse-Ratzka M, et al: Saethre-Chotzen syndrome caused by *TWIST1* gene mutations: functional differentiation from Muenke coronal synostosis syndrome. Eur J Hum Genet 2006;14:39–48.
28 Schibler L, Gibbs L, Benoist-Lasselin C, Decraene C, Martinovic J, et al: New insight on *FGFR3*-related chondrodysplasias molecular physiopathology revealed by human chondrocyte gene expression profiling. PLoS One 2009;4: e7633.
29 Lowry RB, Jabs EW, Graham GE, Gerritsen J, Fleming J: Syndrome of coronal craniosynostosis, Klippel-Feil anomaly, and Sprengel shoulder with and without Pro250Arg mutation in the *FGFR3* gene. Am J Med Genet 2001;104:112–119.
30 Grosso S, Farnetani MA, Berardi R, Bartalini G, Carpentieri M, et al: Medial temporal lobe dysgenesis in Muenke syndrome and hypochondroplasia. Am J Med Genet A 2003;120A:88–91.

31 Shah PS, Siriwardena K, Taylor G, Steele L, Ray P, Blaser S, Chitayat D: Sudden infant death in a patient with *FGFR3* P250R mutation. Am J Med Genet A 2006;140:2794–2796.
32 de Jong T, Bannink N, Bredero-Boelhouwer HH, van Veelen ML, Bartels MC, et al: Long-term functional outcome in 167 patients with syndromic craniosynostosis; defining a syndrome-specific risk profile. J Med Genet 2010; 47:803–808.
33 Webster MK, Donoghue DJ: FGFR activation in skeletal disorders: too much of a good thing. Trends Genet 1997;13: 178–182.
34 L'Hôte CG, Knowles MA: Cell responses to FGFR3 signalling: growth, differentiation and apoptosis. Exp Cell Res 2005; 304:417–431.
35 Ibrahimi OA, Zhang F, Eliseenkova AV, Linhardt RJ, Mohammadi M: Proline to arginine mutations in FGF receptors 1 and 3 result in Pfeiffer and Muenke craniosynostosis syndromes through enhancement of FGF binding affinity. Hum Mol Genet 2004;13:69–78.
36 Bochukova E, Soneji S, Wall S, Wilkie AO: Scalp fibroblasts have a shared expression profile in monogenic craniosynostosis. J Med Genet 2010;47: 803–808.
37 Funato N, Ohtani K, Ohyama K, Kuroda T, Nakamura M: Common regulation of growth arrest and differentiation of osteoblasts by helix-loop-helix factors. Mol Cell Biol 2001;21:7416–7428.

Maximilian Muenke
NIH, MSC 3717
Building 35, Room 1B-203
Bethesda, MD, 20892–3717 (USA)
Tel. +1 301 402 8167, Fax +1 301 496 7184, E-Mail mamuenke@mail.nih.gov

Muenke M, Kress W, Collmann H, Solomon BD (eds): Craniosynostoses: Molecular Genetics, Principles of Diagnosis, and Treatment.
Monogr Hum Genet. Basel, Karger, 2011, vol 19, pp 98–106

Saethre-Chotzen Syndrome: Clinical and Molecular Genetic Aspects

W. Kress[a] · H. Collmann[b]

[a]Institute of Human Genetics, [b]Department of Neurosurgery, Julius-Maximilians University, Würzburg, Germany

Abstract

Saethre-Chotzen syndrome (SCS) is one of the frequent autosomal dominant craniosynostosis syndromes with the following main features: coronal suture fusion resulting in progressive synostosis, dilated parietal foramina, low frontal hairline, hypertelorism, ptosis of upper eyelids, small auricles with prominent anthelical crura, broad or bifid great toe and soft tissue syndactyly, but without primary mental retardation. The most striking difference between FGFR1/2-associated craniosynostoses and SCS is the lack of proptosis due to normally sized orbits in the latter. There is a phenotypic overlap with Muenke syndrome, and the mildest forms of SCS present with only isolated coronal synostosis. SCS shows high penetrance but great variability. It is caused by loss-of-function mutations in the *TWIST1* gene on chromosome 7p21. TWIST1 is an important transcription factor and part of a complicated signaling pathway involved in both early embryogenesis and later on in chondroblast and osteoblast differentiation. The mutational spectrum comprises missense mutations located mainly in the basic helix-loop-helix domain, nonsense mutations, small in-frame duplications, and whole gene deletions. About one-third of mutations are de novo. There is no recognizable genotype-phenotype correlation. The main complication is a high rate of elevated intracranial pressure due to progressive synostosis.

Saethre-Chotzen syndrome (SCS) [MIM 101 400] belongs historically to the acrocephalosyndactylies because its main features include coronal suture synostosis, broad or bifid great toes and soft tissue syndactyly. SCS has an autosomal dominant inheritance with high penetrance but variable expressivity [1], and occurs at an estimated incidence of roughly 1:25,000 to 1:50,000 live births [2]. About 70% of cases are familial. SCS is caused by private heterozygous mutations in the *TWIST1* gene [MIM 601 622], a transcription factor on chromosome 7p21 [3–5]. Phenotypical overlap with Muenke syndrome [MIM 602 849] has been reported [6, 7].

Phenotypic Features

Long before the responsible gene had been identified, the syndrome was recognized as a genetic entity by Haakon Saethre and Fritz Chotzen in the early thirties of the last century (see Chapter 1). During the following decades, the phenotype has been outlined by numerous authors, most comprehensively by Olof Pantke and Michael Cohen [8]. However, authors in the pre-molecular era were not able to clearly differentiate between SCS and Muenke syndrome. Therefore, the reported frequency of features in the early literature has to be examined with reservation.

Patients present with a highly variable phenotype ranging from non-syndromic coronal craniosynostosis to the classical full-blown picture of SCS, both within and between families. The variability is particularly highlighted by a report of a large Indian family harboring a *TWIST1* mutation, which was associated with blepharophimosis, epicanthus inversus, and moderate to severe ptosis in most family members, while in the majority craniosynostosis was absent [9]. The authors suggested an overlap with BPES (blepharophimosis, ptosis, epicanthus inversus syndrome).

The typical features of classical SCS drawn from a cohort of patients with proven *TWIST1* mutations are shown in table 1.

Craniofacial Symptoms

The classical SCS phenotype comprises uni- or bicoronal synostosis causing brachycephaly or plagiocephaly with absent supraorbital ridges (fig. 1a, b). However, as other sutures may additionally be affected, the resultant head shape may vary: a peculiar turricephalic appearance can be noted in patients with additional congenital metopic synostosis (fig. 2), whereas oxycephaly results from progressive multisutural fusion. The latter is a common phenomenon in SCS: in our own study group, 35% of individuals presented with pansynostosis at a median age of 30 months. Progressive multisutural fusion likely explains the high rate of intracranial hypertension developing in childhood [6, 8]. Craniosynostosis may be absent in a small proportion of individuals. Microcephaly (defined as a head circumference below the third centile) has been noted in one-third of individuals. After birth, a midline calvarial defect similar to that observed in patients with Apert syndrome can be observed in some patients. In about half of our own cases, enlarged parietal foramina have been verified (fig. 3) [6].

The typical facial aspect comprises a low frontal hair line, ptosis of one or both eyelids, small palpebral fissures, a deviated nasal septum and anteverted nares in young children, but a prominent nose in adults. Significant tear duct stenosis may lead to epiphora in some patients. The auricles tend to be small, rotated posteriorly, and have prominent anthelical crura (fig. 4) [10]. In some individuals, the external auditory meatus may be stenotic. Mild midface hypoplasia may be noted in some cases (fig. 1c). Intra- and interfamiliar variability of all the above findings is striking.

Table 1. Phenotypic features of proven *TWIST1*-associated SCS (adopted from [6]). The number of individuals investigated for specific features varies from 35 to 71.

Feature	Frequency (%)
Brachycephaly	46
Plagiocephaly	37
Oxycephaly, normal head shape	17
Coronal suture fusion (age <16 years)	96
Progressive synostosis (age <16 years)	82
Multiple suture fusion (age <16 years)	53
Midline calvarial defect (age <6 months)	74
Enlarged parietal foramina	55
Head circumference <3rd centile	39
Evident intracranial hypertension	35
Papilledema/optic nerve atrophy	28
Low-set frontal hairline	55
Hypertelorism	53
Ptosis of upper eyelids	45
Tear duct stenosis	25
Subnormal auricular length	43
Prominent (anti-)helical crura	51
Recurrent middle ear effusions/otitis	63
Mild midfacial retrusion	25
High arched palate	34
Visceral anomalies	18
Soft tissue syndactyly	52
Broad or bifid great toe	55
X-ray: bifid distal phalanx hallucis	44
Cervical vertebral fusion	23
Thoracolumbar scoliosis	11

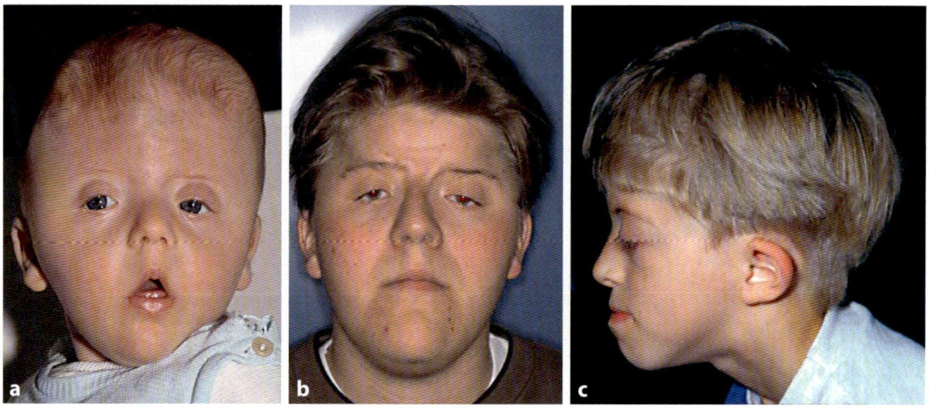

Fig. 1. **a**, **b** Classical SCS, same patient at the age of 5 months and 18 years. **c** Profile of a patient with classical SCS showing midface hypoplasia.

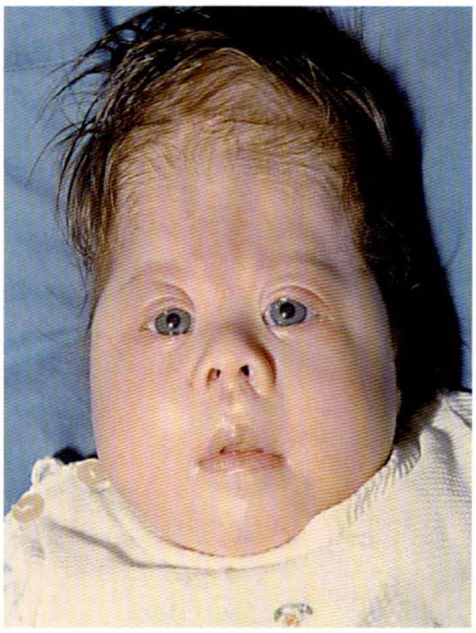

Fig. 2. SCS patient with a turricephalic aspect caused by coronal and metopic synostosis.

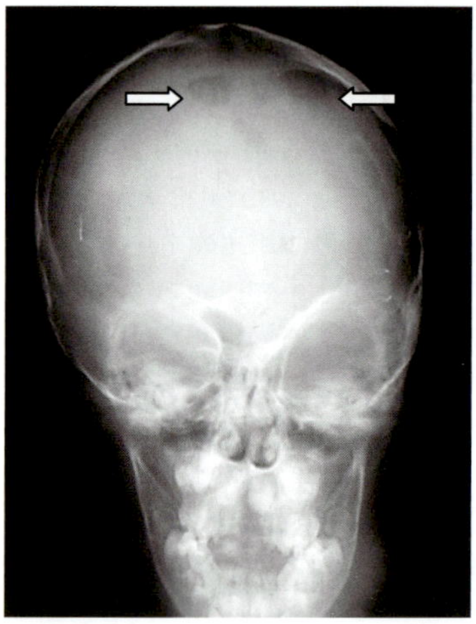

Fig. 3. X-rays of the skull showing open parietal foramina (arrows).

Neurodevelopmental Aspects

Cognitive and motor development is usually within normal limits [6, 8]. There are reports that patients with a microdeletion of the whole gene and neighboring regions may have mental retardation [11]. This was not observed in the 6 families in our series, who harbored deletions between 80 and 6,000 kb [6]. Neuroimaging did not reveal any intracranial abnormalities attributable to the genetic disorder in 49 individuals examined at the craniofacial center of Würzburg. Sensorineural hearing loss is not a feature of SCS (as opposed to Muenke syndrome), but conductive hearing loss due to recurrent middle ear effusions may be a significant problem. This is probably attributable to mild midface retrusion that interferes with tympanic ventilation but usually does not compromise the upper airways.

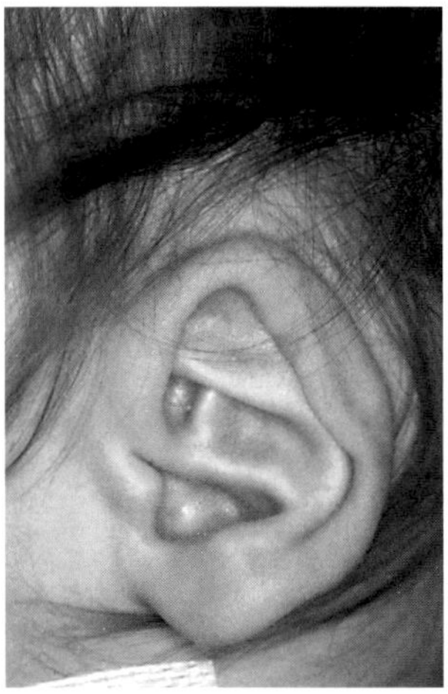

Fig. 4. Typical small ear with prominent helical and anthelical crura.

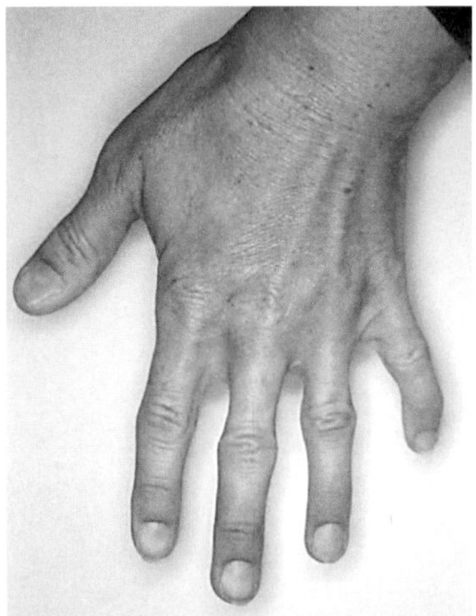

Fig. 5. Cutaneous syndactyly, most prominent between the second and third finger.

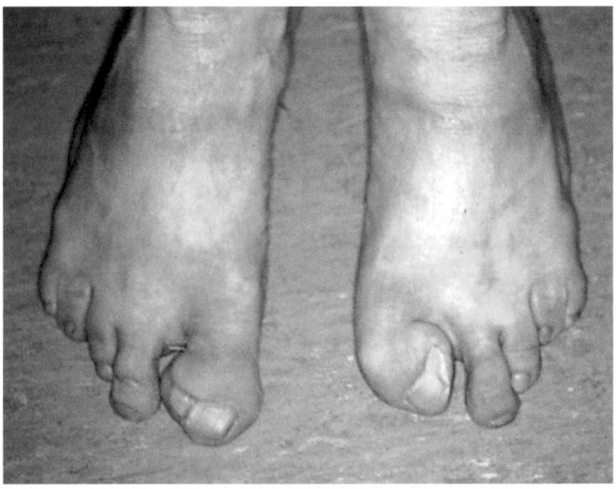

Fig. 6. Double distal phalanx of great toe, varus deviation.

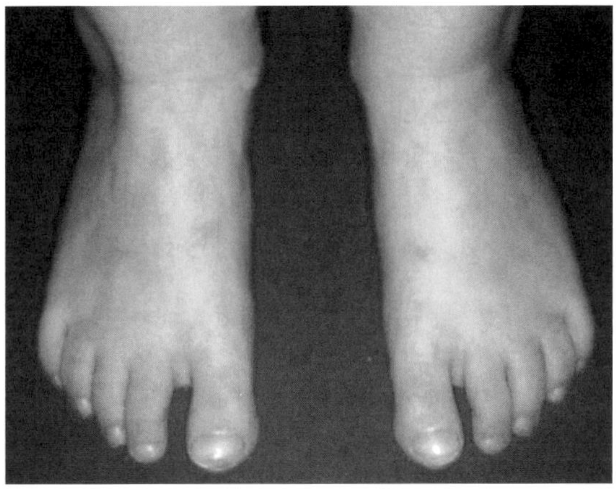

Fig. 7. Broadened terminal phalanx of the great toes.

Extracranial Features

Interdigital webbing of the fingers essentially involves digits 2–5, which however is most obvious in digits 2/3 (fig. 5). The webbing can mimic brachydactyly which is actually a less striking feature. The thumb may be twisted dorsally, resembling a finger. In a few instances, fusion of some carpal (or tarsal) bones has been verified in our own study group [12]. A broad or bifid great toe, often in a valgus position, with a bifid (figs. 6, 8) or partially duplicated distal phalanx (figs. 7, 9) represents abortive preaxial polydactyly, and is nearly diagnostic for SCS. In some cases, evidence of this anomaly can only be drawn from radiographs (fig. 9) [12]. Partial ankylosis of the radioulnar joint may be noted in some patients (fig. 10). Cervical vertebral fusion (fig. 11) is also a fairly common phenotypic feature [8, 12].

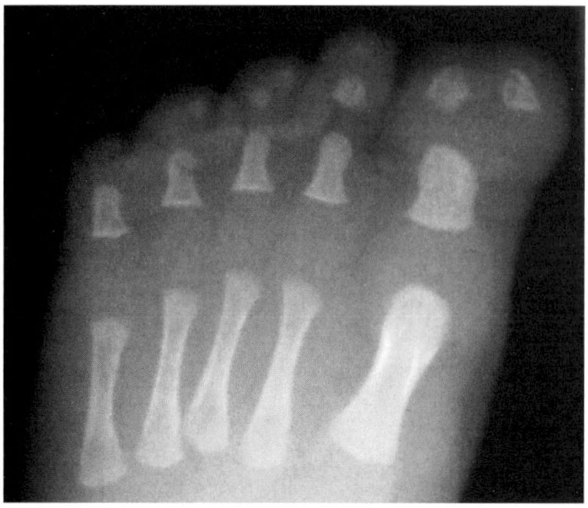

Fig. 8. X-rays showing double distal phalanx of the great toe.

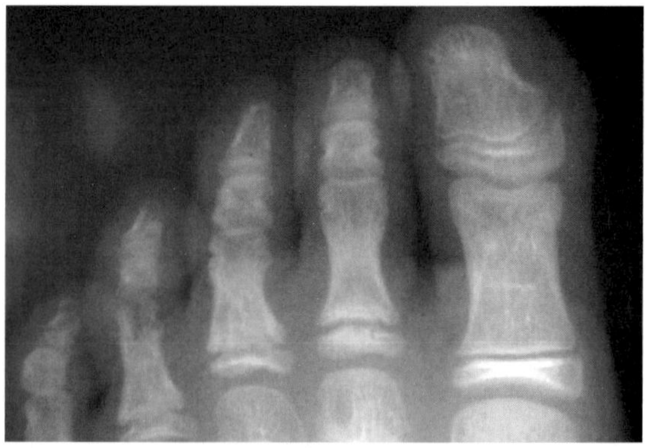

Fig. 9. X-rays showing valgus deviation and broadening of great toe's terminal phalanx.

In a study published in 2007, a high rate of breast cancer was reported in females from SCS families segregating *TWIST1* mutations, suggesting that mutated *TWIST1* may be a breast cancer susceptibility gene [13]. This observation could not be confirmed in a subsequent study [14].

Diagnostic Phenotypic Features
Dilated parietal foramina, severe ptosis of the eye lids, interdigital webbing between digits 2/3 and 3/4, and abortive duplication of the distal phalanx of the great toe may be considered nearly diagnostic for SCS. A low frontal hairline and subnormal ear length are less specific signs.

Distinction from Muenke Syndrome
In view of the high phenotypic variability of both, SCS and Muenke syndrome, there can be no doubt that in former times, these syndromes had been frequently confused. This is readily conceivable for all cases of SCS in which specific signs are absent. Differences between both syndromes predominantly involve function rather than outer appearance. The high rate of intracranial hypertension in SCS, putting the optic nerve at risk, and the generally normal mental development sharply contrasts with a generally normal intracranial pressure, fairly common mental retardation, and a sensory hearing deficit in patients with Muenke syndrome (see Chapter 8). Therefore, separation of these two syndromes is of high clinical importance. As a consequence, testing for the defining Muenke syndrome mutation [7] should be performed in all patients with clinical features suspicious of SCS but without a *TWIST1* mutation.

The SCS Causing Gene *TWIST1*

In 1992, the locus for SCS was located by linkage analysis to chromosome 7p [15].

As described in Chapter 13, this localization was already known from chromosomal aberrations of chromosome 7 in syndromic patients exhibiting an SCS-like phenotype. Using further families and patients with reciprocal translocations, the locus was narrowed down to the 7p21 region. Two groups demonstrated independently that SCS was caused by mutations in the *TWIST1* gene [3, 4].

The *TWIST1* gene and its paralog, *TWIST2*, code for nuclear transcription factors active in

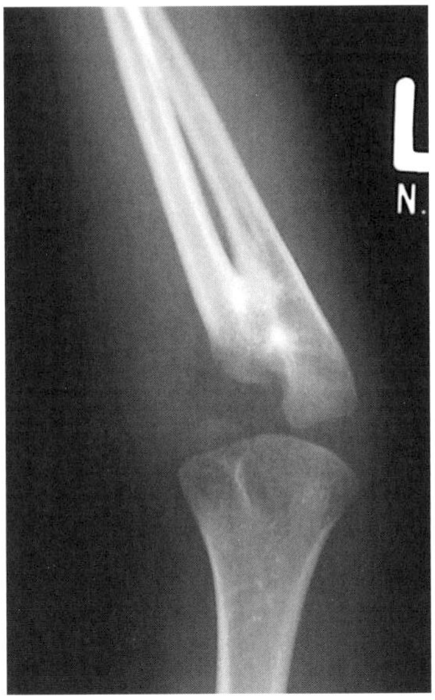

Fig. 10. X-rays showing partial ankylosis of the radioulnar joint.

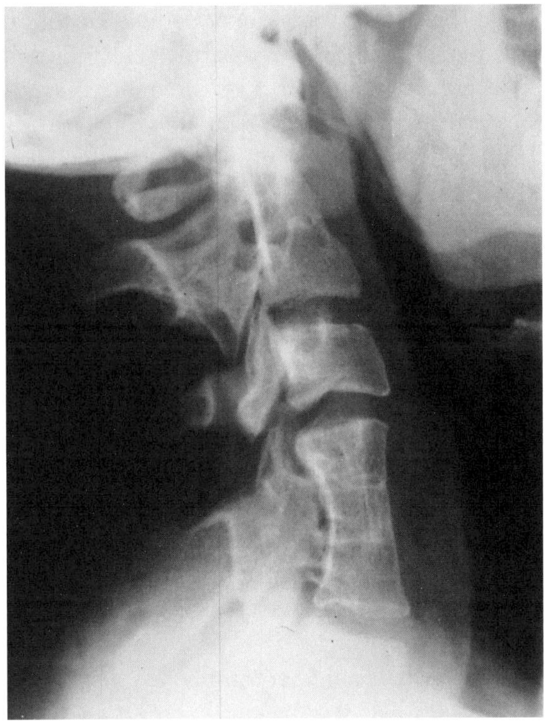

Fig. 11. X-rays of cervical spine showing vertebral fusion.

early embryonic development. There are also 2 paralogs in mice. In zebrafish, the small family of *twist* genes comprises 4 paralogs [16]. The embryonic lethality of *Twist* null-mutants in both vertebrates (mouse) and invertebrates *(Drosophila)* demonstrates that at least 1 functioning *Twist* gene is essential for development and survival. Including information from many species, it is now commonly accepted that the highly conserved *Twist* genes are necessary for differentiation of mesodermal derivatives (mesodermal determining factor, establishing a multiple transcriptional network), and in vertebrates they are also required for the development of the head neural crest. In later stages of development especially, TWIST1 assumes another role (like the FGFRs) in (out)growth, e.g. in cranial sutures and limb buds. Its function and interaction with numerous signaling cofactors in an open suture are discussed in Chapter 4. In the adult organism, the mammalian *Twist* genes are expressed at a basal level in many tissues, and over-expression contributes to tumor progression and metastasis in a variety of cancers [17]. Epithelial to mesenchymal transition and vice versa, an important process in embryogenesis, is repeated in structured epithelial cancer cells. These cells lose polarity and acquire mesenchymal features, allowing for cell movement and forming metastatic tumors.

The large exon 1 of the *TWIST1* gene codes for the important functional domains that are highly conserved between species: the DNA binding domain, the helix-loop-helix (HLH) motif, and the C-terminal domain TWIST box [18]. The presence of these domains assigns the *TWIST* genes to the super-family of bHLH transcription factors (b stands for basic amino acids in the DNA binding domain); they bind to specific DNA sequences called E boxes, forming dimer complexes with a broad set of potential dimer partners. In addition, phosphorylation of conserved threonine and serine residues within TWIST-family proteins leads to a second level of control and organization [19]. Moreover, regulation through phosphorylation sub-localizes proteins in the cell, thereby positioning the TWIST protein (and perhaps its partner) in a functional or non-functional environment.

A complex interaction between phosphorylation and formation of homo- or hetero-dimers with changing partners controls differentiation of mesenchymal cells in the cranial sutures and the limb bud (hand/foot formation), as shown in mice [20]. A minor imbalance of this interaction caused by heterozygous mutations may be the key to the variable expression of phenotype.

TWIST1 Mutational Spectrum

By the end of 2009, 146 different mutations had been registered in the Human Gene Mutation Database (HGMD; https://portal.biobase-international.com/hgmd/pro/all.php) for the *TWIST1* gene. The most common type of mutations are missense/nonsense mutations (approximately 55–65%), followed by small deletions/insertions (approximately 22–28%), and whole gene deletions (approximately 5–15%). The above ranges reflect results from the database and from our own series. No splice mutations were identified, as there is only one coding exon. From the spectrum of mutations, a common functional mechanism could be inferred: haploinsufficiency.

The distribution of mutations within protein domains dependent on the type of mutation is given in table 2. Most mutations are localized in the most important functional bHLH domain and comprise private missense mutations. Recurrent small in-frame-duplications of 21 bp are located in the first helix domain. In the N-terminal part of the gene, nonsense mutations predominate, some of which were found recurrently in unrelated families. The C-terminal gene region contains the TWIST box, a binding region of the transcription factor RUNX2, on which the anti-osteogenic function of the *TWIST* genes is exerted [18]. Additionally, a few missense mutations have been detected within this motif.

Table 2. Distribution of mutations in the *TWIST1* gene and clustering of missense mutations in the functional domains. Mutations from HGMD (Human Gene Mutation Database; https://portal.biobase-international.com/hgmd/pro/all.php).

Gene domain	Numbers of different mutations
N-terminal	11 nonsense mutations 15 small deletions/insertions 2 missense mutations
DNA-binding domain	2 nonsense mutations 8 small deletions 13 missense mutations
HLH motif	5 nonsense mutations 39 missense mutations 8 small deletions/insertions
C-terminal	4 nonsense mutations 4 missense mutations 2 small deletions

No correlation can be established between phenotype and the type or location of mutations in *TWIST1*. Preceding the DNA binding domain, there is a polymorphic stretch of glycines interrupted by one alanine. The default sequence beginning at cDNA position c.244 is $(GGC)_5GCG(GGC)_5$. Variations of this repeat were also detected in healthy controls. There is currently no suggestion that this type of variation could influence the phenotype [6].

Most of the SCS cases are familial, but there are also de novo mutations. From our own cohort, roughly one-third of SCS patients were estimated to carry a de novo mutation.

Mouse Model

Twist-null heterozygous mice are a straightforward animal model for human SCS [2, 21]. Whereas homozygous knockout mice for the *Twist1* gene die during embryogenesis, heterozygous animals exhibit many features seen in human SCS. Carver et al. [2] demonstrated fusion of the coronal suture and other sutural abnormalities, which could only be verified in older mice, but not in newborns or fetuses. Unlike humans, in rodents all but one of the cranial sutures remain patent throughout the life span of the animal, with only the posterior portion of the metopic (interfrontal) suture normally fusing after birth. A duplicated hallux is also observed in some animals, dependent on the genetic background of the mice upon which the *Twist1* mutation is acting. In summary, the mouse model is an important aid in studying the molecular pathology of SCS and could be a target for any treatment trials.

Treatment

Surgical treatment of SCS patients is described in Chapter 17. Intra-cranial hypertension obviously related to progressive synostosis is an important complication of SCS. Attention should be also paid to recurrent middle ear effusions, impending amblyopia resulting from ptosis, tear duct stenosis, and sometimes even airway obstruction due to midface hypoplasia. Vertebral fusions and scoliosis may be present as well. Because of these issues, long-term surveillance must be continued until adolescence. This surveillance should include ophthalmoscopy at 3-month intervals and routine skull X-rays even after successful skull surgery.

References

1 Reardon W, Winter RM: Saethre-Chotzen syndrome. J Med Genet 1994;31:393–396.

2 Carver EA, Oram KF, Gridley T: Craniosynostosis in *Twist* heterozygous mice: a model for Saethre-Chotzen syndrome. Anat Rec 2002;268:90–92.

3 Howard TD, Paznekas WA, Green ED, Chiang LC, Ma N, et al: Mutations in TWIST, a basic helix-loop-helix transcription factor, in Saethre-Chotzen syndrome. Nat Genet 1997;15:36–41.

4 El Ghouzzi V, Le Merrer M, Perrin-Schmitt F, Lajeunie E, Benit P, et al: Mutations of the *TWIST* gene in the Saethre-Chotzen syndrome. Nat Genet 1997;15:42–46.

5 Rose CS, Patel P, Reardon W, Malcolm S, Winter RM: The *TWIST* gene, although not disrupted in Saethre-Chotzen patients with apparently balanced translocations of 7p21, is mutated in familial and sporadic cases. Hum Mol Genet 1997;6:1369–1373.

6 Kress W, Schropp C, Lieb G, Petersen B, Büsse-Ratzka M, et al: Saethre-Chotzen syndrome caused by TWIST 1 gene mutations: functional differentiation from Muenke coronal synostosis syndrome. Eur J Hum Genet 2006;14:39–48.

7 Muenke M, Gripp KW, McDonald-McGinn DM: A unique point mutation in the fibroblast growth factor receptor 3 gene *(FGFR3)* defines a new craniosynostosis syndrome. Am J Hum Genet 1997;60:555–564.

8 Pantke OA, Cohen MM Jr, Witkop CJ Jr, Feingold M, Schaumann B, et al: The Saethre-Chotzen syndrome. Birth Defects Orig Artic Ser 1975;11:190–225.

9 Dollfus H, Biswas P, Kumaramanickavel G, Stoetzel C, Quillet R, et al: Saethre-Chotzen syndrome: noteable intrafamilial phenotypic variability in a large family with Q28X TWIST mutation. Am J Med Genet 2002;109:218–225.

10 Cohen MM: Saethre-Chotzen syndrome; in Cohen MM, Mc Lean RE (eds): Craniosynostosis – Diagnosis, Evaluation, and Management. New York, Oxford University Press, 2000, pp 374–376.

11 Johnson D, Horsley SW, Moloney DM, Oldridge M, Twigg SR, et al: A comprehensive screen for *TWIST* mutations in patients with craniosynostosis identifies a new microdeletion syndrome of chromosome band 7p21.1. Am J Hum Genet 1998;63:1283–1293.

12 Trusen A, Beissert M, Collmann H, Darge K: The pattern of skeletal anomalies in the cervical spine, hands and feet in patients with Saethre-Chotzen syndrome and Muenke-type mutation. Pediatr Radiol 2003;33:168–172.

13 Sahlin P, Windh P, Lauritzen C, Emanuelsson M, Grönberg H, Stenman G: Women wih Saethre-Chotzen syndrome are at increased risk of breast cancer. Genes Chromosomes Cancer 2007;46:656–660.

14 James PA, Culling B, Mullan G, Jenkins M, Elakis G, et al: Breast cancer risk is not increased in individuals with *TWIST1* mutation confirmed Saethre-Chotzen syndrome: an Australian multicenter study. Genes Chromosomes Cancer 2009;48:533–538.

15 Brueton LA, van Herwerden L, Chotai KA, Winter RM: The mapping of a gene for craniosynostosis: evidence for linkage of the Saethre-Chotzen syndrome to distal chromosome 7p. J Med Genet 1992;29:681–685.
16 Germanguz I, Lev D, Waisman T, Kim CH, Gitelman I: Four *twist* genes in zebrafish, four expression patterns. Dev Dyn 2007;236:2615–2626.
17 Yang J, Mani SA, Donaher JL, Ramaswamy S, Itzykson RA, et al: Twist, a master regulator of morphogenesis, plays an essential role in tumor metastasis. Cell 2004;117:927–939.
18 Castanon I, Baylies MK: A Twist in fate: evolutionary comparison of Twist structure and function. Gene 2002;287:11–22.
19 Cai J, Jabs EW: A twisted hand: bHLH protein phosphorylation and dimerization regulate limb development. BioEssays 2005;27:1102–1106.
20 Bialek P, Kern B, Yang X, Schrock M, Sosic D, et al: A twist code determines the onset of osteoblast differentiation. Dev Cell 2004;6:423–435.
21 Bourgeois P, Bolcato-Bellemin A-L, Danse J-M, Bloch-Zupan A, Yoshiba K, et al: The variable expressivity and incomplete penetrance of the twist-null heterozygous mouse phenotype resemble those of human Saethre-Chotzen syndrome. Hum Mol Genet 1998;7:945–949.

Wolfram Kress, PhD, MD
Institute of Human Genetics, Julius-Maximilians University
Biozentrum, Am Hubland
97074 Würzburg (Germany)
Tel. +49 931 318 4062, Fax +49 391 318 4069, E-Mail wkress@biozentrum.uni-wuerzburg.de

Muenke M, Kress W, Collmann H, Solomon BD (eds): Craniosynostoses: Molecular Genetics, Principles of Diagnosis, and Treatment.
Monogr Hum Genet. Basel, Karger, 2011, vol 19, pp 107–118

Craniofrontonasal Syndrome: Molecular Genetics, *EFNB1* Mutations and the Concept of Cellular Interference

I. Wieland

Institute of Human Genetics, University Clinic, Otto-von-Guericke-University, Magdeburg, Germany

Abstract

Craniofrontonasal syndrome (CFNS) is a multiple congenital anomaly syndrome mainly characterized by hypertelorism, a broad or bifid nasal tip, coronal suture synostosis, corpus callosum hypoplasia or agenesis, and developmental delay but without severe mental deficiency. In some patients, cleft lip and palate and a wide spectrum of additional extracranial heterogeneous features have also been described. The pattern of inheritance for this malformation syndrome is quite unusual since females are more severely affected than males. CFNS is caused by heterozygous mutations or deletions in the ephrin-B1 encoding gene *EFNB1* located at Xq12/13. The transmembrane protein ephrin-B1 is a regulator of cell-cell communication involved in diverse cellular functions such as axon guidance, and cell sorting and migration, which best explains the peculiar appearance of CFNS as reflecting false cellular behavior, particularly of cells derived from the neural crest. To date, 129 *EFNB1* mutations including 87 distinct missense, frameshift, nonsense and splice site mutations, as well as 8 gene deletions, have been reported in sporadic and familial patients with a typical phenotype. Among 24 informative parent-offspring trios, 21 (88%) germline mutations were paternally derived. Most mutations disrupt *EFNB1* gene function; however, genotype-phenotype analyses demonstrated a highly variable expressivity independent of both the mutation type, and whether there was a familial or sporadic occurrence. This highly variable expressivity together with the more severe manifestation of CFNS in females than in males provoked the formulation of a novel pathological mechanism: the concept of cellular interference. This concept proposes divergent cellular behavior in heterozygous females as a consequence of random X inactivation of wildtype and mutant *EFNB1* carrying X chromosomes.

Craniofrontonasal syndrome (CFNS [OMIM 304110]) is a subgroup of frontonasal dysplasia first described by Cohen [1]. The condition was simultaneously recognized as frontonasal dysplasia with coronal craniosynostosis [2]. CFNS is an X-linked developmental malformation syndrome with a peculiar inheritance since females are more severely affected than males [3]. CFNS occurs sporadically or in families and is caused by heterozygous mutations in the *EFNB1* gene (OMIM 300035) on chromosome Xq12/13 in the majority of patients [4, 5].

Clinical Features

Patients display a high phenotypic variability; hence, affected individuals show some but not all characteristic features of CFNS [6, 7]. Phenotypic features typically reported in CFNS

Table 1. Clinical features of CFNS

Frequency	Head and neck	Brain and development	Chest, abdomen, genitourinary system	Limbs, nails, and hair
> 50%	Hypertelorism, broad or bifid nasal tip, brachycephaly, coronal suture synostosis, frontal bossing, facial asymmetry, high-arched palate	Normal mental development, strabismus		
10 – 50%	Short neck, webbed neck	Developmental delay, corpus callosum hypoplasia or agenesis	Sprengel anomaly, scoliosis, asymmetric chest, unilateral breast hypoplasia	Asymmetric limbs, cutaneous syndactyly, clinodactyly of the 5th finger, polydactyly, grooved nails, thick and wiry hair, low anterior hair line, widow's peak
Occasionally	Cleft lip and/or palate, cranium bifidum occultum	Sensorineural hearing loss, cerebellar dysplasia, mild learning difficulties	Asymmetry of pectoral muscles, axillary pterygium, diaphragmatic hernia, umbilical hernia, bicornuate uterus, duplication of kidney and uterus	Broad hallux, joint laxity

are summarized in table 1. In a previous review, the frequencies of symptoms were described in more detail based on several studies with and without molecular testing of the underlying *EFNB1* gene defect [8]. The frequencies of clinical features, however, may vary in different study cohorts depending on the selection criteria of patients (such as the prevalence of patients with craniosynostosis and whether or not there is a female bias) and the specifics of the clinical evaluations, such as the use of in-depth diagnostic measurements (e.g. brain magnetic resonance imaging [MRI]).

Craniofacial Symptoms

CFNS is characterized by hypertelorism, the most common dysmorphic feature observed in nearly all affected females and males. Coronal suture synostosis and craniofacial and orbital asymmetry are detected frequently in females but rarely in males. Craniofacial midline defects commonly include a broad or bifid nasal tip, a high-arched palate, and occasionally cleft lip and/or palate and cranium bifidum occultum (fig. 1). Frontonasal dysplasia (FND [OMIM 136760]) has been described as a very heterogeneous group of malformations. Apart from CFNS, causative mutations have been identified only in the aristaless-related ALX homeobox 3 gene *ALX3* [9]. Because of the distinct facial appearance, Twigg et al. [9] proposed frontorhiny for this type of FND. Although there exists clinical overlap with CFNS, craniosynostosis does not

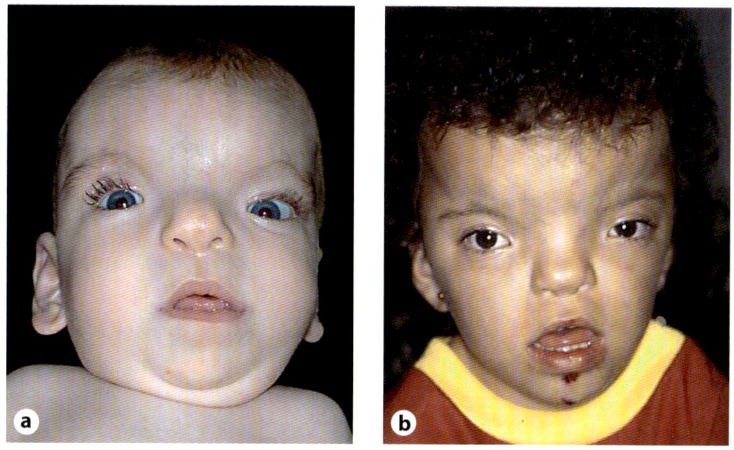

Fig. 1. Facial features of CFNS patients in **a** infancy and **b** childhood. Typical features include hypertelorism, down-slanting palpebral fissures, a broad nasal root, a hypoplastic nasal tip, and a prominent forehead. Facial asymmetry to varying degree is partly due to asymmetric coronal craniosynostosis. Photos courtesy of H. Collmann.

appear to be included in the spectrum of symptoms in frontorhiny. Frontorhiny is inherited in a recessive manner; in fact, all seven *ALX3* mutations identified were found in the homozygous state in children of consanguineous or possibly distant consanguineous parents.

Brain and Psychomotor Developmental Aspects
The most frequent brain abnormality in CFNS manifests as hypoplasia or partial and complete agenesis of the corpus callosum. In a few patients, cerebellar dysplasia and sensorineural hearing loss were diagnosed. Strabismus is a common finding in female patients, and may be partly due to severe hypertelorism. Psychomotor developmental delay was recognized in some patients, but learning disabilities appear to be rather infrequent [5, 10–12]. The majority of patients, including both females and males, demonstrate normal mental performance.

Extracranial Features
Extracranial manifestations of CFNS include body asymmetry, midline defects, and skeletal and dermatological abnormalities, as described in table 1. No major features may be delineated in this category because of the wide spectrum of symptoms and highly variable expressivity. Repeatedly, duplications of the uterus, kidneys, and ureters have been reported. Additionally, either one or a combination of several of the following features may be present in affected individuals: Sprengel anomaly, abnormal clavicles and thorax, scoliosis, pre- and postaxial polydactyly, mild cutaneous syndactyly, clinodactyly of the fifth finger, lower-limb asymmetry, as well as longitudinally grooved nails, and thick wiry hair with a widow's peak, among some from the long list of features described in CFNS patients. Rarely detected manifestations include umbilical and diaphragmatic hernia, sacrococcygeal teratoma, and joint laxity.

Pattern of Inheritance

X-linked Inheritance and Variable Expressivity
CFNS is an X-linked condition, as no instances of male-to-male transmission were reported in pedigrees comprising 3–5 generations, and all daughters of obligate carrier males were affected [3, 6, 11]. In these families, highly variable expressivity of disease symptoms was observed in affected females. Variable expressivity supports X-linked inheritance and a random pattern of

X-inactivation [13]. The latter finding has been demonstrated in patient blood lymphocytes and primary fibroblast cultures by the so-called HUMAR assay [14]. This assay uses the androgen receptor gene that contains a highly polymorphic CAG repeat. Methylation of sensitive *Hpa*II and *Hha*I restriction enzyme sites less than 100 bp flanking the repeat correlates with inactivation of the respective X chromosome in females [15].

CFNS Is a Genetic Paradox

Unlike classical X-linked diseases, CFNS shows a paradoxical inheritance pattern because female patients are severely affected, whereas obligate male carriers are usually mildly affected, often demonstrating only hypertelorism and occasionally cleft lip and/or palate. This peculiar inheritance of CFNS in females versus males led to the proposal of several genetic explanations, with Johnson's metabolic interference theory among the most favored [3, 11]. Johnson [16] proposed that some disorders may only develop in heterozygotes as a consequence of adverse interactions of 2 alleles, rather than a mutant allele acting alone. Such a mechanism results neither in a dominant nor in a recessive inheritance pattern. After detecting the disease-causing gene *EFNB1*, cellular interference (discussed in more detail below) modeled on Johnson's theory was proposed as the main mechanism responsible for disease manifestation in CFNS females [4].

The CFNS Causing Gene *EFNB1*

The major causative gene locus for CFNS was mapped to the pericentromeric region of the X chromosome by haplotype and linkage analysis in a large, 5-generation German family [17]. This localization replaced an earlier proposed mapping interval on Xp22 that has not been confirmed by other research groups [11]. Using a combination of a positional approach and candidate gene strategy, *EFNB1* was believed to be the most promising candidate because Compagni et al. [18] reported targeted inactivation of the mouse homolog *Efnb1* to be associated with a CFNS-like inheritance and phenotype in mice. The *EFNB1* gene is located on the X chromosome at the border region between Xq12 and Xq13, and is subject to random X-inactivation in females [19]. The gene consists of 5 exons spanning approximately 13 kb. Mutations in *EFNB1* were independently identified by 2 research groups [4, 5]. Wieland et al. [4] detected 3 different germline mutations including an intragenic deletion of exons 2–5 and 2 distinct missense mutations in exon 2 of *EFNB1* in 3 unrelated families with CFNS. Twigg et al. [5] described 17 distinct *EFNB1* mutations in 5 unrelated familial and 15 sporadic patients with clinical diagnosis of CFNS. Since then, *EFNB1* mutations have been reported in more than 100 patients with familial or sporadic CFNS.

Ephrin Ligands and Eph Receptors

Ephrins and their receptors control cell-cell communication in diverse cell types and tissues during development and body maintenance. *EFNB1* encodes the transmembrane protein ephrin-B1, which is one of the 8 known ephrin ligands. Ephrin ligands preferentially interact with their cognate Eph receptor tyrosine kinases expressed on opposing cellular compartments. However, Eph receptors show relaxed binding specificity with several ephrin-ligands and vice-versa, hence, Eph/ephrin engagement has been viewed as promiscuous [20–22]. A special property of the Eph/ephrin interaction is bi-directional signaling upon cell-cell contact (fig. 2). Receptor-ligand dimerization and higher-order clustering are essential for activation of the receptor downstream signaling cascade (forward signaling) in the Eph-expressing cell. The reverse signal is transduced into the ephrin-expressing cell (reverse signaling). Forward signaling activates the receptor tyrosine kinase and may proceed

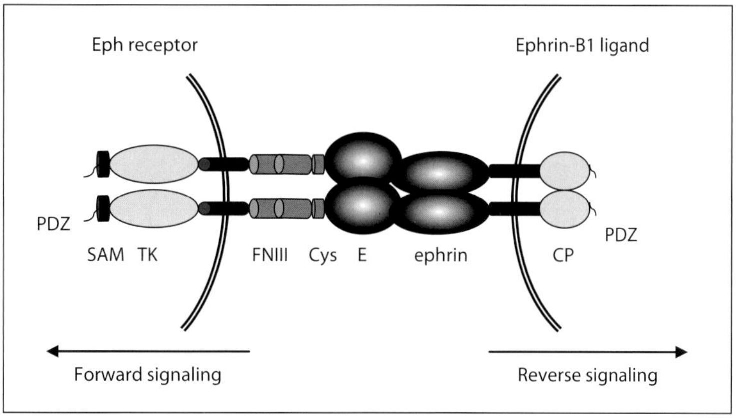

Fig. 2. Bi-directional signaling in the Eph receptor/ephrin system. The domain structure of Eph receptors is depicted by the globular ephrin-binding domain (E), a cystein-rich region (Cys) and two fibronectin III repeats (FNIII) on the extracellular side. The cytoplasmic domains are the tyrosine kinase (TK), a sterile alpha motif (SAM), and the postsynaptic density, disc-large, zona occludens-1 (PDZ) motif. The cognate Eph receptor interacts with the ephrin domain of ephrin-B1 which contains a PDZ domain at the cytoplasmic tail (CP). Contact of Eph receptor-expressing and ephrin-B1 ligand-expressing cells leads to receptor-ligand dimerization and higher-order clustering that is a prerequisite for forward signaling in the Eph receptor-expressing cell and reverse signaling in the ephrin-B1 ligand-expressing cell.

through different pathways leading mostly to cell repulsion, while reverse signaling activates src kinases and subsequent downstream signaling pathways and also seems to affect cell-cell communication through gap junctions [23–29]. In addition, there is evidence for crosstalk to non-Eph/ephrin signaling molecules for both signaling directions, with the receptor and ligand acting independently of each other [28, 30–33]. This highly complex Eph/ephrin system plays guiding roles in cell sorting and migration involved in pattern formation during neural development and tissue morphogenesis. During development of the skull, *EFNB1* appears to be involved in precisely defining the position of the coronal suture at the neural crest/mesoderm tissue boundary, and in prevention of premature fusion of the coronal suture separating the frontal from parietal bones [34–37].

EFNB1 Mutation Spectrum

Germline mutations in *EFNB1* have been described in 129 unrelated patients with familial and sporadic CFNS (fig. 3). Of these, 127 patients were enrolled in 3 larger, clinically well-characterized study cohorts (table 2). Germline mutations in the *EFNB1* gene were responsible for about 80% [5, 12, 38–41] and 50% [42] of CFNS patients. The reason for the difference in the study of Wallis et al. [42] is currently not known. In total, *EFNB1* mutations were detected in 42 (33%) families and 85 (67%) sporadic CFNS patients, indicating a high incidence of de novo mutations (table 2). This has been molecularly proven in 22 families, each consisting of an affected female heterozygous for an *EFNB1* mutation and unaffected parents [5, 12, 25]. Most *EFNB1* mutations are point mutations, small deletions and

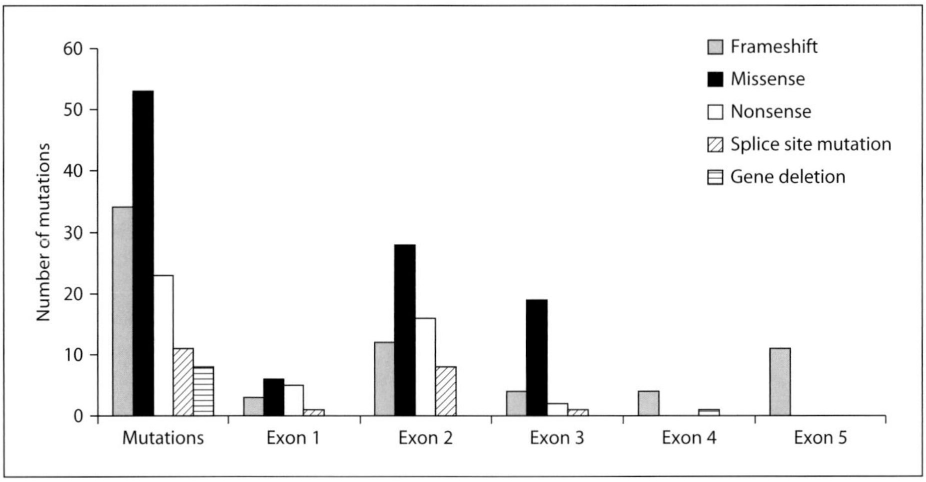

Fig. 3. *EFNB1* mutation spectrum. *EFNB1* mutations have been detected in a total of 129 unrelated patients with sporadic and familial CFNS.

Table 2. Familial versus sporadic occurrence of *EFNB1* mutations in CFNS

	Twigg et al., 2004, 2006	Wieland et al., 2004, 2005, 2007	Wallis et al., 2008	Total
Familial	19	14	9	42 (33%)
Sporadic	40[a]	35[a]	10	85 (67%)

[a]Molecularly proven de novo mutations in 9/40 and 11/35 individuals, respectively.

insertions of single to few nucleotides (94%), whereas partial or complete *EFNB1* gene deletions are less frequent (6%). In the 129 patients, 87 distinct small *EFNB1* mutations have been described, indicating a predominance of private mutations (table 3). Recurrent mutations occurring in more than 3 unrelated patients were missense mutations at amino acid positions p.P54 (p.P54L), p.P119 (p.P119S, p.P119T, p.P119A, p.P119H), and p.G151 (p.G151S, p.G151V, p.G151D), as well as the nonsense mutation p.R66X and splice site mutations at the splice junction of exons 2 and 3. Missense mutations constitute 41% of all mutations, and all of them were detected in exons 1–3, which encode the extracellular domain of ephrin-B1. They substitute highly conserved amino-acid residues important for receptor-ligand interaction and appear to compromise signaling [43]. Nonsense, frameshift, and splice site mutations account for up to 53% of *EFNB1* mutations. They result in premature termination codons (PTCs) either by directly introducing a stop codon or because of aberrant splicing events and changing of the reading frame. PTCs elicit nonsense-mediated mRNA decay (NMD) when occurring in internal exons of *EFNB1* [14]. NMD is a general surveillance mechanism to eliminate aberrant transcripts resulting from incorrect RNA processing [44]. By this mechanism, the synthesis of truncated ephrin-B1 polypeptides exhibiting dominant-

Table 3. Summary of *EFNB1* mutations

EFNB1 mutations	Twigg et al., 2004, 2006	Wieland et al., 2004, 2005, 2007	Wallis et al., 2008	Shotelersuk et al., 2006	Torii et al., 2007	Babbs, 2009	Total
Small mutation	56	45	18	1	1	–	121 (94%)
Gene deletion	3[a]	4[b]	1	–	–	–	8 (6%)
Gene duplication	–	–	–	–	–	1[c]	

[a]Including 1/3 contiguous gene deletions.
[b]Including 3/4 contiguous gene deletions.
[c]Duplication including neighboring genes in a family with Teebi type hypertelorism.

negative functions is prevented. Therefore, these PTC generating *EFNB1* mutations are functionally null mutations. Interestingly, only frameshift mutations were detected in exons 4 and 5 of *EFNB1* encoding the juxtamembrane segment, the transmembrane domain and the highly conserved cytoplasmic tail of ephrin-B1. They may escape NMD, but seem to be incompatible with a stable protein [45]. The clinical phenotypes of the patients harboring small *EFNB1* mutations were not highly suggestive of a genotype-phenotype correlation, although diaphragmatic hernia was diagnosed in 2 females harboring putative truncating ephrin-B1 mutations in exons 4 and 5.

In 3 of the 8 patients, heterozygous *EFNB1* gene deletion was recognized as part of a contiguous gene deletion involving neighboring genes [41]. The estimated deletion sizes were on the order of 0.5 to 1.6 Mb, and included the START domain-containing 8 gene (*STARD8* [OMIM 300689]) in all 3 patients, the oligophrenin-1 gene (*OPHN1* [OMIM 300127]) and praja 1 gene (*PJA1* [OMIM 300420]) in 2 patients and, additionally, the gene encoding ectodysplasin A (*EDA* [OMIM 300451]) in 1 patient (fig. 4). Comparison of the clinical features of patients with partial or complete *EFNB1* gene deletions with those harboring intragenic small mutations revealed no consistent phenotypic differences. However, possible differences such as ventricular enlargement may be attributable to heterozygous deletion of additional genes in a patient with contiguous gene deletion [41]. More recently, an *EFNB1* gene duplication including neighboring genes was identified in a family with Teebi-type hypertelorism [46].

Paternal Origin of Germline EFNB1 Mutations
Our laboratory previously identified an affected mother who transmitted the missense mutation p.P27R to 2 of her children [38]. To investigate the parental origin of this germline mutation, haplotype analysis encompassing the *EFNB1* gene of all available family members was performed. This revealed segregation of the disease, with the haplotype of the maternal grandfather demonstrating that the mutation arose in the paternally inherited *EFNB1* gene. Subsequently, Twigg and coworkers [12] analyzed the parental origin of 20 de novo intragenic and 3 deletion germline mutations by using highly polymorphic microsatellite markers and single nucleotide polymorphisms (SNPs) within the *EFNB1* gene that could be used to trace the parental origin of the germline mutation. Among 17 informative families identified in this analysis, 15 heterozygous mutations (88%) arose from the father. We observed 6 of 7 de novo germline mutations occurring in the paternally derived *EFNB1* gene, which constituted

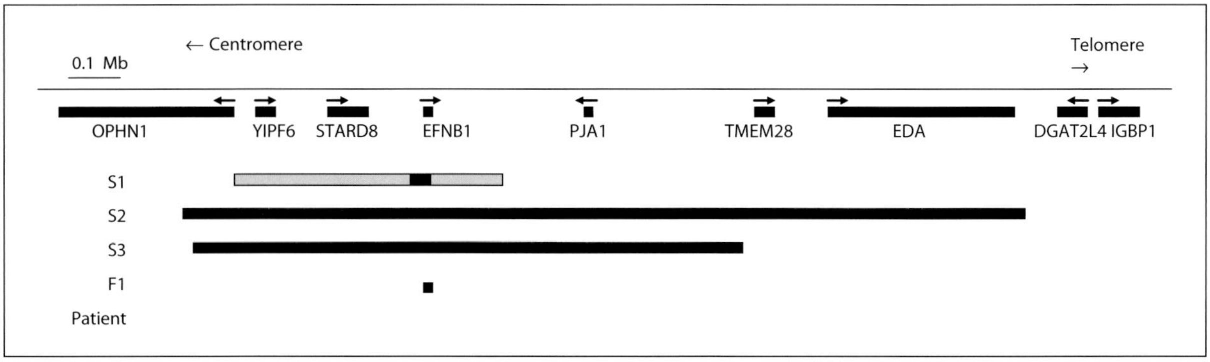

Fig. 4. Schematic illustration of *EFNB1* and contiguous gene deletions in CFNS patients. *EFNB1* neighboring genes are indicated on a scale oriented with respect to the chromosomal centromere and telomere. Arrows above each gene symbol indicate the direction of gene transcription. The minimal region of deletion detected in 3 sporadic (S1–S3) and 1 familial (F1) CFNS patient is shown by black bars.

4 intragenic small *EFNB1* mutations and 3 gene deletions [41, unpublished results]. In contrast to other craniosynostosis-associated mutations (i.e. in *FGFR2*), no significant paternal-age effect has been recognized [47]. The predominance of paternally arising germline *EFNB1* mutations has also been used as an explanation why males are apparently underrepresented in CFNS pedigrees, which frequently comprise just 2 generations of a mother and her offspring. It has been proposed that the paternal origin of de novo germline *EFNB1* mutations affects only the daughters in the next generation, who experience lower reproductive fitness. This agrees well with the observation that molecularly proven CFNS has been diagnosed twice as often in sporadic female patients than in CFNS families.

In contrast to the prevalence of paternally derived germline mutations, postzygotic *EFNB1* mutations as reflected by somatic mosaicism were preferentially observed (5/6) in female carriers [12]. This has been established by quantification of *EFNB1* mutations in DNA from blood, hair roots, and buccal swaps. However, the level of mosaicism in any of the tissues analyzed was poorly correlated with clinical features of the probands, which aids neither in disease identification nor prognostic correlations, but may help to estimate sibling recurrence risk for genetic counseling.

Sex-Dependent Manifestation and Proposed Pathomechanism in CFNS

CFNS in Male Carriers

Hemizygous *EFNB1* carrier males show milder and fewer malformations compared to heterozygous females (the genetic paradox). Clinical features in males frequently include hypertelorism and occasionally craniofacial anomalies like a high-arched palate, cleft lip and/or palate, and a bifid nasal tip [6, 7, 42]. Additional CFNS features are observed rarely and include congenital diaphragmatic hernia and sacrococcygeal teratoma [6, 48]. In hemizygous males, only a single cell population exists with regard to ephrin-B1, and there is no evidence for an ephrin homologous gene on the Y chromosome to compensate for an *EFNB1* mutation on the X chromosome. According to Johnson's theory, the mild manifestation of CFNS in males is due to the hemizygous state. In addition, ephrin-B1 deficiency may be compensated at discrete developmental stages by the promiscuity of ephrin receptors and their ligands, e.g. opposing Eph-receptor expressing cells will choose another ephrin ligand rather than the preferred ephrin-B1. However, not all effects of ephrin-B1 mediated forward and reverse signaling seem to be compensated by this mechanism, as exemplified by the high frequency of hypertelorism in hemizygous males.

The Concept of Cellular Interference

The severe manifestations of CFNS in heterozygous females have been explained as being a consequence of the random X-inactivation of wildtype and mutant *EFNB1*-carrying X chromosomes [4, 13]. This random X-inactivation results in a cellular mosaic consisting of 2 cell populations regarding ephrin-B1 expression: cells expressing the wildtype ephrin-B1 and cells that are deficient for functional ephrin-B1 (fig. 5). Clonal expansions from primary fibroblasts of a heterozygous female demonstrated that it is possible to separate the wildtype and mutant phenotypes in cell culture [14]. Since loss-of-function of the *EFNB1* gene rather than intragenic dominant-negative mutations per se are the most likely cause of CFNS, bi-directional signaling will only be driven by ephrin-B1-expressing cells upon cell-cell contact with opposing Eph receptor-expressing cells. In the mosaic females, mutant cells will interfere with the function of wildtype cell populations causing cellular interference. Presumably, this will lead to divergent cell sorting and migration, ultimately resulting in indistinct tissue border definition and premature fusion of the coronal suture [36]. Experimental support for such a pathogenic mechanism is derived from *Efnb1*-knock-out mice and in vitro studies with zebrafish embryos showing that extensive cell intermingling occurred in ephrin-B1-deficient cellular compartments [34, 36, 49, 50]. In heterozygous *Efnb1*-knock-out mice, divergent cell populations apparently lead to cell sorting defects at chondrogenic condensations, resulting in segmentation defects of the axial and appendicular skeleton and in defects of neural crest cell migration responsible for craniofacial development [18, 51, 28].

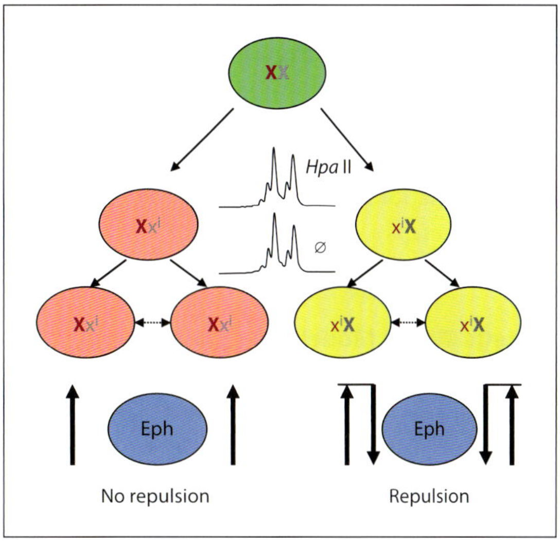

Fig. 5. The model of cellular interference. In heterozygous CFNS females, one of the X chromosomes carries a mutant *EFNB1* gene (shown in red) and the other the wildtype homolog (shown in gray). During early cleavage divisions of the zygote (green), one of the X chromosomes becomes randomly heterochromatic for reasons of dosage compensation in mammals. This X inactivation functionally silences most of the genes and once established, it is transmitted from one cell to all the daughter cells. In CFNS females, we observe random X inactivation of either the X chromosome harboring the wildtype (pink cells) or mutant (yellow cells) *EFNB1* gene (shown by the insets from the HUMAR assay). Cells with the mutant *EFNB1* gene on their active X chromosome (pink cells) will not display functional ephrin-B1 on their cell surface. These cells are not capable of ephrin-B1-mediated bi-directional signaling upon encounter with Eph receptor expressing cells (blue cells). In contrast, cells expressing wildtype ephrin-B1 (yellow cells) will be able to mediate bi-directional signaling resulting in cell repulsion. This cellular interference of mutant and wildtype ephrin-B1-expressing cells has been proposed to perturb cell-cell communication and the formation of distinct tissue borders.

The concept of cellular interference appears not to be unique to CFNS. Epilepsy and mental retardation limited to females (EFMR, OMIM 300088) is an X-linked disorder that affects females, while male carriers are unaffected. EFMR is caused by heterozygous mutations in the *PCDH19* gene encoding the cell-cell adhesion molecule protocadherin 19 [52]. As in CFNS, somatic mosaicism for *PCDH19* may cause cellular interference leading to malformations in the brain and to the development of epilepsy [52, 53].

Genetic Mouse Models for CFNS

Targeted inactivation of the X-linked ephrin-B1 gene in a mouse model was first reported by Compagni et al. (2003), who observed an unusual severity of phenotype in heterozygous mutant female mice, reminiscent of findings described in human CFNS patients [18]. A high percentage of hemizygous males and heterozygous females died prenatally, some also postnatally, apparently due to multiple defects including incomplete body wall closure, cleft palate, and shortening of the skull. Surviving ephrin-B1 mutant mice displayed skeletal abnormalities, in particular asymmetric arrangement of sternocostal connections and fused sternae. Preaxial polydactyly was exclusively seen in heterozygous female mice, which was attributed to mosaic expression of wildtype and mutant ephrin-B1 in heterozygous animals. Subsequently, Davy et al. (2004) reasoned that the high percentage of cleft palate in ephrin-B1-deficient animals could be due to deficiencies of neural crest cells in the regulation of craniofacial development [51]. Conditional ablation of ephrin-B1 from neural crest cells demonstrated that ephrin-B1 acts autonomously and controls neural crest cell migration. The presence of coronal craniosynostosis was not reported in any of the ephrin-B1 deficient mice. Unfortunately, it is not clear whether this reflects the difficulties in diagnosing the phenotype in the mouse, or whether it is a rare event in this species, as has been demonstrated in the genetic mouse model for the Muenke craniosynostosis syndrome [54].

Acknowledgements

The author thanks colleagues, clinicians and patients and their families for their participation, contribution of information and support, and apologizes to all colleagues whose work was not cited due to the conciseness of this monograph.

References

1 Cohen MM Jr: Craniofrontonasal dysplasia. Birth Defects Orig Art Ser 1979;15: 85–89.
2 Slover R, Sujansky E: Frontonasal dysplasia with coronal craniosynostosis in three sibs. Birth Defects Orig Art Ser 1979;15:75–83.
3 Rollnick B, Day D, Tissot R, Kaye C: A pedigree possible evidence for the metabolic interference hypothesis. Am J Hum Genet 1981;33:823–826.
4 Wieland I, Jakubiczka S, Muschke P, Cohen M, Thiele H, et al: Mutations of the ephrin-B1 gene cause craniofrontonasal syndrome. Am J Hum Genet 2004; 74:1209–1215.
5 Twigg SRF, Kan R, Babbs C, Bochukova EG, Robertson SP, et al: Mutations of ephrin-B1 (*EFNB1*), a marker of tissue boundary formation, cause craniofrontonasal syndrome. Proc Natl Acad Sci USA 2004;101:8652–8657.
6 Morris CA, Palumbos JC, Carey JC: Delineation of the male phenotype in craniofrontonasal syndrome. Am J Med Genet 1987;27:623–631.
7 Kere J, Ritvanen A, Martinnen E, Kaitila I: Craniofrontonasal dysostosis: variable expression in a three-generation family. Clin Genet 1990;38:441–446.
8 Wieacker P, Wieland I: Clinical and genetic aspects of craniofrontonasal syndrome: Towards resolving a genetic paradox. Mol Gen Metabol 2005;86:110–116.
9 Twigg SRF, Versnel SL, Nürnberg G, Lees MM, Bhat M, et al: Frontorhiny, a distinctive presentation of frontonasal dysplasia caused by recessive mutations in the *ALX3* homeobox gene. Am J Hum Genet 2009;84:698–705.
10 Saavedra D, Richieri-Costa A, Guion-Almeida ML, Cohen MM: Craniofrontonasal syndrome: Study of 41 patients. Am J Med Genet 1996;61:147–151.
11 Feldman GJ, Ward DE, Lajeunie-Renier E, Saavedra D, Robin NH, et al: A novel phenotypic pattern in X-linked inheritance: Craniofrontonasal syndrome maps to Xp22. Hum Mol Genet 1997;6: 1937–1941.

12 Twigg SRF, Matsumoto K, Kidd AMJ, Goriely A, Taylor IB, et al: The origin of *EFNB1* mutations in craniofrontonasal syndrome: frequent mosaicism and explanation of the paucity of carrier males. Am J Hum Genet 2006;78:999–1010.

13 Migeon BR: Females are mosaics: X inactivation and sex differences in disease. (Oxford University Press, Oxford/New York 2007).

14 Wieland I, Makarov R, Reardon W, Tinschert S, Goldenberg A, Thierry P, Wieacker P: Dissecting the molecular mechanisms in craniofrontonasal syndrome: differential mRNA expression of mutant *EFNB1* and the cellular mosaic. Eur J Hum Genet 2008;16:184–191.

15 Allen RC, Zoghbi HY, Moseley AB, Rosenblatt HM, Belmont JW: Methylation of *Hpa*II and *Hha*I sites near the polymorphic CAG repeat in the human androgen-receptor gene correlates with X chromosome inactivation. Am J Hum Genet 1992;51:1229–1239.

16 Johnson WG: Metabolic interference and +– heterozygote: a hypothetical form of simple inheritance which is neither dominant nor recessive. Am J Hum Genet 1980;32:374–386.

17 Wieland I, Jakubiczka S, Muschke P, Wolf A, Gerlach L, Krawczak M, Wieacker P: Mapping of a further locus for X-linked craniofrontonasal syndrome. Cytogenet Genome Res 2002;99: 285–288.

18 Compagni A, Logan M, Klein R, Adams R: Control of skeletal patterning by ephrinB1-EphB interactions. Dev Cell 2003;5:217–230.

19 Carrel L, Willard HF: X-inactivation profile reveals extensive variability in X-linked gene expression in females. Nature 2005;434:400–404.

20 Klein R: Eph/ephrin signaling in morphogenesis, neural development and plasticity. Curr Opin Cell Biol 2004;16: 580–589.

21 Pasquale EB: Eph receptor signalling casts a wide net on cell behaviour. Nat Rev Mol Cell Biol 2005;6:462–475.

22 Poliakov A, Cotrina M, Wilkinson DG: Diverse roles of Eph receptors and ephrins in the regulation of cell migration and tissue assembly. Dev Cell 2004;7: 465–480.

23 Kalo MS, Yu H-H, Pasquale EB: In vivo tyrosine phosphorylation sites of activated ephrin-B1 and EphB2 from neural tissue. J Biol Chem 2001;276:38940–38948.

24 Lu Q, Sun EE, Klein RS, Flanagan JG: Ephrin-b reverse signaling is mediated by a novel PDZ-RGS protein and selectively inhibits G protein-coupled chemoattraction. Cell 2001;105:69–79.

25 Cowan CA, Henkemeyer M: The SH2/SH3 adaptor Grb4 transduces B-ephrin reverse signals. Nature 2001;413:174–179.

26 Zimmer M, Palmer A, Köhler J, Klein R: EphB-ephrinB bi-directional endocytosis terminates adhesion allowing contact mediated repulsion. Nat Cell Biol 2003;5: 869–878.

27 Marston DJ, Dickinson S, Nobes CD: Rac-dependent trans-endocytosis of ephrinBs regulates Eph-ephrin contact repulsion. Nat Cell Biol 2003;5:879–888.

28 Davy A, Bush JO, Soriano P: Inhibition of gap junction communication at ectopic Eph/ephrin boundaries underlies craniofrontonasal syndrome. Plos Biol 2006;4:e315.

29 Bong Y-S, Lee H-S, Carim-Todd L, Mood K, Nishanian TG, Tessarollo L, Daar IO: EphrinB1 signals from the cell surface to the nucleus by recruitment of STAT3. Proc Natl Acad Sci USA 2007;104: 17305–17310.

30 Dalva MB, Takasu MA, Lin MZ, Shamah SM, Hu L, Gale NW, Greenberg ME: EphB receptors interact with NMDA receptors and regulate excitatory synapse formation. Cell 2000;103:945–956.

31 Tanaka M, Kamata R, Sakai R: Phosphorylation of ephrin-B1 via the interaction with claudin following cell-cell contact formation. EMBO J 2005;24:3700–3711.

32 Schmitt AM, Shi J, Wolf AM, Lu CC, King LA, Zou Y: Wnt-Ryk signalling mediates medial-lateral retinotectal topographic mapping. Nature 2006;439:31–37.

33 Lee HS, Nishanian TG, Mood K, Bong YS, Daar IO: EphrinB1 controls cell-cell junctions through the Par polarity complex. Nat Cell Biol 2008;10:979–986.

34 Morriss-Kay GM, Wilkie AOM: Growth of the normal skull vault and its alteration in craniosynostosis: insights from human genetics and experimental studies. J Anat 2005;207:637–653.

35 Mundy GR, Elefteriou F: Boning up on ephrin signaling. Cell 2006;126:441–443.

36 Merril AE, Bochukova EG, Brugger SM, Ishii M, Pilz DT, et al: Cell mixing at a neural crest – mesoderm boundary and deficient ephrin-Eph signaling in the pathogenesis of craniosynostosis. Hum Mol Gen 2006;15:1319–1328.

37 Edwards CM, Mundy GR: Eph receptors and ephrin signaling pathways: a role in bone homeostasis. Int J Med Sci 2008;5: 263–272.

38 Wieland I, Reardon W, Jakubiczka S, Franco B, Kress W, et al: Twenty-six novel *EFNB1* mutations in familial and sporadic craniofrontonasal syndrome (CFNS). Hum Mut 2005;26:113–118.

39 Shotelersuk V, Siriwan P, Ausavarat S: A novel mutation in EFNB1, probably with a dominant negative effect, underlying craniofrontonasal syndrome. Cleft Palate Craniofac J 2006;43:152–154.

40 Torii C, Izumi K, Nakajima H, Takahashi T, Kosaki K: EFNB1 mutation at the ephrin ligand-receptor dimerization interface in a patient with craniofrontonasal syndrome. Congenit Anom (Kyoto) 2007;47:49–52.

41 Wieland I, Weidner C, Ciccone R, Lapi E, McDonald-McGinn D, et al: Contiguous gene deletions involving *EFNB1*, *OPHN1*, *PJA1* and *EDA* in patients with craniofrontonasal syndrome. Clin Genet 2007;72:506–516.

42 Wallis D, Lacbawan F, Jain M, Der Kaloustian VM, Steiner CE, et al: Additional *EFNB1* mutations in craniofrontonasal syndrome. Am J Med Genet 2008;146:2008–2012.

43 Nikolov DB, Li C, Barton WA, Himanen J-P: Crystal structure of the ephrin-B1 ectodomain: Implications for receptor recognition and signaling. Biochemistry 2005;44:10947–10953.

44 Maquat LE: Nonsense-mediated mRNA decay: Splicing, translation and mRNA dynamics. Nat Rev Mol Cell Biol 2004;5: 89–99.

45 Makarov R, Steiner B, Preisler-Adams S, Rauch A, Wieacker P, Wieland I: Expression and functional analysis of EFNB1 mutations in craniofrontonasal syndrome. Eur Hum Genet Conf 2009; P02.168.

46 Babbs C, Stewart H, Williams L, Connell L, Goriely A, et al: Duplication of the *EFNB1* gene in familial hypertelorism: imbalance in ephrin-B1 expression and abnormal phenotypes in humans and mice. Eur Hum Genet Conf 2009;C04.6.

47 Moloney DM, Slaney SF, Oldridge M, Wall SA, Sahlin P, Stenman G, Wilkie AOM: Exclusive paternal origin of new mutations in Apert syndrome. Nat Genet 1996;13:48–53.
48 Vasudevan PC, Twigg SR, Mulliken JB, Cook JA, Quarrell OW, Wilkie AOM: Expanding the phenotype of craniofrontonasal syndrome: two unrelated boys with *EFNB1* mutations and congenital diaphragmatic hernia. Eur J Hum Genet 2006;14:887–888.
49 Xu Q, Mellitzer G, Robinson V, Wilkinson DG: In vivo cell sorting in complementary segmental domains mediated by Eph receptors and ephrins. Nature 1999;399:267–271.
50 Mellitzer G, Xu Q, Wilkinson DG: Eph receptors and ephrins restrict cell intermingling and communication. Nature 1999;400:77–81.
51 Davy A, Aubin J, Soriano P: Ephrin-B1 forward and reverse signaling are required during mouse development. Genes Dev 2004;18:572–583.
52 Dibbens LM, Tarpey PS, Hynes K, Bayly M, Scheffer IE, et al: X-linked protocadherin 19 mutations cause female-limited epilepsy and cognitive impairment. Nat Genet 2008;40:776–781.
53 Depienne C, Bouteiller D, Keren B, Cheuret E, Poirier K, et al: Sporadic infantile epileptic encephalopathy caused by mutations in PCDH19 resembles Dravet syndrome but mainly affects females. Plos Genet 2009;5:e1000381.
54 Twigg SRF, Healy C, Babbs C, Sharpe JA, Wood WG, et al: Skeletal analysis of the Fgfr3 (P244R) mouse, a genetic model for the Muenke craniosynostosis syndrome. Dev Dyn 2009;238:331–342.

Ilse Wieland
Institut für Humangenetik, Universitätsklinikum
Otto-von-Guericke-Universität
Leipziger Str. 44, 39210 Magdeburg (Germany)
Tel. +49 391 67 15381, Fax +49 391 67 15066, E-Mail ilse.wieland@med.ovgu.de

Muenke M, Kress W, Collmann H, Solomon BD (eds): Craniosynostoses: Molecular Genetics, Principles of Diagnosis, and Treatment. Monogr Hum Genet. Basel, Karger, 2011, vol 19, pp 119–142

Uncommon Craniosynostosis Syndromes: A Review of Thirteen Conditions

M.S. Raam[a,b] · M. Muenke[a]

[a]Medical Genetics Branch, National Human Genome Research Institute, National Institutes of Health, Bethesda, Md., [b]HHMI-NIH Research Scholars Program, Howard Hughes Medical Institute, Chevy Chase, Md., USA

Abstract

Uncommon craniosynostosis syndromes, while individually less well characterized than more common conditions such as Apert, Crouzon, Pfeiffer, Muenke, and Saethre-Chotzen syndromes, comprise a significant proportion of craniosynostosis cases when considered in sum. Thirteen of these rare syndromes are covered here with respect to nosology, associated clinical characteristics, and molecular genetics. They were selected for discussion in this chapter due to recent molecular advances therein that can significantly enhance clinicians' ability to diagnose and counsel patients with these syndromes. The syndromes discussed here include Antley-Bixler syndrome, Baller-Gerold syndrome, Beare-Stevenson cutis gyrata syndrome, Bohring-Opitz syndrome, C (Opitz trigonocephaly) syndrome, Carpenter syndrome, Crouzon syndrome with acanthosis nigricans, Jackson-Weiss syndrome, Jacobsen syndrome, Loeys-Dietz syndrome type I, osteoglophonic dysplasia, P450 oxidoreductase deficiency, and Shprintzen-Goldberg syndrome.

Syndromic craniosynostosis comprises approximately 15% of craniosynostosis cases, with well over 180 syndromes identified to date [1]. Although much attention is given to several well-characterized craniosynostosis syndromes, including Apert syndrome, Crouzon syndrome, Pfeiffer syndrome, Muenke syndrome, and Saethre-Chotzen syndrome (see individual chapters on each in this volume), the vast majority of craniosynostosis syndromes are less well characterized and/or individually involve a comparatively small number of patients (see partial list in table 1). Despite these aspects of uncommon craniosynostosis syndromes, they comprise a significant proportion of craniosynostosis cases when considered in aggregate [2]. Additionally, the clinical issues observed in some uncommon syndromes differ from those encountered in the major syndromes: mental retardation and perinatal death, for instance, are seen more often in several uncommon syndromes, shifting focus away from simple surgical correction and creating a greater emphasis on prenatal diagnosis, psychomotor development, and genetic counseling [2]. Perhaps most importantly, description and delineation of uncommon craniosynostosis syndromes allow clinicians to better treat and counsel the significant numbers of families of patients with conditions that are not well understood.

Cohen Jr. and MacLean have provided a comprehensive discussion of the process of syndrome delineation, particularly with respect to craniosynostosis syndromes [2]. Based on whether or not a syndrome has an identifiable cause, it can be categorized as a syndrome of unknown genesis

Table 1. Partial list of uncommon craniosynostosis syndromes. Syndromes covered in this chapter are bolded and MIM numbers are provided wherever available. Although the text of this chapter covers relatively well-described syndromes for which underlying molecular bases are known, this list is provided as a starting point to demonstrate that the vast majority of the uncommon craniosynostosis syndromes are described in very few patients, do not clearly demonstrate Mendelian genetics, do not have a known underlying molecular basis, and/or are not clearly distinguishable from other syndromes. Better molecular characterization of patients and greater correlation between molecular findings and syndrome delineation can narrow this rather unwieldy list of syndromes to one that is more useful to clinicians and patients. (Adapted from Table 31-1, p. 385, Chapter 31, in [147] with permission from Oxford University Press, Inc.)

MIM number	Uncommon craniosynostosis syndromes
	Acrocephalospondylosyndactyly
201050	Acrocraniofacial dysostosis
%201550	Adducted thumbs (Christian) syndrome
#207410	**Antley-Bixler syndrome**
	Armendares syndrome
#218600	**Baller-Gerold syndrome**
	Baraitser syndrome
#123790	**Beare-Stevenson cutis gyrata syndrome**
	Berant syndrome
	Blair/Pakistan syndrome
#605039	**Bohring-Opitz syndrome**
#211750	**C (Opitz trigonocephaly) syndrome**
	CAP syndrome
	COH syndrome
	Calabro syndrome
302030	Calvarial hyperostosis
#201000	**Carpenter syndrome**
%605627	Cerebrooculonasal syndrome
	Cerebrotrichofacial syndrome
601853	Cerebellotrigeminal dermal dysplasia (Gómez-López-Hernández syndrome)
241519	Chitayat hypophosphatemia syndrome
112240	Cole-Carpenter syndrome
#218330, #613610	Cranioectodermal dysplasia
218350	Craniofacial dyssynostosis
	Craniofaciocervical osteoglyphic dysplasia
602558	Craniomicromelic syndrome
	Cranio-oculo-arthrogrypotic syndrome
123050	Craniorhiny
	Craniosyndactyly/intestinal atresia syndrome
603595	Craniosynostosis with ectopia lentis
#604757	Craniosynostosis, Boston type
%601222	Craniosynostosis, Philadelphia type
#612247	**Crouzon syndrome with acanthosis nigricans**
218670	Craniotelencephalic dysplasia
	Curry Carpenter-like syndrome

Table 1. Continued

MIM number	Uncommon craniosynostosis syndromes
601707	Curry-Jones syndrome
%224690	Ear, patella, short stature (Meier-Gorlin) syndrome
200995	Elejalde syndrome
	Fontaine-Farriaux syndrome
#190440	Frydman trigonocephaly syndrome
	Fryns craniosynostosis syndrome
601370	Genoa syndrome
233500	Gorlin-Chaudhry-Moss syndrome
	Hall syndrome
#235510	Hennekam lymphangiectasia-lymphedema syndrome
#133701	Hereditary multiple exostoses, type II
	Herrmann syndrome
	Hersh syndrome
601379	Hunter-McAlpine syndrome
%241310	Hypomandibular faciocranial syndrome
	Idaho syndrome
#123150	**Jackson-Weiss syndrome**
#147791	**Jacobsen syndrome**
123155	Jones craniosynostosis/Dandy-Walker syndrome
	Kozlowski craniosynostosis syndrome
	Kreiborg/Pakistan syndrome
	Lampert syndrome
218649	Lin-Gettig syndrome
#609192, #610168	**Loeys-Dietz syndrome, type I**
	Lowry syndrome
600252	Lowry-MacLean syndrome
	Mehta syndrome
257920	Michels syndrome
%251230	Microcephaly-micromelia (Ives-Houston) syndrome
602361	Osteocraniostenosis/gracile bone dysplasia
#166250	**Osteoglophonic dysplasia**
#201750	**P450 oxidoreductase deficiency**
	Passos-Bueno craniosynostosis/cataracts syndrome
218450	Pfeiffer-type cardiocranial syndrome
	Pfeiffer-type dolichocephalosyndactyly
	Richieri-Costa overgrowth syndrome
	Sagittal synostosis/auricular anomalies syndrome
101120	Sakati syndrome
	Salinas syndrome
	San Francisco syndrome

Table 1. Continued

MIM number	Uncommon craniosynostosis syndromes
251240	Say-Barber syndrome
314320	Say-Meyer trigonocephaly syndrome
	Say-Poznanski syndrome
312830	SCARF syndrome
#210600	Seckel syndrome
#182212	**Shprintzen-Goldberg syndrome**
	Speare-Mickle syndrome
602611	Spondyloepiphyseal dysplasia/craniosynostosis syndrome
	Ventruto syndrome
	Wisconsin syndrome

or as a syndrome of known genesis. Syndromes of unknown genesis can be further subdivided into syndromes with a provisionally unique pattern, in which a unique combination of anomalies has so far been observed in only 1 patient, and syndromes with a recurrent pattern, in which similar anomalies have been observed in 2 or more unrelated patients. Syndromes of known genesis can be further subdivided into those thought to have a monogenic cause, those with an identified chromosomal cause, those in which a specific enzymatic defect has been implicated, and those in which specific teratogens or environmental factors are causative. As of 1991, when 90 craniosynostosis syndromes had been identified, 40 syndromes were syndromes with mostly unidentified monogenic causes, 24 were syndromes of unknown genesis, 16 were syndromes with an identified chromosomal cause, and 4 were environmentally induced disorders [2].

Given the impressive spectrum of tools for molecular analysis available to clinicians today, it is possible for the entire delineation of a new syndrome to occur in 1 step, bypassing the typical progression from syndromes with provisionally unique patterns to syndromes with recurrent patterns to syndromes of known genesis. One example of this occurred in 1996 and 1997, when Muenke syndrome was described as a new syndrome and was simultaneously associated with a specific point mutation in *FGFR3* [3, 4]. Nevertheless, most craniosynostosis syndromes were initially identified decades ago purely on a phenotypic basis, as syndromes with provisionally unique patterns or syndromes with recurrent patterns, and the etiologies of many of these syndromes have not been further clarified since then. In the meantime, the number of patients described as having each syndrome has typically increased over time, based on the phenotypic similarity of these new patients to the first patients described, leading to issues such as artificial homogeneity of patients and undue emphasis on the most severe aspects of a given syndrome [2]. Thus, there is significant subjectivity regarding lumping and splitting of syndromes and regarding whether or not certain patients should be included in specific syndromes.

In this chapter, the considerably large list of uncommon craniosynostosis syndromes is narrowed to 13 syndromes that are covered here with regard to their nosology, associated clinical characteristics, inheritance patterns, molecular genetics, and treatment paradigms. These 13 syndromes include former syndromes of unknown genesis for which a potential molecular cause has recently been identified, as well as syndromes in which a monogenic cause was previously proposed to exist and has recently been identified as a specific gene. These particular syndromes were chosen for discussion in this chapter because these recent molecular discoveries have important and novel ramifications for clinical diagnosis and genetic counseling in these disorders, and because these discoveries can potentially reduce some of the confusion that has resulted from the initially subjective nature of the delineation of these entities. Also in this chapter, figures 1–12 accompany the textual descriptions and provide visual depictions of each of the disorders covered here.

Antley-Bixler Syndrome (MIM #207410) P450 Oxidoreductase (POR) Deficiency (MIM #201750)

Antley-Bixler syndrome (ABS) is traditionally thought to consist of multiple specific malformations of the skeleton and cartilage, but exact descriptions of the nosology and molecular genetics of the condition have been elusive for many years. Moreover, as described later in this section, recent evidence shows that what is traditionally termed 'ABS' may, in fact, represent 2 disorders with distinct etiologies. To enable the reader to better understand the evolving characterization of these 2 disorders, a chronologic narrative is presented here.

Since the initial descriptions of ABS in 1975 [5] and 1980 [6], several new cases have been reported: a 2001 review by Lee et al. described 34 patients diagnosed with ABS [7]. In terms of the skeletal phenotype of these patients, several features have occurred with almost uniform consistency. The 2001 review notes a high occurrence of craniosynostosis (27/34 patients), radiohumeral synostosis (30/34), and multiple joint contractures (28/34), as well as components of a characteristic craniofacial phenotype including brachycephaly (29/34), midface hypoplasia (31/34), frontal bossing (28/34), ocular proptosis (30/34), dysplastic ears (33/34), and a depressed nasal bridge (31/34) [7]. While femoral bowing was included in the original phenotype [6], 12/34 patients reviewed by Lee et al. had straight femurs; moreover, patterns of elbow joint synostosis other than radiohumeral synostosis have also been seen [8, 9]. Of relevance to the molecular genetics causing the phenotype, discussed next, genital anomalies were found in 15/34 patients, with findings including clitoromegaly, fused labia, and hypoplastic labia majora [7]. Photographs of a patient demonstrating the skeletal phenotype can be seen in figures 1a and 1b, while this patient's genital anomalies are shown in figure 1c.

Two major issues have shaped our current understanding of the molecular genetics behind this entity. First, due to subjectivity regarding the diagnostic criteria for ABS, there has been debate in the literature regarding whether mutations in *FGFR2* are associated with ABS. In 1998, a de novo p.Ser351Cys mutation in *FGFR2* was found in 1 patient clinically diagnosed with ABS whose principal features included craniosynostosis and elbow joint synostosis [10]. While several authors contended that these features are sufficient to diagnose ABS [7, 9], others did not agree that ABS was the correct diagnosis [11, 12], with some pointing out that the combination is not specific to ABS and can occasionally be found in other craniosynostosis syndromes [13, 14]. In 2004, it was asserted that no patient with classical ABS thus far had demonstrated an *FGFR* mutation [13], although some of the patients initially discussed by Reardon et al. [14] and expanded upon by Huang et al. [15] appear to demonstrate the *FGFR2* p.Ser351Cys mutation with femoral bowing, fractures, and/or choanal stenosis in addition to craniosynostosis, midface hypoplasia, and elbow joint synostosis.

Second, questions have arisen as to whether this entity is, in fact, 2 disorders with separate etiologies: a newer but fairly well-supported view thus far. In 2000, Reardon et al. demonstrated that 7/16 patients diagnosed with ABS displayed abnormal steroid biochemistry and that 5 of these

7 also demonstrated abnormal female genitalia (predominantly clitoromegaly and fused labia) [14]. The abnormal steroid biochemistry was characterized by aberrant serum or urine concentrations of several steroid metabolites, including 17-hydroxyprogesterone, cortisol, pregnanetriol, aldosterone, and others [14]. Of note, while 7/16 patients were also found to have mutations in *FGFR2*, they tended not to overlap with those patients who had abnormal steroid biochemistry [14]. Subsequent work implicated the cytochrome P450 system and specifically the gene for P450 oxidoreductase *(POR)* in the abnormal steroid biochemistry that was observed [16–19], further supported by the fact that malformations resembling ABS were found in infants of mothers receiving fluconazole, a selective inhibitor of P450 enzymes [20, 21]. This led to the postulate that 'ABS' is, in fact, 2 separate disorders, and that the ABS phenotype with abnormal steroidogenesis is caused by autosomal recessive mutations in *POR* ('POR deficiency') and is associated with genital abnormalities, while the ABS phenotype without abnormal steroidogenesis or genital abnormalities is autosomal dominant and *FGFR*-associated [15, 17]. The postulate was corroborated by data from Huang et al., who found that recessive *POR* mutations and dominant *FGFR* mutations segregated completely in a cohort of 32 individuals with the skeletal phenotype, and that individuals with *POR* mutations could be morphologically distinguished from those with *FGFR* mutations by the presence of genital abnormalities [15].

In light of the molecular findings detailed above, Huang et al. emphasize that clinically distinguishing between classical ABS and POR deficiency is essential, as different etiologies, patterns of inheritance, risk factors, and management practices apply to these conditions [15]. For instance, patients with POR deficiency have been observed to die suddenly and inexplicably, to require steroid hormone supplementation, and to be at risk for adrenal insufficiency and Addisonian crisis during illness or surgery [14, 15]. Clinical management of patients with a diagnosis of ABS should therefore include an endocrinologic evaluation of the cortisol response to stress and the adrenal and gonadal synthesis of C21 and C19 steroids [15].

An additional focus of clinical management of patients with the skeletal phenotype is the management of choanal atresia and stenosis, which were found in 19/34 patients reviewed by Lee et al. and which can cause upper respiratory obstruction in neonates [7]. This is a major factor in the recommendation that a guarded prognosis should be given to patients with the skeletal phenotype, as only one third of the 34 patients reviewed by Lee et al. were alive in 2001, with 10 children dying during the first year of life due to respiratory distress [7, 22]. To prevent respiratory complications in patients with choanal atresia or stenosis, early tracheotomy is often preferred, as the midface deformities can complicate efforts to dilate

Composite 1, Figs. 1–7. Permission to republish these photographs has been obtained from BMJ Publishing Group, Ltd. (figs. 1, 3, 4), Elsevier (fig. 6), John Wiley & Sons (figs. 2, 5), and Medknow Publications and Media, Pvt. Ltd. (fig. 7).

Fig. 1. Patient initially diagnosed with Antley-Bixler syndrome [14] and later found to have POR deficiency [15]. The patient has the Antley-Bixler skeletal phenotype, demonstrating a characteristic craniofacial appearance (**a**), fixed elbow joint (**b**), and genital anomalies, including clitoromegaly and hooded prepuce (**c**).

Fig. 2. Patient diagnosed with Beare-Stevenson cutis gyrata syndrome [51]. **a** Cloverleaf skull, cutis gyratum of the frontal area, and marked proptosis; **b** Deep vertical pre-auricular skin furrow; **c** Large protruding umbilicus; **d** Deep skin corrugations on the soles of the feet.

Fig. 3. Two siblings diagnosed with Baller-Gerold syndrome [35]. **a–c** 16-week-old fetus displaying mild brachycephaly, radial aplasia, and oligodactyly. **d–f** Newborn with marked brachycephaly and facial dysmorphic characteristics, including a small mouth, short nose, short palpebral fissures with telecanthus, bulging forehead, and widely opened anterior fontanelle.

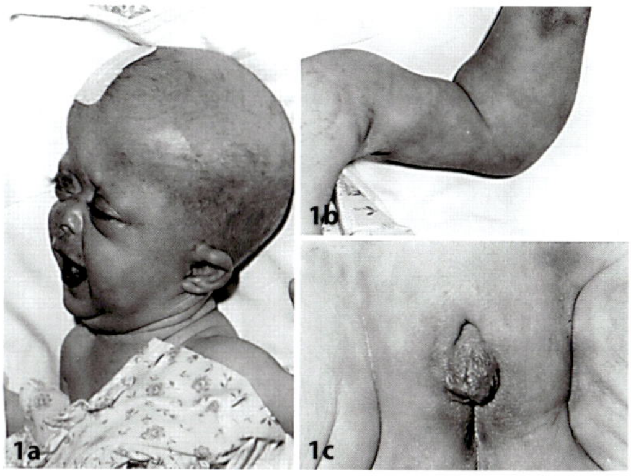

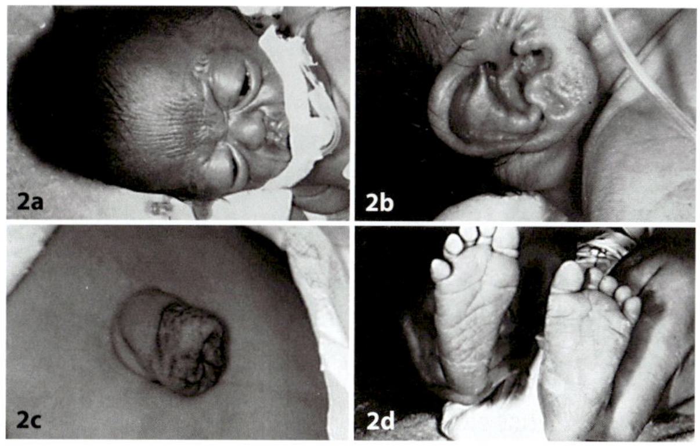

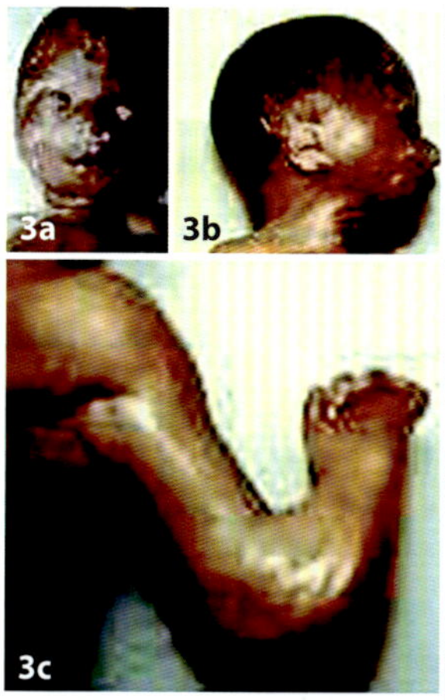

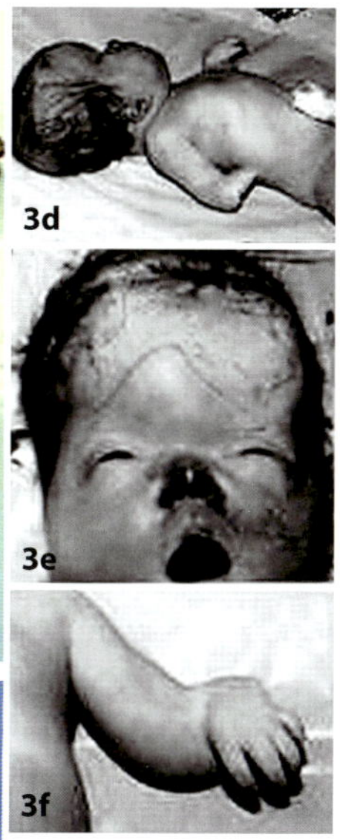

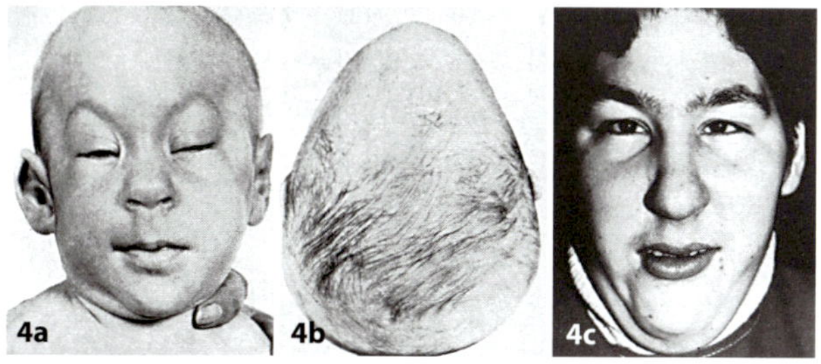

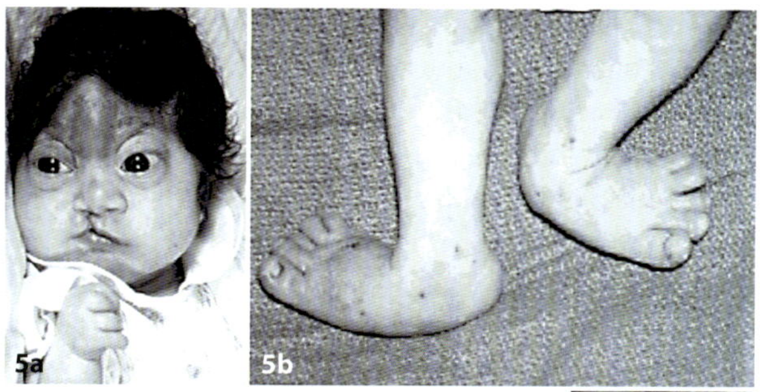

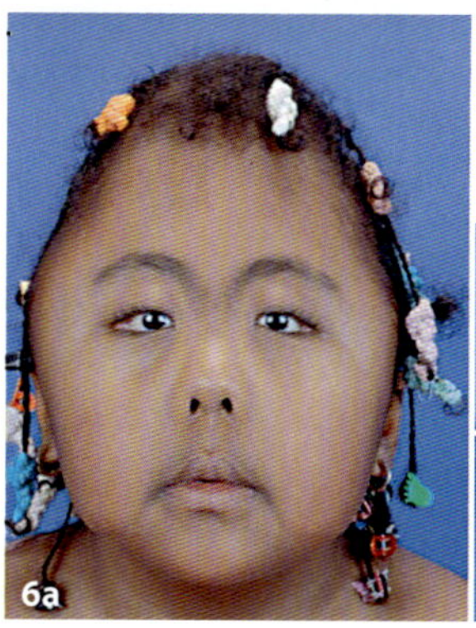

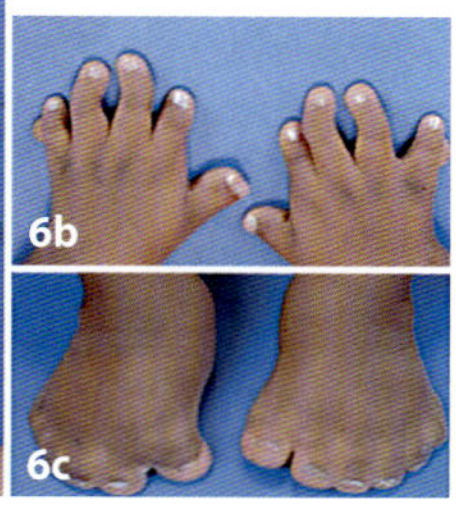

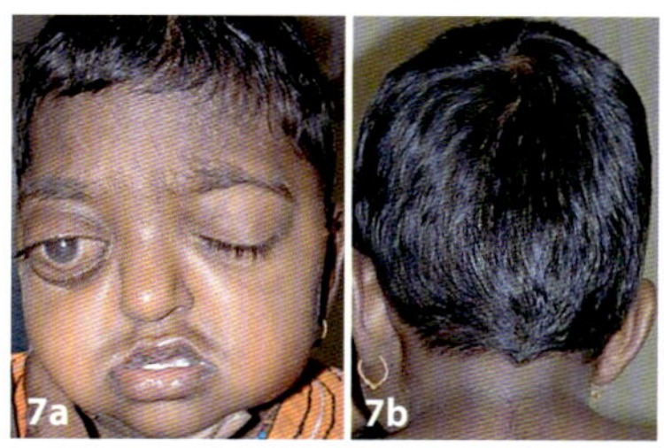

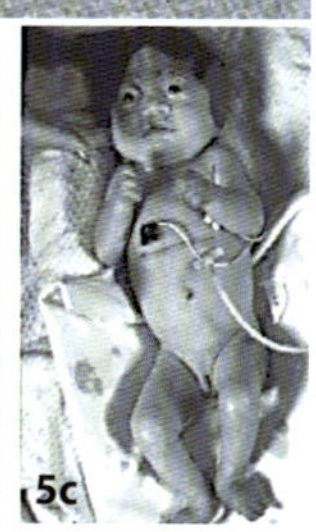

Fig. 4. Patient diagnosed with C (Opitz trigonocephaly) syndrome [67]. Facial appearance at 5 months (**a**) and 19 years (**c**); skull shape at 5 months (**b**).

Fig. 5. Patient diagnosed with Bohring-Opitz syndrome [59]. **a** Prominent forehead with glabellar capillary hemangioma and hirsutism, prominent eyes, and cleft lip; **b** Foot deformity; **c** Multiple contractures and cutis marmorata.

Fig. 6. Siblings affected by Carpenter syndrome [71]. **a** Metopic ridge and temporal bulging secondary to multisuture synostosis, arched eyebrows, epicanthic folds, and anteverted nares; **b**, **c** Broad thumbs and halluces with syndactyly, brachydactyly, clinodactyly, and polydactyly (postaxial in hands, central in feet).

Fig. 7. Patient diagnosed with Crouzon syndrome with acanthosis nigricans [148]. **a** Frog-like facies, hypertelorism, tower-shaped skull, dull look, and hyperpigmentation on forehead; **b** Thick, velvety, hyperpigmented skin of the neck.

the posterior choanae [7]. A good prognosis with the possibility of normal intellectual development can be achieved in some cases with early and effective management of craniosynostosis and respiratory dysfunction, but issues such as neurologic impairment, hearing deficits, and scoliosis have been noted in some survivors [22].

Baller-Gerold Syndrome (MIM #218600)

Baller-Gerold syndrome (BGS), cardinal features of which include craniosynostosis and radial aplasia or hypoplasia, demonstrates the need for a careful clinical workup due to its phenotypic overlap with a number of other entities. Here, an overview of BGS is presented, followed by description of this phenotypic overlap and clinical recommendations.

The original patients were described by Baller and Gerold in 1950 and 1959, respectively; they included a young adult female with acrocephaly, oxycephaly, and bilateral radial aplasia born to third cousins [23], and 2 sibs demonstrating tower skull, ulnar hypoplasia, and radial aplasia [24]. Since that time, over 20 cases have been reported with a presumptive diagnosis of BGS. In a 1994 review by Ramos Fuentes et al., 22/22 patients had craniosynostosis (predominantly of the coronal sutures and resulting in turribrachicephaly), 21/22 had absent or hypoplastic thumbs, 17/22 had absence or hypoplasia of one or both radii, and 22/22 were reported to have other upper extremity defects, including abnormal fingers, abnormal ulnae, or metacarpal anomalies [25]. Facial anomalies were present in 18/22 patients, with low-set or posteriorly rotated ears (14/22) and micrognathia (11/22) listed as the most common of these. Outside the craniofacial spectrum, some patients also had an imperforate or anteriorly displaced anus (9/22), vertebral anomalies (7/22), lower limb anomalies (7/22), ocular anomalies (9/22), growth retardation (13/20), and neurologic impairment (8/16), as well as other, less common anomalies [25]. Figure 3 shows 2 patients demonstrating many of these features of BGS. The proportions of these features should be interpreted with caution, though, as other syndromes may not have been adequately excluded during the diagnostic workup in some of the earlier patients. With respect to the inheritance pattern, observations of parental consanguinity suggested autosomal recessive inheritance [23, 26, 27], although Galea and Tolmie raised the prospect of genetic heterogeneity and cautioned against assuming this to be the sole inheritance pattern [28].

Phenotypic overlap with a number of other entities has been observed, leading some to question whether BGS is a distinct entity and to recommend reducing its scope to a more narrow phenotype [29–32]. Huson et al. reported a patient with major skeletal features of Baller-Gerold syndrome, but whose facial appearance and cytogenetic results showing premature chromosome separation ultimately led to a diagnosis of Roberts-SC phocomelia syndrome (MIM #268300) [32]. Another set of clinical entities with a close phenotypic overlap includes BGS, Fanconi anemia (MIM #227650), and VACTERL association (MIM #192350): 4 individuals with a diagnosis of BGS (one of whom was initially diagnosed with VACTERL association even prior to this) were rediagnosed with Fanconi anemia after thrombocytopenia and/or positive chromosome breakage studies were observed [30, 33, 34]. Overlap of BGS with Saethre-Chotzen syndrome (MIM #101400) was suggested when a patient with craniosynostosis and unilateral radial aplasia with no other malformations and negative chromosome breakage studies was found to have a p.Glu181Stop mutation in the *TWIST* gene, which is implicated in Saethre-Chotzen syndrome [31]. Thus, proper clinical management of a patient with suspected BGS should include hematologic workup, specific chromosomal analysis checking for premature chromosome separation and chromosome breakage, and sequencing of *FGFR1, FGFR2, FGFR3*, or *TWIST* genes if clinical findings are compatible with other disorders characterized by mutations in those genes [29, 31, 32, 35]. Proper separation of the nosologic entities mentioned here is crucial for effective genetic counseling due to the different inheritance patterns of each [31].

In 2006, causal mutations in *RECQL4* were discovered in patients within 2 families who were initially diagnosed with and subsequently reassessed for BGS. This is of particular significance because yet another group of entities that BGS has been observed to overlap with includes Rothmund-Thomson syndrome (RTS; MIM #268400) [29, 36, 37] and RAPADILINO syndrome (MIM #266280) [35], both of which are also associated with mutations in *RECQL4* [38–40]. Due to this commonality, van Maldegrem et al. have suggested that BGS, RTS, and RAPADILINO syndrome form a clinical spectrum of related etiology, with core criteria including radial ray defects, growth deficiency, facial dysmorphia, gastrointestinal disturbances, and patellar abnormalities, and specific features more particular to each syndrome: examples include craniosynostosis in BGS; palatal abnormalities and joint abnormalities in RTS; and dental/nail abnormalities, cataracts, and sparse hair in RAPADILINO syndrome [35]. Thus, *RECQL4* sequencing is also warranted upon observation of malformation syndromes involving craniosynostosis and radial ray aplasia [35].

Beare-Stevenson Cutis Gyrata Syndrome (MIM #123790)

Beare-Stevenson cutis gyrata syndrome (BSS), first described by Beare et al. in 1969 [41] and Stevenson et al. in 1978 [42], has been reported in a total of 24 patients since that time. The syndrome was further delineated in 1992 by Hall et al., who described the cardinal features as consisting of craniofacial anomalies, predominantly craniosynostosis with cloverleaf skull; cutis verticis gyrata; ear defects; acanthosis nigricans; anogenital anomalies; skin tags; and prominent umbilical stump [43]. Photographs of a patient with many of these features can be found in figure 2. Cutis verticis gyrata is a hallmark dermatologic finding of BSS, manifesting as coarse furrowing of the skin caused by excessive skin buckling [44]. On the cellular level, this quality of the skin is secondary to an increase in dermal collagen, fibroblasts, and adnexal structures [44]. While the term 'cutis verticis gyrata' typically refers to the scalp alone, the furrowing in BSS extends to other areas of the body, including the back, abdomen, and limbs [43].

Three different mutations in *FGFR2* have been identified in patients with BSS. In 1996, Przylepa et al. sequenced *FGFR2* in 5 BSS patients, including the original patient reported by Stevenson et al. in 1978, finding a p.Tyr375Cys mutation in 2 patients and a p.Ser372Cys mutation in a third patient (the patient of Stevenson et al. was negative) [45]. Including these patients, the p.Tyr375Cys mutation has since been reported in a total of 9 unrelated patients [45–51], while the p.Ser372Cys mutation has been reported twice [45, 52]. A third mutation was identified in 2009 when Slavotinek et al. reported a c.1506del63 mutation in a patient with BSS, an exonic deletion resulting in the loss of amino acids 287–308 of the protein [53].

Slavotinek et al. compiled clinical characteristics on the 12 patients with *FGFR2* mutations identified thus far [53]. Of the patients with the p.Tyr375Cys mutation, prominent features included fused cranial sutures (9/9; often causing cloverleaf skull), ocular proptosis (9/9), hypertelorism (7/9), choanal atresia (6/9), Arnold-Chiari malformation (5/9), cutis gyrata (9/9) with preauricular (7/9) or limb (5/9) skin furrows, skin tags (5/9), prominent umbilicus (8/9), and anterior/imperforate anus (5/9). Features common to both patients with the p.Ser372Cys mutation included proptosis, hypertelorism, midface hypoplasia, cutis gyrata, nail hypoplasia, and prominent umbilicus. The patient with the 21-amino acid deletion displayed all of the features above as well as several findings uncommonly observed in BSS, such as neonatal teeth, partial anodontia, external auditory canal atresia, mild optic nerve hypoplasia, orofacial clefting, and hypospadias.

A guarded prognosis should generally be given to BSS patients. In the compilation of clinical characteristics in BSS patients with mutations, 5/12 patients required a tracheostomy for respiratory obstruction, 5/12 patients required a ventriculoperitoneal shunt for hydrocephalus, and 6/10 patients died before 2 years of age [53]. Two groups have discussed their experiences with airway management and challenging intubations in the perioperative care of patients with BSS [54, 55]. Hall et al. noted that patient performance seemed to be related to whether or not the patient had cloverleaf skull [43].

C (Opitz Trigonocephaly) Syndrome (MIM #211750) Bohring-Opitz Syndrome (MIM #605039)

C syndrome, referred to hereafter as COTS, was first described by Opitz et al. in 1969, who named the condition after the initial letter of the surname of 2 affected siblings with multiple congenital anomalies and mental retardation [56]. While trigonocephaly is one distinctive feature of the syndrome, leading to the alternate designation 'Opitz trigonocephaly syndrome,' the full syndrome additionally consists of anomalies in a number of different organ systems, including characteristic craniofacial anomalies, limb defects, visceral defects, capillary hemangiomata, redundant skin, developmental abnormalities, and congenital heart defects [57]. The prevalence of the syndrome has been estimated to be between 1:800,000 and 1:1,000,000, but due to a high mortality rate, it may be more common in fetuses and deceased infants [58].

Approximately 3 dozen cases have been reported since the original case report, although disputes regarding the exact nosology of the condition have resulted in some cases being reclassified [58]. Most prominently, a separate condition named Bohring-Opitz syndrome (BOS) was proposed due to descriptions of several patients whose features were reminiscent of COTS but still clinically distinguishable [59]. In a 2007 article, Kaname et al. compiled clinical characteristics of COTS and BOS cases in the literature [57]. Craniofacial features common to both COTS and BOS include trigonocephaly (23/23 COTS patients; 13/13 BOS patients), upslanting palpebral fissures (22/23; 13/13), strabismus (16/22; 8/8), depressed nasal bridge (15/22; 13/13), anomalous and posteriorly angulated ears (18/21; 12/13), and wide alveolar ridges (10/18; 4/6). Non-craniofacial findings seen in both COTS and BOS include capillary hemangiomata (9/17; 13/13), joint contractures (7/21; 13/13), developmental abnormalities (18/19; 9/9), and congenital heart anomalies (11/22; 5/11). Only COTS patients had epicanthal folds (20/22) and redundant skin (14/20), while only BOS patients demonstrated prominent eyes (13/13), agenesis of the corpus callosum (7/10), intrauterine growth retardation (12/13), failure to thrive (11/11), cleft lip/palate, retinal involvement, flexion deformities of upper limbs, dislocation of radial heads, and forehead hirsutism [57, 59]. For further comparison, figure 4 shows characteristics of a patient diagnosed with COTS, while figure 5 demonstrates several features unique to BOS. In addition to the diagnostic overlap between COTS and BOS, overlap has been also noted between COTS and Kabuki syndrome [60], CHARGE association [61], Váradi-Papp syndrome [62, 63], and other chromosomal syndromes, including duplication-deficiency of chromosome 3 [64] and partial trisomy/tetrasomy 13 [65]; this highlights the need to perform cytogenetic studies on patients with suspected COTS. Extensive details on pathologic findings in COTS were published in 2006 by Opitz et al. [58].

Prior to the implication of a gene in this condition, several hypotheses were advanced by Opitz et al. with respect to the developmental pathology of COTS [58]. Due to the prevalence of midline malformations affecting many structures, including the central nervous system, they proposed that these malformations occur during blastogenesis and that mutant genetic events affect the primary developmental field. Redundant skin and joint anomalies were suggested to occur due to either resorbed lymphedema or a primary connective tissue dysplasia, the latter of which may also explain cranial suture anomalies. The presence of unusual vascular anomalies in several patients led to the proposal that cardiovascular findings may represent more than nonspecific sentinel defects.

Two loci for COTS were proposed in 2006 when Chinen et al. reported a patient with mild COTS and a de novo, apparently balanced reciprocal translocation described as t(3;18)(q13.13;q12.1) [66]. Upon further investigation, Kaname et al. discovered that the *CD96 (TACTILE)* gene, encoding a member of the immunoglobulin superfamily, was located at the 3q13.13 breakpoint; they subsequently identified a p.Thr280Met mutation in this gene in 1 patient with BOS [57]. In vitro experiments showed that cells with the p.Thr280Met mutation in *CD96* were deficient in adhesion and growth, suggesting that *CD96* is important for cell-matrix adhesion [57]. Thus, although COTS and BOS have been differentiated based on phenotype, the fact that *CD96* may be implicated in both conditions raises the questions of whether the 2 syndromes are allelic and whether they represent a gradient of severity [57]. This molecular discovery also raises important questions with respect to inheritance patterns: while autosomal recessive inheritance was previously postulated based on consanguineous matings, affected siblings born to unaffected parents, and the equal sex ratio [67], germline mosaicism has also been postulated [57], and the fact that the mutations identified in *CD96* have been heterozygous suggests autosomal dominant inheritance [57]. Therefore, the syndrome appears to be genetically heterogeneous and a simple prediction of recurrence risk may be difficult.

Carpenter Syndrome (MIM #201000)

Carpenter syndrome, also referred to as acrocephalopolysyndactyly type II, is principally characterized by craniosynostosis, obesity, polydactyly, and soft tissue syndactyly, and was first recognized as a syndrome with autosomal recessive inheritance in Temtamy's review of 13 patients in 1966 [68]. The number of cases in the literature has steadily risen since then: a 1987 review by Cohen et al. compiled 39 cases [69], and a total of over 70 cases have been reported to date.

In the review of 39 cases by Cohen et al., common features included obesity (25/26 patients), thick neck (27/27), syndactyly of the hands (25/30) and feet (33/34), polydactyly of the hands (10/15) and feet (25/26), and brachy- or agenesis mesophalangy of the hands (25/25) and feet (20/20). Sagittal and lambdoidal sutures were typically observed to close first, with the coronal suture closing last; calvarial shapes were described as variable, supported by a recent retrospective review of 3 siblings in which diverse craniofacial anatomical variation was observed [70]. Obesity predominantly involved the trunk, proximal limb, face, and neck. Some craniofacial findings included low-set or malformed ears (24/25), dystopia canthorum (30/31), epicanthal folds (22/25), and flat nasal bridge (22/27). Abnormalities were also found in the oral cavity (23/23), genitourinary system (18/22), and cardiovascular system (14/28). Fifteen of 24 patients were reported as having mental retardation, with IQs of all 24 patients ranging from 52 to 104 [69]. Several of the above features of patients with Carpenter syndrome are demonstrated in figure 6.

A molecular etiology has been recently identified for this syndrome: a linkage analysis performed in 2007 using a large family allowed the disease locus to be mapped to 6p12.1–q12, and sequencing of genes within this region in affected family members revealed a p.Leu145Stop mutation in *RAB23* (*ras*-like in rat brain 23) [71]. The mutation spectrum in *RAB23* was expanded using a total of 15 independent Carpenter syndrome families, with 4 truncating mutations and 1 missense mutation identified [71]. As *RAB23* is a negative regulator of hedgehog signaling, specifically regulating Gli transcription factor processing, the authors suggest that hedgehog signaling may play a role in cranial suture biogenesis or in obesity [71]. Moreover, due to the requirement for cholesterol in hedgehog signaling [72], a pathophysiological link may exist between Carpenter syndrome and other craniosynostosis syndromes with disrupted steroid metabolism, such as POR deficiency [71].

With respect to clinical management, an issue of particular importance in this condition is management of the anatomically altered airway caused by dental abnormalities, thick neck, facial hypoplasia, hypertrophic tonsils, and/or hypoplastic mandible or maxilla [73, 74]. Other anesthetic considerations call for ECG and echocardiogram in patients diagnosed with Carpenter syndrome, as well as the ascertainment of hydrocephalus and increased intracranial pressure [74]. Taravath and Tonsgard documented cerebral malformations in a patient with Carpenter syndrome, highlighting the need for cranial imaging studies to clarify the etiology of neurologic impairment in craniosynostosis syndromes [75]. Hearing loss has been reported in some cases, demonstrated in 1 case by an auditory brainstem response test [73]. Several authors have commented on the feasibility of diagnosing Carpenter syndrome in utero [76, 77].

Crouzon Syndrome with Acanthosis Nigricans (MIM #612247)

Crouzon syndrome with acanthosis nigricans (CAN) is considered to be distinct from Crouzon syndrome, with a separate molecular etiology and phenotype [78, 79]. Due to the cardinal features of a Crouzonoid phenotype and acanthosis nigricans (AN) as well as occasionally observed jaw cementomas and alterations of the vertebral column, a new name was devised by one author to distinguish this syndrome from Crouzon syndrome, leading to the alternate designation of 'Crouzonodermoskeletal syndrome' [79].

A recent review by Arnaud-López et al. analyzed clinical features in 35 patients reported in the literature, describing several features prominent in the syndrome and highlighting several important differences from the phenotypes of Crouzon syndrome and isolated AN, respectively [78]. All patients demonstrated AN, craniosynostosis involving multiple cranial sutures, and several associated facial features, including downslanting palpebral fissures, exophthalmos, ocular hypertelorism, midface hypoplasia, convex nose, and posteriorly rotated ears. In addition, a female preponderance was reported. In contrast to patients with Crouzon syndrome, patients with CAN had a lower frequency of neurologic impairment (only 2/35 patients had mental retardation), hearing loss (5/35 patients), and Chiari malformations (8/35 patients). Moreover, some contend that the presence of multiple suture craniosynostosis, choanal atresia, and hydrocephalus in patients with Crouzon syndrome should suggest a diagnosis of CAN [80]. Abnormalities of bone have been postulated to be part of the syndrome [79]; although not all patients may have been examined in sufficient detail, only 7/35 patients demonstrated abnormalities of vertebrae and only 2/35 patients had odontogenic tumors. AN manifested differently in patients with CAN than in other conditions with isolated AN, occurring at an earlier age of onset (within the first decade for 20/25 patients) and with a more widespread distribution, involving the neck, axillae, perioral region, eyelids, inguinal region, and perianal region [78]. Figure 7 includes photographs of a patient with CAN, demonstrating the craniofacial features as well as the unusual distribution of AN.

In 1995, Meyers et al. observed a p.Ala391Glu mutation in the transmembrane domain of *FGFR3* in 3 unrelated families with CAN; the mutation was not observed in 29 unrelated patients with Crouzon syndrome or in 50 unrelated ethnically matched controls [81]. This establishes a different genetic etiology for CAN than for Crouzon syndrome, as Crouzon syndrome is associated with mutations in *FGFR2* [82]. The location of this mutation within *FGFR3* is also significant because it is only 11 and 16 amino acids away from the p.Gly380Arg and p.Gly375Cys mutations that are known to cause achondroplasia [83–85]. Schweitzer et al. reviewed skeletal findings in 6 patients with the p.Ala391Glu mutation and diagnoses of CAN, including 3 originally described by Meyers et al., and found subtle radiographic findings of achondroplasia in all 6, including slightly broadened and shortened metacarpals and phalanges (still within normal limits), shortened vertebral bodies along the anterior-posterior axis, caudal interpediculate narrowing of the spine, and narrow sacrosciatic notches [80]. The prevalence of these findings in patients with CAN is unknown, due to uncertainty whether skeletal findings were sufficiently explored in all patients, and Arnaud-López et al. advise that management of all patients with CAN should include dental panorex films, measurements of interpediculate narrowing on X-ray, and identification of silent odontogenic tumors and subtle vertebral anomalies [78].

Jackson-Weiss Syndrome (MIM #123150)

Jackson-Weiss syndrome (JWS) is principally characterized by foot abnormalities and/or craniofacial anomalies. Jackson et al. originally described the syndrome in 1976, identifying 138 affected individuals in a large Amish kindred [86]. An autosomal dominant inheritance pattern was ascribed to the phenotype, and the syndrome was distinguished from Pfeiffer syndrome due to the absence of thumb anomalies in the former [86].

A particularly striking feature of the original family is the tremendous intrafamilial variability with respect to the phenotypic expression. While all affected individuals in the original family demonstrated some abnormality of the feet, either clinically or radiographically, only some affected individuals had craniosynostosis, acrocephaly, proptosis, and/or midface hypoplasia (fig. 8a); others did not demonstrate any craniofacial aberrations. The range of foot abnormalities observed in various affected individuals, some of which are displayed in figures 8b–f, included broad medially deviated great toes (up to 90° in 1 individual), fused tarsal bones, broad short first metatarsals, deformities of the second and third metatarsals, broad proximal phalanges of the great toes, calcaneocuboid fusion, and coalition of the navicular and first cuneiform bones. Intelligence appeared to be normal, and hand anomalies were not typically observed. Other branches of the same family were reported by Cross and Opitz [87] as well as by Heike et al. [88]. Cross and Opitz had previously thought that their branch demonstrated autosomal recessive inheritance and had also noted mental retardation [87], perhaps implying a more complex genetic mechanism in at least this branch of the family. Heike et al. noted extensions to the phenotype, including a leg length discrepancy and unilateral absence of the fifth digital ray in the left foot of their proband [88].

Additional cases, mostly sporadic, were reported as JWS cases by several authors [89–94], but these diagnoses are unconvincing due to the absence of radiographic evidence in most cases and the strong possibility that they instead have Pfeiffer syndrome [88, 95]. Heike et al. noted that foot radiographs are an essential component of the JWS diagnosis, as clinical examination can be misleading [88].

The high degree of variable expressivity in the original JWS family led Jackson et al. to postulate that some of the acrocephalosyndactyly syndromes might also be associated with high variability if extremely large families with those conditions were identified, as with JWS; nevertheless, Cohen Jr. cautions against conflating JWS with these other syndromes, noting that large families with Pfeiffer syndrome and Crouzon syndrome tend to 'breed true' [96]. There is disagreement within the literature regarding whether wide intrafamilial variability is the defining characteristic of JWS and whether JWS can occur sporadically [97, 98].

In 1994, Li et al. performed linkage and haplotype analyses using the original JWS family and localized the JWS locus to between 10q23 and 10q26 [99]; that same year, Jabs et al. identified a p.Ala344Gly mutation in *FGFR2* present in all of the affected members of the original JWS family [100] (this mutation has also been erroneously reported as p.Ala342Gly and p.Arg344Gly [101]). Upon the discovery of a new branch of the original family by Heike et al., the p.Ala344Gly mutation was also found in affected members of that branch [88]. Curiously, the same mutation was also found in a family clinically diagnosed with Crouzon syndrome [89]. A number of other mutations in *FGFR2* have been described in the patients with doubtful JWS diagnoses described above; these include p.Cys278Phe [92], p.Gln289Pro [90], p.Cys342Arg [91], p.Cys342Ser [94], and p.Pro252Arg [93]. All of these mutations are also found in families with Crouzon and/or Pfeiffer syndromes [95].

Jacobsen Syndrome (MIM #147791)

Jacobsen syndrome (JS), originally described by Jacobsen et al. in 1973 [102], is mainly associated with growth retardation, psychomotor retardation, and facial dysmorphism [103], although a high degree of phenotypic variability is present due to its status as a contiguous gene deletion syndrome [104]. It is also known as chromosome 11q deletion syndrome due to its association with terminal deletions in the long arm of chromosome 11 [105, 106]. Over 200 cases have been described in the literature thus far [103], most of which have been delineated in a retrospective manner via case reports.

Grossfeld et al. published a prospective study of 110 cases in 2004, with patients included in the study based on molecular ascertainment of terminal 11q deletions [107]; this is a useful source for information on the typical clinical features included in JS. The most commonly observed finding was thrombocytopenia (64/68 patients), with 13/14 patients additionally characterized as possibly having Paris-Trousseau syndrome, an inherited entity consisting of thrombocytopenia,

Composite 2, Figs. 8–12. Permission to republish these images has been obtained from BMJ Publishing Group, Ltd. (fig. 10a–c), Elsevier (fig. 10d–e), John Wiley & Sons (figs. 8, 9c–f, 11), Nature Publishing Group (fig. 12), and BioMed Central (fig. 9a, b).

Fig. 8. Related patients diagnosed with Jackson-Weiss syndrome [88]. **a** Proband at 10 weeks of age, with acrocephaly, bitemporal widening, flattening of brows, and mild zygomatic flattening. **b** Diagram of normal anatomic relationships of the foot, anteroposterior view, with medial cuneiform (m.c.), navicular (n.), cuboid (c.), and calcaneus (cal.) bones labeled. **c, d** Foot radiographs in the anteroposterior view of the proband's maternal grandfather (**c**), showing fusion of the navicular and medial cuneiform bones, fusion of the cuboid and calcaneus bones, broad-based and short first metatarsal and phalanges, and fibrous fusion of the second and third metatarsals and of the proband's maternal uncle (**d**), showing multiple tarsal coalitions. **e** Diagram of normal anatomic relationships of the foot, oblique view, with bones labeled as in **b**. **f** Foot radiograph in the oblique view of a different maternal uncle of the proband, showing fusions of the navicular bone with the medial cuneiform bone, the calcaneus with the cuboid bone, and possible fusion of the calcaneus and navicular bones.

Fig. 9. Patients diagnosed with Jacobsen syndrome (**a, b** from [103]; **c–f** from [107]). **a, b** Facial dysmorphism, frontal view. **c–f** Serial photographs of one patient at 5 weeks (**c**), 7 months (**d**), and 5 years (**e, f**).

Fig. 10. Patients diagnosed with osteoglophonic dysplasia (**a–c** from [125]; **d, e** from [124]). **a** Hypertelorism and anteverted nostrils, **b** frontal bossing and severe mandibular prognathism and **c** dwarfism at age 21 years in the same patient. **d** Lower leg radiograph of a different patient, showing severe lesions at the metaphyses, shortened bone length, and decreased mineral density. **e** Femoral radiograph of a different patient, with arrow showing a lesion at the metaphysis.

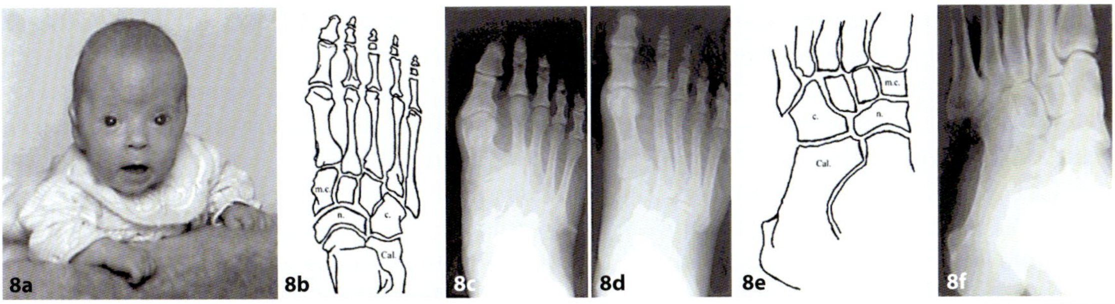

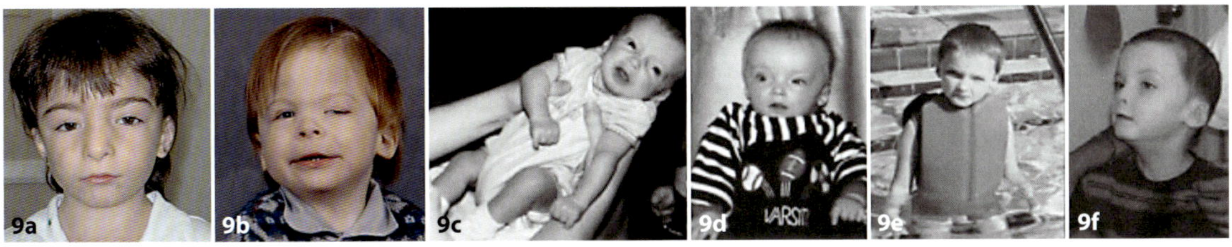

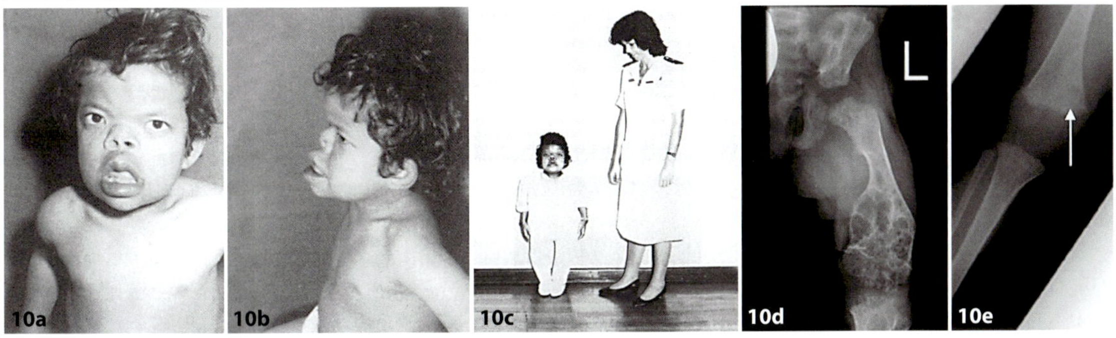

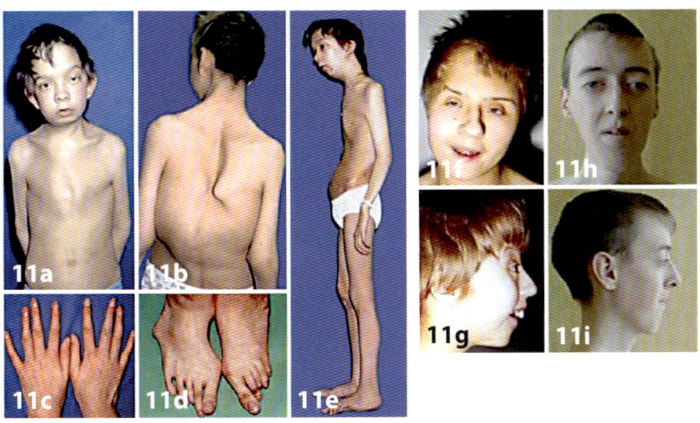

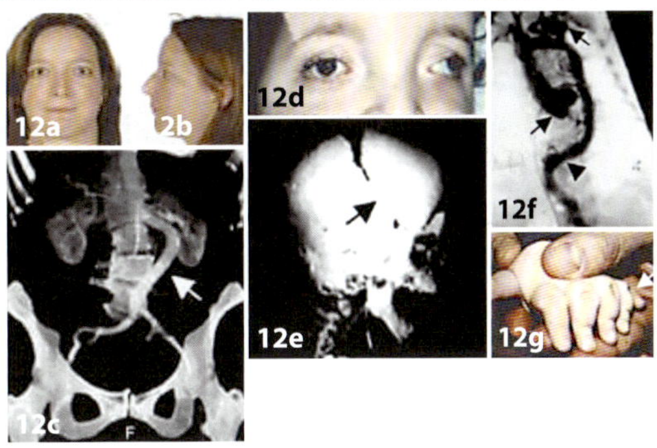

Fig. 11. Patients diagnosed with Shprintzen-Goldberg syndrome [128]. **a**–**e** Physical characteristics of a patient demonstrating dolichocephaly, high prominent forehead, hypertelorism, ptosis, exophthalmos, strabismus, maxillary hypoplasia, micrognathia, low-set posteriorly rotated ears, microcephaly, arachnodactyly, scoliosis, pectus deformity, and cubitus valgus. **f**–**i** Frontal and side views of 2 other patients who also presented with craniosynostosis; status post-repair (**f**, **g**), repair status not specified (**h**, **i**).

Fig. 12. Patients diagnosed with Loeys-Dietz syndrome [129]. **a**, **b** Frontal and side views of a patient demonstrating hypertelorism and malar flattening. **c** Radiographic evidence of a tortuous abdominal aorta in the same patient. **d**–**g** Patient demonstrating marked hypertelorism and exotropia (**d**), premature fusion of the coronal suture (**e**), marked tortuosity of the aorta (arrow head) and aneurysms of the aortic root and subclavian artery (arrows) (**f**) and 6th digit on the left hand (**g**).

platelet inclusion bodies, and dysmegakaryopoiesis [108]. Other common features included developmental delay (11/13 patients), short stature (25/37, with IGF-1 deficiency in 4/8 with short stature), undescended testes (18/31), and congenital heart disease (52/93; mostly ventricular septal defects and left-sided valvular obstruction). In 36 patients for whom a comprehensive morphologic examination was performed, common dysmorphic features, shown in figure 9, included ocular hypertelorism (92%), broad nasal bridge (91%), thin upper lip (84%), downslanting palpebral fissures (83%), low-set or malformed ears (81%), toe anomalies (83%), and syndactyly of the hands (72%). The frequency of trigonocephaly has varied across studies; in some cohorts, trigonocephaly was observed with a frequency of less than 50% [103, 107], while in other cohorts, it has been reported to be one of the most common features of the syndrome [106]. This variation may be explained by differences in breakpoints of patients within these cohorts, discussed below.

In 1986, Fryns et al. identified a deletion of 11q24.1 causing the JS phenotype in 2 patients [105]; after more detailed breakpoint mapping studies were performed in JS patients, JS is now thought of as a contiguous gene deletion syndrome predominantly involving terminal deletions at 11q [104]. After mapping 23 JS breakpoints, Tunnacliffe et al. determined that the breakpoints all fell within the 11q23.3–q24.2 interval, which spans 13.5 Mb and contains 100 genes [104]. Notably, while chromosomal breakage events in many diseases have typically been thought to occur de novo, a minority (around 10%) of JS breakpoints were observed to cluster within the 11q23.3 region, which contains *FRA11B*, a folate-sensitive fragile site caused by a $(CCG)_n$ trinucleotide repeat expansion; this raised the prospect that some JS cases may be caused by inheritance of a fragile site followed by chromosomal breakage at that site [104, 109, 110].

An ongoing effort currently aims at clarifying genotype-phenotype correlations using breakpoints identified in patients. Grossfeld et al. identified critical regions for 14 phenotypic and cognitive functional components of the JS clinical spectrum: the smallest such region spanned 6.8 Mb, from D11S1351 to the telomere, and was associated with Paris-Trousseau syndrome, undescended testes, pyloric stenosis, and mental retardation [107]; additional work has implicated *FLI1* in thrombocytopenia in JS [111, 112]. Penny et al. hypothesized that a gene influencing calvarial suture closure exists between D11S1316 and D11S912, corresponding to a region within distal 11q23.3 and proximal 11q24.1 and possibly also explaining digit anomalies [106]. Other regions have been hypothesized to explain cardiac defects [113], cognitive defects [114], and ocular coloboma [107], although some predictions regarding cardiac defects, with regard to the candidate gene *JAM3*, have produced negative results to date [115].

Clinical management of patients with JS includes many components that are common to the management of all patients with craniosynostosis, but several recommendations have been put forth to address unique issues found in JS [103]. Severe cardiac malformations can occur during the neonatal period, necessitating cardiac surgery; moreover, hematologic defects can cause bleeding during infancy and must be taken into account before surgical interventions. In addition to cardiac and hematologic evaluations, recommended evaluations include an immunologic assessment, an endocrine evaluation due to the presence of short stature in many patients, and an abdominal ultrasound to exclude pyloric stenosis and malformations of the kidney and urinary tract. More details can be found in the 2009 review by Mattina et al. [103].

Osteoglophonic Dysplasia (MIM #166250)

Osteoglophonic dysplasia (OGD) principally consists of characteristic craniofacial abnormalities, rhizomelic dwarfism, and non-ossifying bone lesions. While the syndrome was initially given its name to evoke the 'hollowed-out' nature of the metaphyses [116], Greenberg and Lewis point out that the root of the Greek verb γλυφειν, meaning 'to hollow out,' persists in English as '-glyph,' suggesting that the true name of the disorder should be 'osteoglyphic dysplasia' or 'osteoglyphidic dysplasia' [117]. Nevertheless, these names have not enjoyed popular usage in the literature to date.

At least 14 OGD cases have been reported in the literature thus far, 8 of which were reviewed by Sklower Brooks et al. in 1996 [118]. Craniofacial anomalies (fig. 10a, b) include craniosynostosis (8/8 patients, mostly involving the coronal sutures), abnormal skull shape at birth (8/8), and notable mandibular prognathism (6/6), as well as nasal obstruction/breathing difficulty (8/8), hypertelorism (6/6), unerupted teeth (6/6), anteverted nares (5/5), frontal bossing (4/5), and ocular proptosis (4/6). Distinctive findings outside the craniofacial region (fig. 10c–e) include rhizomelic dwarfism (8/8), cystic metaphyseal defects (8/8) that resolve in patients surviving to adulthood, and platyspondyly (4/6). Life expectancy appears to correlate with the severity of craniofacial abnormalities with respect to their impact on feeding and breathing [118]; while some patients died in infancy [119, 120], others survived to adulthood [121–123]. Developmental delay (5/5) is common in OGD, but intelligence remains normal [118], as demonstrated by adult patients who worked in careers such as drafting and machining [121, 122]. While most cases have occurred sporadically, some familial cases have been noted, leading some to suggest the possibility of autosomal dominant inheritance [118, 121, 124, 125].

From a biochemical standpoint, laboratory studies of serum calcium, phosphorus, and alkaline phosphatase have typically been normal [118, 125], although 3 out of 4 patients reported by White et al. were hypophosphatemic secondary to renal phosphate wasting [124]. As it had previously been observed that patients with fibrous dysplasia of bone have nonossifying lesions similar to those in OGD, and the levels of the fibroblast growth factor 23 (FGF23) phosphaturic factor produced by the lesions in those patients correlate with renal phosphate wasting, White et al. postulated that hypophosphatemia in OGD is also a result of FGF23 production from the nonossifying lesions, successfully demonstrating elevated serum FGF23 levels in 1 OGD patient [124]. It has also been noted that there is phenotypic similarity between OGD and hypophosphatasia, a distinct bone metabolic disorder [125].

Four patients with OGD were sequenced in 2005 by White et al., who identified 3 different activating mutations in *FGFR1*: a p.Tyr374Cys mutation (originally reported as p.Tyr372Cys) in an affected father and son within 1 kindred, as well as p.Asn330Ile and p.Cys381Arg (originally p.Cys379Arg) mutations, respectively, in 2 sporadic OGD patients [124]. The most recent amino acid position numbers are current as per GenBank accession number AAA35958 [126]. These mutations were not found in normal family members or in normal control populations. Farrow et al. additionally identified the p.Tyr374Cys mutation in Beighton's original patient reported in 1980 [116], and found the p.Asn330Ile mutation in another patient [126]. The p.Tyr374Cys mutation is of interest because analogous mutations in *FGFR2* and *FGFR3* cause Beare-Stevenson cutis gyrata syndrome and thanatophoric dysplasia type I, respectively. Similarly, *FGFR2* and *FGFR3* mutations analogous to the p.Asn330Ile mutation cause Crouzon syndrome and hypochondroplasia, respectively, while mutations in *FGFR3* analogous to the p.Cys381Arg mutation cause over 90% of achondroplastic dwarfism [124, 126]. Finally, the fact that the OGD mutations are present in *FGFR1* is surprising, as most major craniosynostosis syndromes are associated with *FGFR2* mutations and syndromes with short stature are usually associated with *FGFR3* mutations [126]. Thus, White et al. postulated that *FGFR1* fulfills a critical, as-yet-unknown role in the modulation of bone elongation [124].

Shprintzen-Goldberg Syndrome (MIM #182212)
Loeys-Dietz Syndrome, Types IA and IB (MIM #609192, MIM #610168)

Shprintzen-Goldberg syndrome (SGS), originally described in 1981 [127], is principally characterized by craniosynostosis and a marfanoid habitus, but lack of a single pathognomonic feature and the presence of phenotypic overlap with a number of different disorders has led to confusion regarding whether SGS is a unique pathogenic entity [128]. A related disorder named Loeys-Dietz syndrome type I was described in 2005; the associated phenotype, also comprising craniosynostosis and a marfanoid habitus, has been observed to overlap considerably with that of SGS [129]. Compounding this uncertainty, it is still unclear whether the 2 disorders share a common etiology, as detailed later in this section. Nonetheless, the continuing clarification of these syndromes is helpful in expanding the clinical spectrum and known molecular etiologies of disorders associated with a marfanoid phenotype beyond the well-characterized Marfan syndrome and homocystinuria.

Over 40 SGS cases have been described in the literature to date, most of which were reported to occur sporadically. In the 3 familial cases that have been observed, the inheritance pattern has not been precisely determined [128, 130]. Two recent comprehensive clinical analyses of patients with SGS are those by Greally et al. in 1998 [131] and Robinson et al. in 2005 [128]. According to Robinson et al., craniofacial findings identified in over two thirds of reported SGS patients include micrognathia (33/37 patients), low-set posteriorly rotated ears (32/37), downslanting palpebral fissures (31/37), high arched palate (30/37), dolichocephaly (28/37), hypertelorism (28/37), and exophthalmos (29/37), with craniosynostosis confirmed in 18/37 patients. Common skeletal anomalies include arachnodactyly (34/37) and pectus deformity (30/37), with moderately common findings including camptodactyly (24/37), scoliosis (23/37), and joint hypermobility (21/37). Cardiovascular manifestations occur with moderate frequency, consisting of mitral valve prolapse (13/37) and aortic root dilatation (8/37), and neurologic findings include hypotonia (26/37) and developmental delay (32/37) with mild to severe neurologic impairment.

SGS was postulated by some to consist of 2 subtypes, one of which encompasses craniosynostosis, marfanoid habitus, mental retardation, and a normal aortic root, and the other of which comprises craniosynostosis, marfanoid habitus, normal intelligence, and aortic root anomalies [130, 132]. Greally et al. and Robinson et al. noted that while several radiographic abnormalities were identified in patients in the former category, whether the 2 subtypes were genuinely different was not conclusively known at the time [128, 131].

In 2005, the issue was compounded further when Loeys et al. described 10 families with Loeys-Dietz syndrome type I (LDSI), a disorder similar to the second proposed subtype of SGS. Loeys et al. noted that the principal distinguishing criteria between LDSI and SGS consisted of cardiovascular findings, as LDSI patients have cleft palate, arterial tortuosity, vascular pathology, and aortic aneurysms and dissections outside the aortic root, all of which are not typically seen in SGS [129]. In general, common cardiovascular anomalies in LDSI include aortic root aneurysms (39/40), aneurysms of other vessels (21/40), and arterial tortuosity (21/25), while craniofacial anomalies in LDSI include hypertelorism (36/40), cleft palate or abnormal uvula (36/40), craniosynostosis (19/40), malar hypoplasia (24/40), retrognathia (20/40), and blue sclerae (16/40) [133]. Skeletal anomalies in LDSI are similar to those in SGS, including arachnodactyly (28/40), pectus deformity (27/40), scoliosis (20/40), and joint laxity (27/40) [133]. Notably uncommon findings in LDSI include ectopia lentis (0/40) and developmental delay (6/40). For further comparison, figure 11 includes photographs of patients diagnosed with SGS, while figure 12 includes photographs and radiographs demonstrating several features unique to LDSI. Despite the phenotypic overlap between LDSI, SGS, and Marfan syndrome, it is still clinically important to distinguish between the three, as the risk of early-occurring aggressive aortic pathology, including aortic dissection and rupture, is increased in LDSI when compared to those in SGS and in Marfan syndrome [133–135]. Other syndromes from which it is important to distinguish SGS include congenital contractural arachnodactyly, homocystinuria, Lujan-Fryns syndrome, Antley-Bixler syndrome, and Idaho syndrome II [128, 136].

Mutations contributing to the pathogenesis of SGS and LDSI have been identified, but the etiology of LDSI has been elucidated more clearly. Due to the hypothesis that loss-of-function mutations in *TGFBR2*, which encodes a transforming growth factor beta (TGF-β) receptor, phenocopy Marfan syndrome, and due to the implication of TGF-β signaling in vascular and craniofacial processes in animal models, Loeys et al. sequenced the original 10 LDS families for mutations in *TGFBR1* and *TGFBR2*, identifying unique, heterozygous *TGFBR1* mutations in 4 families and *TGFBR2* mutations in 6 families [129]. A follow-up study in 2006 showed that of 52 families with LDS, 29 *TGFBR2* mutations and 13 *TGFBR1* mutations were found, with 64% of these occurring de novo and most occurring as missense mutations in or near the serine-threonine kinase domains of the receptor [133]. A 2006 study by Singh et al. showed that in 41 patients with a tentative diagnosis of Marfan syndrome or who satisfied the Ghent nosology for Marfan syndrome, 7 mutations were identified in *TGFBR1* and *TGFBR2*, and upon reexamination, several patients with the mutations were found to have signs of LDS, revealing clinical overlap between Marfan syndrome and LDS [137]. A 2009 study found clinical differences between patients with *TGFBR1* and *TGFBR2* mutations, showing that those with *TGFBR2* mutations are more likely to dissect at aortic diameters less than 5.0 cm than those with *TGFBR1* mutations [138] (5.0 cm is a clinically significant diameter, above which surgical repair may be warranted).

With respect to the molecular genetics of SGS, in 1996, Sood et al. identified 2 purported mutations in *FBN1*, the same gene implicated in Marfan syndrome, while studying patients with SGS [139]. One of these, a p.Pro1148Ala substitution, was later found to be a polymorphic variant [140, 141]. The other mutation, a p.Cys1223Tyr change, had previously been found in Marfan syndrome [142] and is similar to a p.Cys1221Tyr mutation subsequently found in an SGS patient reported by Kosaki et al. [143]. Despite screening in additional patients, no other mutations in *FBN1* have been identified, leading some to suggest that while *FBN1* mutations may cause clinical signs of SGS, they are not a major cause of SGS [135]. Additionally, based on the suggestion that SGS, like LDSI, may be caused by mutations in genes coding for TGF-β receptors [129], 3 groups have reported mutations in *TGFBR1* and *TGFBR2* in patients they believe to be affected by SGS. Kosaki et al. discovered a splicing defect in *TGFBR2*, reported as IVS5–2A>G [143], but Robinson et al. note that the patient is equally likely to have LDSI [135]. Van Steensel et al. identified a p.Thr516Lys mutation in the catalytic domain of *TGFBR2*, and also stated that because their patient only demonstrated aortic dilatation at the root, with no other vascular anomalies, they believe a diagnosis of SGS is appropriate [144]. Stheneur et al. identified a p.Glu245Gly change in a purported SGS patient, but did not provide specific details on whether a diagnosis of LDSI would have been more appropriate [145].

In the future, it is possible that the nomenclature of syndromes with Marfan-like findings will change, with these syndromes transforming from independent entities into an aggregate spectrum of diseases associated with TGF-β signaling [146]. Nevertheless, aberrant TGF-β signaling is much more firmly implicated in the pathogenesis of

LDSI than in the pathogenesis of SGS, so additional clarification of the molecular causes of SGS is necessary before the 2 entities are linked in this manner.

Acknowledgements

This work was supported by the Division of Intramural Research, National Human Genome Research Institute, National Institutes of Health, Department of Health and Human Services, United States of America.

References

1 Kimonis V, Gold J-A, Hoffman TL, Panchal J, Boyadjiev SA: Genetics of craniosynostosis. Semin Pediatr Neurol 2007;14:150–161.

2 Cohen MM Jr, MacLean RE: Anatomic, genetic, nosologic, diagnostic, and psychosocial considerations; in Cohen MM Jr, MacLean RE (eds): Craniosynostosis: Diagnosis, Evaluation, and Management, 2nd ed. New York, Oxford University Press, 2000, pp 119–146.

3 Bellus GA, Gaudenz K, Zackai EH, Clarke LA, Szabo J, et al: Identical mutations in three different fibroblast growth factor receptor genes in autosomal dominant craniosynostosis syndromes. Nat Genet 1996;14:174–176.

4 Muenke M, Gripp KW, McDonald-McGinn DM, Gaudenz K, Whitaker LA, et al: A unique point mutation in the fibroblast growth factor receptor 3 gene *(FGFR3)* defines a new craniosynostosis syndrome. Am J Hum Genet 1997;60:555–564.

5 Antley R, Bixler D: Trapezoidocephaly, midfacial hypoplasia, and cartilage abnormalities with multiple synostoses and skeletal fractures. Birth Defects Orig Artic Ser 1975;11:397–401.

6 DeLozier CD, Antley RM, Williams R, Green N, Heller RM, et al: The syndrome of multisynostotic osteodysgenesis with long-bone fractures. Am J Med Genet 1980;7:391–403.

7 Lee H-J, Cho D-Y, Tsai F-J, Shen W-C: Antley-Bixler syndrome, description of two new cases and review of the literature. Pediatr Neurosurg 2001;34:33–39.

8 Crisponi G, Porcu C, Piu ME: Antley-Bixler syndrome: Case report and review of the literature. Clin Dysmorphol 1997;6:61–68.

9 Kitoh H, Nogami H, Oki T, Arao K, Nagasaka M, Tanaka Y: Antley-Bixler syndrome: a disorder characterized by congenital synostosis of the elbow joint and the cranial suture. J Pediatr Orthoped 1996;16:243–246.

10 Chun K, Siegel-Bartelt J, Chitayat D, Phillips J, Ray PN: *FGFR2* mutation associated with clinical manifestations consistent with Antley-Bixler syndrome. Am J Med Genet 1998;77:219–224.

11 Gorlin RJ: Patient described by Chun et al. may not present Antley-Bixler syndrome. Am J Med Genet 1999;83:64.

12 Gripp KW, Zackai EH, Cohen MM Jr: Not Antley-Bixler syndrome. Am J Med Genet 1999;83:65–66.

13 Cohen MM Jr: FGFs/FGFRs and associated disorders; in Epstein CJ, Erickson RP, Wynshaw-Boris A (eds): Inborn Errors of Development: The Molecular Basis of Clinical Disorders of Morphogenesis. Oxford, Oxford University Press, 2004, pp 380–400.

14 Reardon W, Smith A, Honour JW, Hindmarsh P, Das D, et al: Evidence for digenic inheritance in some cases of Antley-Bixler syndrome? J Med Genet 2000;37:26–32.

15 Huang N, Pandey AV, Agrawal V, Reardon W, Lapunzina PD, et al: Diversity and function of mutations in P450 oxidoreductase in patients with Antley-Bixler syndrome and disordered steroidogenesis. Am J Hum Genet 2005;76:729–749.

16 Flück CE, Tajima T, Pandey AV, Arlt W, Okuhara K, et al: Mutant P450 oxidoreductase causes disordered steroidogenesis with and without Antley-Bixler syndrome. Nat Genet 2004;36:228–230.

17 Adachi M, Tachibana K, Asakura Y, Yamamoto T, Hanaki K, Oka A: Compound heterozygous mutations of cytochrome P450 oxidoreductase gene *(POR)* in two patients with Antley-Bixler syndrome. Am J Med Genet A 2004;128A:333–339.

18 Fukami M, Horikawa R, Nagai T, Tanaka T, Naiki Y, et al: Cytochrome P450 oxidoreductase gene mutations and Antley-Bixler syndrome with abnormal genitalia and/or impaired steroidogenesis: molecular and clinical studies in 10 patients. J Clin Endocr Metab 2005;90:414–426.

19 Kelley RI, Kratz LE, Glaser RL, Netzloff ML, Wolf LM, Jabs EW: Abnormal sterol metabolism in a patient with Antley-Bixler syndrome and ambiguous genitalia. Am J Med Genet A 2002;110:95–102.

20 Aleck KA, Bartley DL: Multiple malformation syndrome following fluconazole use in pregnancy: report of an additional patient. Am J Med Genet 1997;72:253–256.

21 Lopez-Rangel E, van Allen MI: Prenatal exposure to fluconazole: an identifiable dysmorphic phenotype. Birth Defects Res A 2005;73:919–923.

22 Hassell S, Butler MG: Antley-Bixler syndrome: report of a patient and review of literature. Clin Genet 1994;46:372–376.

23 Baller F: Radiusaplasie und Inzucht. Z Menschl Vererbungs Konstit Lehre 1950;29:782–790.

24 Gerold M: Frakturheilung bei einem seltenen Fall kongenitaler Anomalie der oberen Gliedmaßen. Zbl Chir 1959;84:831–834.

25 Ramos Fuentes FJ, Nicholson L, Scott CI Jr: Phenotypic variability in the Baller-Gerold syndrome: report of a mildly affected patient and review of the literature. Eur J Pediatr 1994;153:483–487.

26 Pelias MZ, Superneau DW, Thurmon TF: Brief clinical report: a sixth report (eighth case) of craniosynostosis-radial aplasia (Baller-Gerold) syndrome. Am J Med Genet 1981;10:133–139.

27 Boudreaux JM, Colon MA, Lorusso GD, Parro EA, Pelias MZ: Baller-Gerold syndrome: an 11th case of craniosynostosis and radial aplasia. Am J Med Genet 1990;37:447–450.

28 Galea P, Tolmie JL: Normal growth and development in a child with Baller-Gerold syndrome (craniosynostosis and radial aplasia). J Med Genet 1990;27:784–787.
29 Cohen MM Jr, Toriello HV: Is there a Baller-Gerold syndrome? Am J Med Genet 1996;61:63–64.
30 Quarrell OWJ, Maltby EL, Harrison CJ: Baller-Gerold syndrome and Fanconi anemia. Am J Med Genet 1998;75:228–229.
31 Gripp KW, Stolle CA, Celle L, McDonald-McGinn DM, Whitaker LA, Zackai EH: *TWIST* gene mutation in a patient with radial aplasia and craniosynostosis: further evidence for heterogeneity of Baller-Gerold syndrome. Am J Med Genet 1999;82:170–176.
32 Huson SM, Rodgers CS, Hall CM, Winter RM: The Baller-Gerold syndrome: phenotypic and cytogenetic overlap with Roberts syndrome. J Med Genet 1990;27:371–375.
33 Farrell SA, Paes BA, Lewis MES: Fanconi anemia in a child previously diagnosed as Baller-Gerold syndrome. Am J Med Genet 1994;50:98–99.
34 Rossbach H-C, Sutcliffe MJ, Haag MM, Grana NH, Rossi AR, Barbosa JL: Fanconi anemia in brothers initially diagnosed with VACTERL association with hydrocephalus, and subsequently with Baller-Gerold syndrome. Am J Med Genet 1996;61:65–67.
35 van Maldergem L, Siitonen HA, Jalkh N, Chouery E, de Roy M, et al: Revisiting the craniosynostosis-radial ray hypoplasia association: Baller-Gerold syndrome caused by mutations in the *RECQL4* gene. J Med Genet 2006;43:148–152.
36 Mégarbané A, Melki I, Souraty N, Gerbaka J, Ghouzzi VE, et al: Overlap between Baller-Gerold and Rothmund-Thomson syndrome. Clin Dysmorphol 2000;9:303–305.
37 Preis S, Majewski F, Korholz D, Gobel U: Osteosarcoma in a 16-year-old boy with Baller-Gerold syndrome. Clin Dysmorphol 1995;4:161–168.
38 Siitonen HA, Kopra O, Kääriäinen H, Haravuori H, Winter RM, et al: Molecular defect of RAPADILINO syndrome expands the phenotype spectrum of *RECQL* diseases. Hum Mol Genet 2003;12:2837–2844.
39 Siitonen HA, Sotkasiira J, Biervliet M, Benmansour A, Capri Y, et al: The mutation spectrum in *RECQL4* diseases. Eur J Hum Genet 2009;17:151–158.
40 Wang LL, Gannavarupu A, Kozinetz CA, Levy ML, Lewis RA, et al: Association between osteosarcoma and deleterious mutations in the *RECQL4* gene in Rothmund-Thomson syndrome. J Natl Cancer Inst 2003;95:669–674.
41 Beare JM, Dodge JA, Nevin NC: Cutis gyratum, acanthosis nigricans and other congenital anomalies. A new syndrome. Br J Dermatol 1969;81:241–247.
42 Stevenson RE, Ferlauto GJ, Taylor HA: Cutis gyratum and acanthosis nigricans associated with other anomalies: a distinctive syndrome. J Pediatr 1978;92:950–952.
43 Hall BD, Cadle RG, Golabi M, Morris CA, Cohen MM Jr: Beare-Stevenson cutis gyrata syndrome. Am J Med Genet 1992;44:82–89.
44 Izakovic J, Leitner S, Schachner LA: What syndrome is this? Beare-Stevenson cutis gyrata syndrome. Pediatr Dermatol 2003;20:358–360.
45 Przylepa KA, Paznekas W, Zhang M, Golabi M, Bias W, et al: Fibroblast growth factor receptor 2 mutations in Beare-Stevenson cutis gyrata syndrome. Nat Genet 1996;13:492–494.
46 Akai T, Iizuka H, Kishibe M, Kawakami S, Kobayashi A, Ozawa T: A case of Beare-Stevenson cutis gyrata syndrome confirmed by mutation analysis of the fibroblast growth factor receptor 2 gene. Pediatr Neurosurg 2002;37:97–99.
47 Eun S-H, Ha KS, Je B-K, Lee ES, Choi BM, et al: The first Korean case of Beare-Stevenson syndrome with a Tyr375Cys mutation in the fibroblast growth factor receptor 2 gene. J Korean Med Sci 2007;22:352–356.
48 Krepelová A, Baxová A, Calda P, Plavka R, Kapras J: *FGFR2* gene mutation (Tyr375Cys) in a new case of Beare-Stevenson syndrome. Am J Med Genet A 1998;76:362–364.
49 McGaughran J, Sinnott S, Susman R, Buckley MF, Elakis G, et al: A case of Beare-Stevenson syndrome with a broad spectrum of features and a review of the *FGFR2* Y375C mutation phenotype. Clin Dysmorphol 2006;15:89–93.
50 Vargas RA, Maegawa GH, Taucher SC, Leite JC, Sanz P, et al: Beare-Stevenson syndrome: two South American patients with *FGFR2* analysis. Am J Med Genet A 2003;121A:41–46.
51 Wang T-J, Huang C-B, Tsai F-J, Wu J-Y, Lai R-B, Hsiao M: Mutation in the *FGFR2* gene in a Taiwanese patient with Beare-Stevenson cutis gyrata syndrome. Clin Genet 2002;61:218–221.
52 Fonseca R, Costa-Lima MA, Cosentino V, Orioli IM: Second case of Beare-Stevenson syndrome with an *FGFR2* Ser372Cys mutation. Am J Med Genet A 2008;146A:658–660.
53 Slavotinek A, Crawford H, Golabi M, Tao C, Perry H, et al: Novel *FGFR2* deletion in a patient with Beare-Stevenson-like syndrome. Am J Med Genet A 2009;149A:1814–1817.
54 Upmeyer S, Bothwell M, Tobias JD: Perioperative care of a patient with Beare-Stevenson syndrome. Pediatr Anesth 2005;15:1131–1136.
55 Erol DD, Eser O: The expected difficult intubation of a patient with Beare-Stevenson syndrome. Pediatr Anesth 2006;16:801.
56 Opitz JM, Johnson RC, McCreadie SR, Smith DW: The C syndrome of multiple congenital anomalies. Birth Defects Orig Art Ser 1969;5:161–166.
57 Kaname T, Yanagi K, Chinen Y, Makita Y, Okamoto N, et al: Mutations in *CD96*, a member of the immunoglobulin superfamily, cause a form of the C (Opitz trigonocephaly) syndrome. Am J Hum Genet 2007;81:835–841.
58 Opitz JM, Putnam AR, Comstock JM, Chin S, Byrne JLB, et al: Mortality and pathological findings in C (Opitz trigonocephaly) syndrome. Fetal Pediatr Pathol 2006;25:211–231.
59 Bohring A, Silengo M, Lerone M, Superneau DW, Spaich C, et al: Severe end of Opitz trigonocephaly (C) syndrome or new syndrome? Am J Med Genet 1999;85:438–446.
60 David G, Sillence D, Hardwick R, Opitz JM: A case of Kabuki (Niikawa-Kuroki) syndrome associated with manifestations resembling C-trigonocephaly syndrome. Am J Med Genet A 2004;130A:389–392.
61 Fryns JP, Snoeck L, Kleczkowska A, van den Berghe H: Opitz trigonocephaly syndrome and terminal transverse limb reduction defects. Helv Paediatr Acta 1985;40:485–488.
62 Cleper R, Kauschansky A, Varsano I, Frydman M: Váradi syndrome (OFD VI) or Opitz trigonocephaly syndrome: overlapping manifestations in two cousins. Am J Med Genet 1993;47:451–455.

63 Sabry MA, Al Saleh Q, Farah S, Obenbergerova D, Simeonov S, et al: Another Arab patient with overlap of Váradi-Papp/Opitz trigonocephaly syndromes? Am J Med Genet 1997;68:54–57.
64 Preus M, Vekemans M, Kaplan P: Diagnosis of chromosome 3 duplication q23→qter, deletion p25→pter in a patient with the C (trigonocephaly) syndrome. Am J Med Genet 1986;23:935–943.
65 Chu TW, Teebi AS, Gibson L, Breg WR, Yang-Feng TL: FISH diagnosis of partial trisomy 13 and tetrasomy 13 in a patient with severe trigonocephaly (C) phenotype. Am J Med Genet 1994;52:92–96.
66 Chinen Y, Kaname T, Yanagi K, Saito N, Naritomi K, Ohta T: Opitz trigonocephaly C syndrome in a boy with a de novo balanced reciprocal translocation t(3;18)(q13.13;q12.1). Am J Med Genet A 2006;140A:1655–1657.
67 Sargent C, Burn J, Baraitser M, Pembrey ME: Trigonocephaly and the Opitz C syndrome. J Med Genet 1985;22:39–45.
68 Temtamy SA: Carpenter's syndrome: acrocephalopolysyndactyly. An autosomal recessive syndrome. J Pediatr 1966;69:111–120.
69 Cohen DM, Green JG, Miller J, Gorlin RJ, Reed JA: Acrocephalopolysyndactyly type II–Carpenter syndrome: clinical spectrum and an attempt at unification with Goodman and Summit syndromes. Am J Med Genet 1987;28:311–324.
70 Perlyn CA, Marsh JL: Craniofacial dysmorphology of Carpenter syndrome: lessons from three affected siblings. Plast Reconstr Surg 2008;121:971–981.
71 Jenkins D, Seelow D, Jehee FS, Perlyn CA, Alonso LG, et al: *RAB23* mutations in Carpenter syndrome imply an unexpected role for Hedgehog signaling in cranial-suture development and obesity. Am J Hum Genet 2007;80:1162–1170.
72 Cooper MK, Wassif CA, Krakowiak PA, Taipale J, Gong R, et al: A defective response to Hedgehog signaling in disorders of cholesterol biosynthesis. Nat Genet 2003;33:508–513.
73 Tarhan E, Oğuz H, Şafak MA, Samim E: The Carpenter syndrome phenotype. Int J Pediatr Otorhinolaryngol 2004;68:353–357.
74 Batra YK, Rajeev S, Nishtala S, Grover G: Anesthetic implications of Carpenter syndrome (Acrocephalopolysyndactyly type II). Pediatr Anesth 2008;18:1235–1237.
75 Taravath S, Tonsgard JH: Cerebral malformations in Carpenter syndrome. Pediatr Neurol 1993;9:230–234.
76 Ashby T, Rouse GA, de Lange M: Prenatal sonographic diagnosis of Carpenter syndrome. J Ultrasound Med 1994;13:905–909.
77 Balci S, Önol B, Eryilmaz M, Haytoglu T: A case of Carpenter syndrome diagnosed in a 20-week-old fetus with postmortem examination. Clin Genet 1997;51:412–416.
78 Arnaud-López L, Fragoso R, Mantilla-Capacho J, Narros-Núñez P: Crouzon with acanthosis nigricans. Further delineation of the syndrome. Clin Genet 2007;72:405–410.
79 Cohen MM Jr: Let's call it 'Crouzonodermoskeletal syndrome' so we won't be prisoners of our own conventional terminology. Am J Med Genet 1999;84:74.
80 Schweitzer DN, Graham JM Jr, Lachman RS, Jabs EW, Okajima K, et al: Subtle radiographic findings of achondroplasia in patients with Crouzon syndrome with acanthosis nigricans due to an Ala391Glu substitution in *FGFR3*. Am J Med Genet 2001;98:75–91.
81 Meyers GA, Orlow SJ, Munro IR, Przylepa KA, Jabs EW: Fibroblast growth factor receptor 3 *(FGFR3)* transmembrane mutation in Crouzon syndrome with acanthosis nigricans. Nat Genet 1995;11:462–464.
82 Reardon W, Winter RM, Rutland P, Pulleyn LJ, Jones BM, Malcolm S: Mutations in the fibroblast growth factor receptor 2 gene cause Crouzon syndrome. Nat Genet 1994;8:98–103.
83 Shiang R, Thompson LM, Zhu Y-Z, Church DM, Fielder TJ, et al: Mutations in the transmembrane domain of *FGFR3* cause the most common genetic form of dwarfism, achondroplasia. Cell 1994;78:335–342.
84 Superti-Furga A, Eich G, Bucher HU, Wisser J, Giedion A, et al: A glycine 375-to-cysteine substitution in the transmembrane domain of the fibroblast growth factor receptor-3 in a newborn with achondroplasia. Eur J Pediatr 1995;154:215–219.
85 Rousseau F, Bonaventure J, Legeal-Mallet L, Pelet A, Rozet J-M, et al: Mutations in the gene encoding fibroblast growth factor receptor-3 in achondroplasia. Nature 1994;371:252–254.
86 Jackson CE, Weiss L, Reynolds WA, Forman TF, Peterson JA: Craniosynostosis, midfacial hypoplasia, and foot abnormalities: an autosomal dominant phenotype in a large Amish kindred. J Pediatr 1976;88:963–968.
87 Cross HE, Opitz JM: Craniosynostosis in the Amish. J Pediatr 1969;75:1037–1044.
88 Heike C, Seto M, Hing A, Palidin A, Hu FZ, et al: Century of Jackson-Weiss syndrome: further definition of clinical and radiographic findings in 'lost' descendants of the original kindred. Am J Med Genet 2001;100:315–324.
89 Gorry MC, Preston RA, White GJ, Zhang Y, Singhai VK, et al: Crouzon syndrome: mutations in two spliceoforms of *FGFR2* and a common point mutation shared with Jackson-Weiss syndrome. Hum Mol Genet 1995;4:1387–1390.
90 Meyers GA, Day D, Goldberg R, Daentl DL, Przylepa KA, et al: *FGFR2* exon IIIa and IIIc mutations in Crouzon, Jackson-Weiss, and Pfeiffer syndromes: evidence for missense changes, insertions, and a deletion due to alternative RNA splicing. Am J Hum Genet 1996;58:491–498.
91 Park W-J, Meyers GA, Li X, Theda C, Day D, et al: Novel *FGFR2* mutations in Crouzon and Jackson-Weiss syndromes show allelic heterogeneity and phenotypic variability. Hum Mol Genet 1995;4:1229–1233.
92 Passos-Bueno MR, Sertié AL, Richieri-Costa A, Alonso LG, Zatz M, et al: Description of a new mutation and characterization of *FGFR1*, *FGFR2*, and *FGFR3* mutations among Brazilian patients with syndromic craniosynostoses. Am J Med Genet 1998;78:237–241.
93 Roscioli T, Flanagan S, Kumar P, Masel J, Gattas M, et al: Clinical findings in a patient with *FGFR1* P252R mutation and comparison with the literature. Am J Med Genet 2000;93:22–28.
94 Tartaglia M, Di Rocco C, Lajeunie E, Valeri S, Velardi F, Battaglia PA: Jackson-Weiss syndrome: identification of two novel *FGFR2* missense mutations shared with Crouzon and Pfeiffer craniosynostotic disorders. Hum Genet 1997;101:47–50.
95 Cohen MM Jr: Jackson-Weiss syndrome. Am J Med Genet 2001;100:325–329.
96 Cohen MM Jr: Craniosynostoses: phenotypic/molecular correlations. Am J Med Genet 1995;56:334–339.

97 Winter RM, Reardon W: Lumpers, splitters, and FGFRs. Am J Med Genet 1996;63:501–502.
98 Cohen MM Jr: A matter of reading English. Am J Med Genet 1996;63:503–504.
99 Li X, Lewanda AF, Eluma F, Jerald H, Choi H, et al: Two craniosynostotic syndrome loci, Crouzon and Jackson-Weiss, map to chromosome 10q23–q26. Genomics 1994;22:418–424.
100 Jabs EW, Li X, Scott AF, Meyers G, Chen W, et al: Jackson-Weiss and Crouzon syndromes are allelic with mutations in fibroblast growth factor receptor 2. Nat Genet 1994;8:275–279.
101 Jabs EW: Correction: Jackson-Weiss and Crouzon syndromes are allelic with mutations in fibroblast growth factor receptor 2. Nat Genet 1995;9:451.
102 Jacobsen P, Hauge M, Henningsen K, Hobolth N, Mikkelsen M, Philip J: An (11;21) translocation in four generations with chromosome 11 abnormalities in the offspring. A clinical, cytogenetical, and gene marker study. Hum Hered 1973;23:568–585.
103 Mattina T, Perrotta CS, Grossfeld P: Jacobsen syndrome. Orphanet J Rare Dis 2009;4:9.
104 Tunnacliffe A, Jones C, Le Paslier D, Todd R, Cherif D, et al: Localization of Jacobsen syndrome breakpoints on a 40-Mb physical map of distal chromosome 11q. Genome Res 1999;9:44–52.
105 Fryns JP, Kleczkowska A, Buttiens M, Marien P, van den Berghe H: Distal 11q monosomy. The typical 11q monosomy syndrome is due to deletion of subband 11q24.1. Clin Genet 1986;30:255–260.
106 Penny LA, Dell'Aquila M, Jones MC, Bergoffen J, Cunniff C, et al: Clinical and molecular characterization of patients with distal 11q deletions. Am J Hum Genet 1995;56:676–683.
107 Grossfeld PD, Mattina T, Lai Z, Favier R, Jones KL, et al: The 11q terminal deletion disorder: a prospective study of 110 cases. Am J Med Genet 2004;129A:51–61.
108 Krishnamurti L, Neglia JP, Nagarajan R, Berry SA, Lohr J, et al: Paris-Trousseau syndrome platelets in a child with Jacobsen's syndrome. Am J Hematol 2001;66:295–299.
109 Jones C, Slijepcevic P, Marsh S, Baker E, Langdon WY, et al: Physical linkage of the fragile site *FRA11B* and a Jacobsen syndrome chromosome deletion breakpoint in 11q23.3. Hum Mol Genet 1994; 3:2123–2130.
110 Jones C, Müllenbach R, Grossfeld P, Auer R, Favier R, et al: Co-localisation of CCG repeats and chromosome deletion breakpoints in Jacobsen syndrome: evidence for a common mechanism of chromosome breakage. Hum Mol Genet 2000; 9:1201–1208.
111 Hart A, Melet F, Grossfeld P, Chien K, Jones C, et al: *Fli-1* is required for murine vascular and megakaryocytic development and is hemizygously deleted in patients with thrombocytopenia. Immunity 2000;13:167–177.
112 Raslova H, Komura E, le Couédic JP, Larbret F, Debili N, et al: *FLI1* monoallelic expression combined with its hemizygous loss underlies Paris-Trousseau/Jacobsen thrombopenia. J Clin Invest 2004;114:77–84.
113 Phillips HM, Renforth GL, Spalluto C, Hearn T, Curtis ARJ, et al: Narrowing the critical region within 11q24–qter for hypoplastic left heart and identification of a candidate gene, *JAM3*, expressed during cardiogenesis. Genomics 2002; 79:475–478.
114 Coldren CD, Lai Z, Shragg P, Rossi E, Glidewell SC, et al: Chromosomal microarray mapping suggests a role for BSX and neurogranin in neurocognitive and behavioral defects in the 11q terminal deletion disorder (Jacobsen syndrome). Neurogenetics 2008;10:89–95.
115 Ye M, Hamzeh R, Geddis A, Varki N, Perryman MB, Grossfeld P: Deletion of *JAM-C*, a candidate gene for heart defects in Jacobsen syndrome, results in a normal cardiac phenotype in mice. Am J Med Genet A 2009;149A:1438–1443.
116 Beighton P, Cremin BJ, Kozlowski K: Osteoglophonic dwarfism. Pediatr Radiol 1980;10:46–50.
117 Greenberg F, Lewis RA: Osteoglophonic dysplasia. J Med Genet 1990;27:213–216.
118 Sklower Brooks S, Kassner G, Qazi Q, Keogh MJ, Gorlin RJ: Osteoglophonic dysplasia: review and further delineation of the syndrome. Am J Med Genet 1996; 66:154–162.
119 Santos H, Campos P, Alves R, Torrado A: Osteoglophonic dysplasia: a new case. Eur J Pediatr 1988;147:547–549.
120 Stöß H, Sieber E, Tietze HU: Osteoglophone Skelettdysplasie: Variante einer generalisierten fibrösen Dysplasie? Pathologe 1991;12:161–166.
121 Kelley RI, Borns PF, Nichols D, Zackai EH: Osteoglophonic dwarfism in two generations. J Med Genet 1983;20:436–440.
122 Fairbank T: An Atlas of General Affections of the Skeleton. Edinburgh, Livingstone, 1959.
123 Roberts TS, Stephen L, Beighton P: Osteoglophonic dysplasia: dental and orthodontic implications. Orthod Craniofac Res 2006;9:153–156.
124 White KE, Cabral JM, Davis SI, Fishburn T, Evans WE, et al: Mutations that cause osteoglophonic dysplasia define novel roles for *FGFR1* in bone elongation. Am J Hum Genet 2005;76:361–367.
125 Beighton P: Osteoglophonic dysplasia. J Med Genet 1989;26:572–576.
126 Farrow EG, Davis SI, Mooney SD, Beighton P, Mascarenhas L, et al: Extended mutational analyses of *FGFR1* in osteoglophonic dysplasia. Am J Med Genet A 2006;140A:537–539.
127 Sugarman G, Vogel MW: Craniofacial and musculoskeletal abnormalities. A questionable connective tissue disease. Synd Iden 1981;7:16–17.
128 Robinson PN, Neumann LM, Demuth S, Enders H, Jung U, et al: Shprintzen-Goldberg syndrome: fourteen new patients and a clinical analysis. Am J Med Genet A 2005;135A:251–262.
129 Loeys BL, Chen J, Neptune ER, Judge DP, Podowski M, et al: A syndrome of altered cardiovascular, craniofacial, neurocognitive and skeletal development caused by mutations in *TGFBR1* and *TGFBR2*. Nat Genet 2005;37:275–281.
130 Adès LC, Morris LL, Power RG, Wilson M, Haan EA, et al: Distinct skeletal abnormalities in four girls with Shprintzen-Goldberg syndrome. Am J Med Genet 1995;57:565–572.
131 Greally MT, Carey JC, Milewicz DM, Hudgins L, Goldberg RB, et al: Shprintzen-Goldberg syndrome: a clinical analysis. Am J Med Genet 1998;76: 202–212.
132 Mégarbané A, Hokayem N: Craniosynostosis and marfanoid habitus without mental retardation: report of a third case. Am J Med Genet 1998;77:170–171.
133 Loeys BL, Schwarze U, Holm T, Callewaert BL, Thomas GH, et al: Aneurysm syndromes caused by mutations in the TGF-β receptor. N Engl J Med 2006;355: 788–798.
134 Aalberts JJJ, van den Berg MP, Bergman JEH, du Marchie Sarvaas GJ, Post JG, et al: The many faces of aggressive aortic pathology: Loeys-Dietz syndrome. Neth Heart J 2008;16:299–304.

135 Robinson PN, Neumann LM, Tinschert S: Response to Kosaki et al., 'Molecular pathology of Shprintzen-Goldberg syndrome'. Am J Med Genet A 2006;140A: 109–110.
136 Lee YCG, Wilson CJ, Winship IM, Veale AG: Marfanoid habitus, dysmorphic features, and web neck. South Med J 2000;93:1197–1200.
137 Singh KK, Rommel K, Mishra A, Karck M, Haverich A, et al: *TGFBR1* and *TGFBR2* mutations in patients with features of Marfan syndrome and Loeys-Dietz syndrome. Hum Mutat 2006;27: 770–777.
138 Tran-Fadulu V, Pannu H, Kim DH, Vick III GW, Lonsford CM, et al: Analysis of multigenerational families with thoracic aortic aneurysms and dissections due to *TGFBR1* or *TGFBR2* mutations. J Med Genet 2009;46:607–613.
139 Sood S, Eldadah ZA, Krause WL, McIntosh I, Dietz HC: Mutation in *fibrillin-1* and the Marfanoid-craniosynostosis (Shprintzen-Goldberg) syndrome. Nat Genet 1996;12:209–211.
140 Watanabe Y, Yano S, Koga Y, Yukizane S, Nishiyori A, et al: P1148A in fibrillin-1 is not a mutation leading to Shprintzen-Goldberg syndrome. Hum Mutat 1997; 10:326–327.
141 Whiteman P, Downing AK, Handford PA: NMR analysis of cbEGF domains gives new insights into the structural consequences of a P1148A substitution in fibrillin-1. Protein Eng 1998;11:957–959.
142 Hewett DR, Lynch JR, Child A, Sykes BC: A new missense mutation of fibrillin in a patient with Marfan syndrome. J Med Genet 1994;31:338–339.
143 Kosaki K, Takahashi D, Udaka T, Kosaki R, Matsumoto M, et al: Molecular pathology of Shprintzen-Goldberg syndrome. Am J Med Genet A 2006;140A: 104–108.
144 van Steensel MAM, van Geel M, Parren LJMT, Schrander-Stumpel CTRM, Marcus-Soekarman D: Shprintzen-Goldberg syndrome associated with a novel missense mutation in *TGFBR2*. Exp Dermatol 2008;17:362–365.
145 Stheneur C, Collod-Béroud G, Faivre L, Gouya L, Sultan G, et al: Identification of 23 *TGFBR2* and 6 *TGFBR1* gene mutations and genotype-phenotype investigations in 457 patients with Marfan syndrome type I and II, Loeys-Dietz syndrome and related disorders. Hum Mutat 2008;29:E284–E295.
146 Adès LC, Sullivan K, Biggin A, Haan EA, Brett M, et al: *FBN1*, *TGFBR1*, and the Marfan-craniosynostosis/mental retardation disorders revisited. Am J Med Genet A 2006;140A:1047–1058.
147 Cohen MM Jr: Other syndromes with craniosynostosis; in Cohen MM Jr, MacLean RE (eds): Craniosynostosis: Diagnosis, Evaluation, and Management, 2nd ed. New York, Oxford University Press, 2000, pp 385–440.
148 Gupta AK, Koley S, Choudhary S, Bhake A, Saoji V, Salodkar A: A rare association of acanthosis nigricans with Crouzon syndrome. Indian J Dermatol Venereol Leprol 2010;76:65–67.

Maximilian Muenke
Building 35, Room 1B203
35 Convent Drive, MSC 3717
Bethesda, MD, 20892-3717 (USA)
Tel. +1 301 402 8167, Fax +1 301 496 7184, E-Mail muenke@nih.gov

Muenke M, Kress W, Collmann H, Solomon BD (eds): Craniosynostoses: Molecular Genetics, Principles of Diagnosis, and Treatment.
Monogr Hum Genet. Basel, Karger, 2011, vol 19, pp 143–151

Metopic Craniosynostosis Syndrome Due to Mutations in *GLI3*

D.M. McDonald-McGinn[a] · H. Feret[a] · H.-D. Nah[b] · E.H. Zackai[a,c]

[a]Division of Human Genetics, Department of Pediatrics, Children's Hospital of Philadelphia, [b]Division of Plastic and Reconstructive Surgery, Department of Surgery, The Children's Hospital of Philadelphia, [c]Departments of Obstetrics and Gynecology and Genetics, University of Pennsylvania School of Medicine, Philadelphia, Pa., USA

Abstract

We summarize the novel association of trigonocephaly and polysyndactyly in 3 unrelated patients due to mutations within the *GLI3* gene. *GLI3* acts as a downstream mediator of the Sonic hedgehog signal-transduction pathway which is essential for early development; playing a role in cell growth, specialization, and patterning of structures such as the brain and limbs. *GLI3* mutations have been identified in patients with Pallister Hall, Greig cephalopolysyndactyly (GCPS), postaxial polydactyly type A1, preaxial polydactyly type IV, and in 1 patient with acrocallosal syndrome (ACLS). Until recently, trigonocephaly has not been associated with abnormalities of *GLI3* and craniosynostosis is not a common feature of GCPS. However, there have been 2 prior reports of patients presenting with trigonocephaly, polysyndactyly, and agenesis of the corpus callosum, one of whom had a father with polysyndactyly. Both were originally considered GCPS, with the simplex case later considered ACLS. In retrospect, these 2 patients, with clinical diagnoses, and the 3 patients recently reported, with confirmed mutations, likely demonstrate a rare presentation of GCPS and highlight the extensive variability observed among patients with *GLI3* mutations.

Premature fusion of the metopic suture and its resultant abnormal head shape is also referred to as trigonocephaly because of the triangular appearance of the forehead when examined from above. Trigonocephaly may occur as an isolated malformation or as part of a multiple anomaly syndrome, with single gene, chromosomal, and teratogenic etiologies [1]. Examples of syndromic metopic craniosynostosis include: valproic acid embryopathy [2]; chromosomal aneuploidy such as deletions of 9p and 11q [3, 4]; and several previously described malformation syndromes whose molecular basis has yet to be defined including Frydman syndrome, with proposed autosomal dominant inheritance and normal intelligence [5]; Opitz C trigonocephaly syndrome, with additional anomalies including polydactyly and an inheritance pattern which is still unclear [4, 6]; Say-Meyer trigonocephaly syndrome, which includes short stature and developmental delay [4, 7]; and autosomal dominant trigonocephaly [8]. In addition, trigonocephaly has occasionally been observed in association with well described craniosynostosis conditions such as Crouzon syndrome due to a mutation in *FGFR2* [9]; Muenke syndrome due to the Pro250Arg mutation in *FGFR3* [10]; and Saethre-Chotzen syndrome prior to the availability of mutational analysis/microdeletion testing [11–13]. Moreover, a child with non-syndromic trigonocephaly was recently reported with an unusual mutation in the

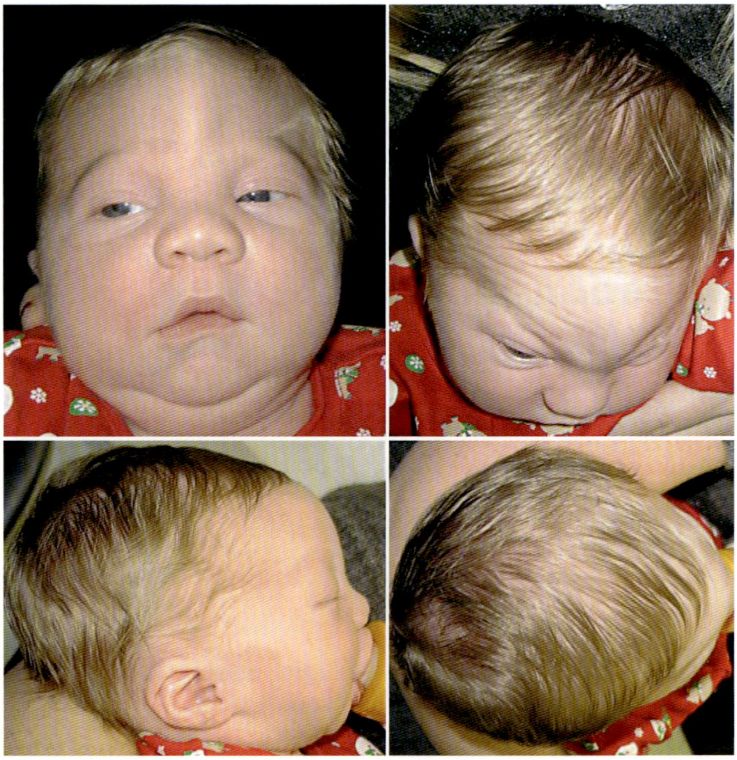

Fig. 1. Anterior-posterior view (AP), lateral and oblique cranial views of patient 1 at 2.5 weeks of age demonstrating trigonocephaly.

IgIII loop domain of *FGFR1* (Ile300Trp) [14]. However, no mutations were subsequently identified in 81 patients with both syndromic and nonsyndromic trigonocephaly screened for this unusual *FGFR1* mutation [15].

Greig cephalopolysyndactyly syndrome (GCPS; OMIM 175700) is a condition defined by Biesecker [16] as the constellation of true hypertelorism, macrocephaly and extremity involvement including preaxial polydactyly with cutaneous syndactyly of at least one limb or mixed pre- and postaxial polydactyly. GCPS is caused by mutations in the *GLI3* gene, located on chromosome 7p13. Craniosynostosis is not considered a common feature of GCPS [17], although in 1986, when reviewing the existing literature of GCPS, Cohen and MacLean stated that, 'absence of craniosynostosis occurs most commonly but craniosynostosis has been reported in approximately 5% of affected individuals and appears to be a low frequency finding' [18]. In a cohort of patients with trigonocephaly, Kini et al. [19] recently identified one patient with GCPS and a *GLI3* mutation, though no further clinical information was provided. However, in reviewing the prior literature, there had been no patients reported with craniosynostosis, including trigonocephaly, and a confirmed *GLI3* mutation, a fact which was later recognized by Cohen and MacLean [13]. Here, we further report 2 additional unrelated patients with metopic craniosynostosis syndrome and extremity involvement, with confirmed mutations in *GLI3* [20].

Case Reports

Patient 1

A male proband presented in infancy due metopic craniosynostosis (fig. 1) and 4 extremity

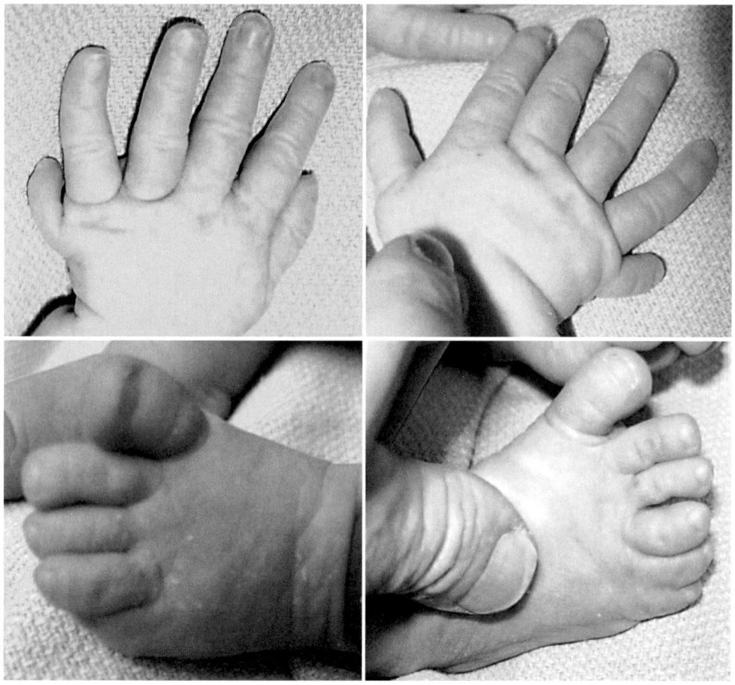

Fig. 2. AP hands and feet demonstrating 4 extremity postaxial polydactyly with cutaneous syndactyly of toes 5 and 6 in patient 1.

postaxial polydactyly (fig. 2). His length measured at approximately the 90th percentile for age, head circumference was 85th percentile, and interpupillary distance was 50th percentile. The trigonocephaly was appreciable with upslanting palpebral fissures. Full digit postaxial polydactyly of all 4 extremities was noted. In addition, the distal phalanges of both thumbs appeared broad (fig. 3). Premature fusion of the metopic suture was confirmed by 3-D CT scan (fig. 4). Follow-up developmental history at 14 months revealed no abnormalities. Family history was noncontributory.

Based on the premise that the patient seemingly had 2 separate entities (metopic suture fusion and postaxial polydactyly) the following laboratory studies were obtained: SNP array and *TWIST1* mutational analysis (Saethre-Chotzen testing) due to the trigonocephaly, as well as *GLI3* sequencing in light of the extremity findings. Both the array and *TWIST1* studies were normal, however the *GLI3* analysis revealed an apparently de novo novel frameshift mutation in exon 14 (c.4542_4545del CCAC) resulting in premature protein termination (p.His1515ProfsX3) [20].

Patient 2

A male proband presented during infancy due to a history of metopic craniosynostosis (fig. 5) and 4 extremity anomalies (fig. 6). On physical examination, his height was approximately 25th percentile for age, head circumference was 60th percentile, and interpupillary distance was 97th percentile. He had apparent trigonocephaly. His extremities were notable for bilateral complete cutaneous syndactyly of the 3rd and 4th fingers; duplication of the great toe on the right with soft tissue syndactyly of toes 2 and 3; and medial deviation of the great toe on the left. Premature fusion of the metopic suture was confirmed by 3-D

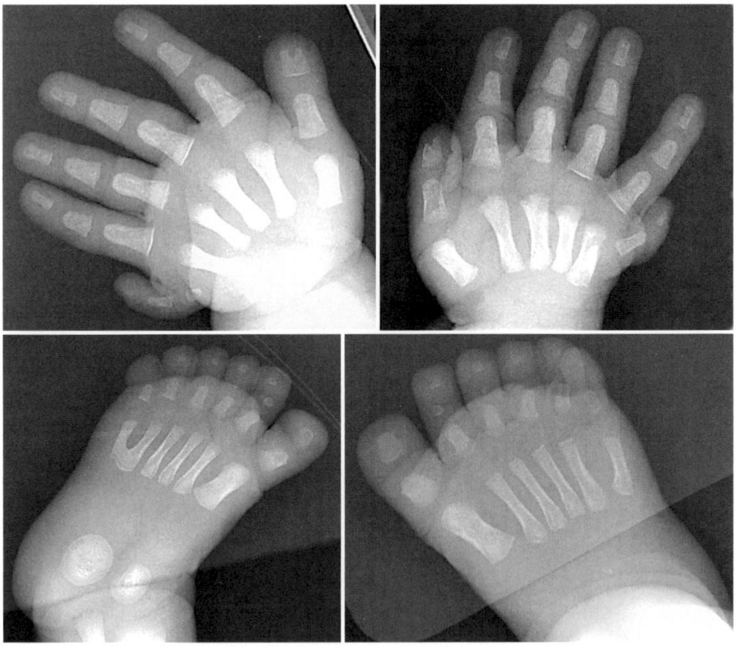

Fig. 3. Patient 1 radiographs demonstrating 4 extremity polydactyly. Note, bifid thumbs and Y-shaped metatarsal on the left.

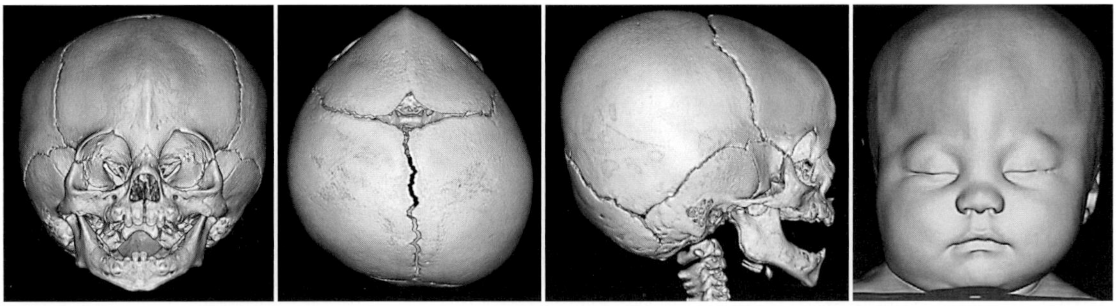

Fig. 4. AP, oblique, and lateral views with simulated reconstruction using 3-D CT scan imaging confirming metopic craniosynostosis in patient 1.

CT scan (fig. 7). Formal IQ testing and follow-up through adolescence revealed no signs of developmental or cognitive impairment. Family history was noncontributory.

Initially viewing the metopic synostosis and extremity findings as 2 separate entities, laboratory testing included a high resolution karyotype and analyses of the *FGFR*s and *TWIST1*. These studies were normal with the exception of identifying a paternally inherited 21 base pair duplication between nucleotides 243 and 277 of the *TWIST* gene resulting in an in-frame insertion of 7 amino acids N terminal to the DNA binding domain. This finding has subsequently been classified as a polymorphism [21]. Thereafter the identification of the *GLI3* mutation in our patient 1

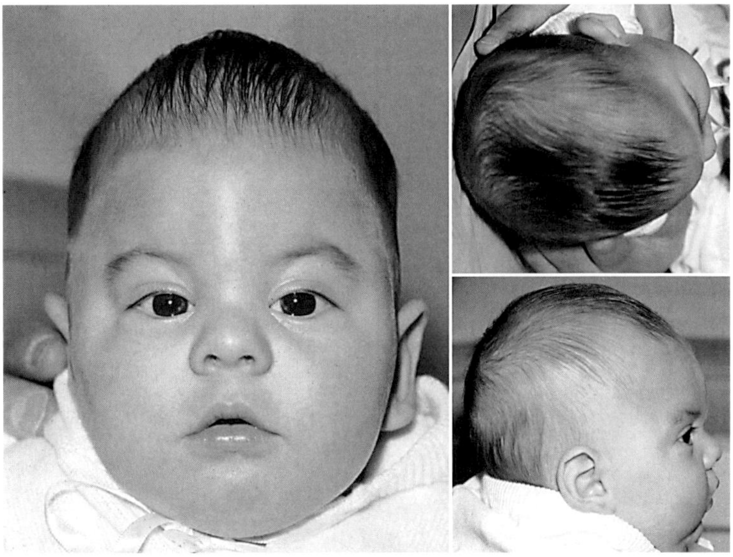

Fig. 5. AP, lateral and oblique cranial views of patient 2 at 4 months of age demonstrating trigonocephaly.

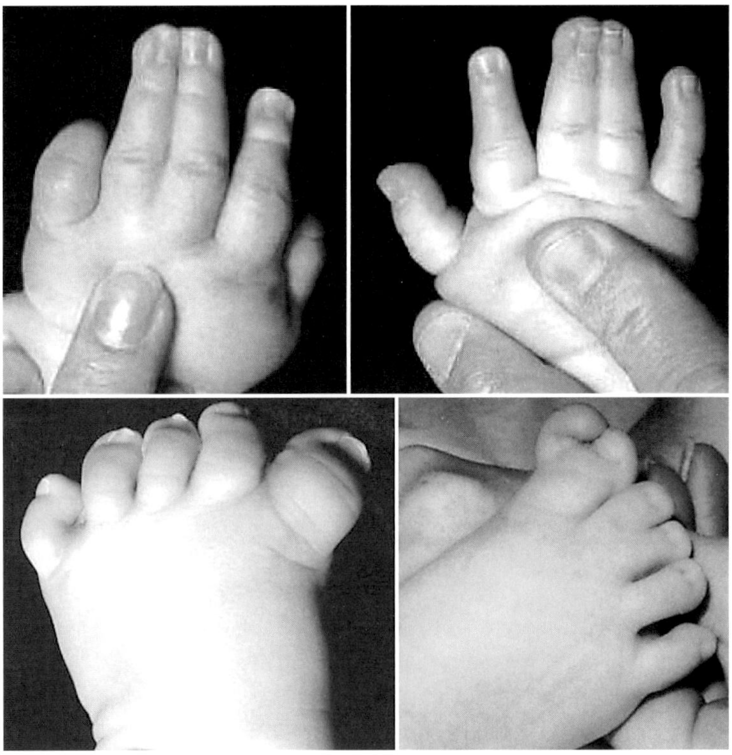

Fig. 6. AP hands and feet demonstrating cutaneous syndactyly of fingers 3 and 4; preaxial polydactyly and 2–3 cutaneous syndactyly of the right foot; and a medially deviated great toe on the left foot in patient 2.

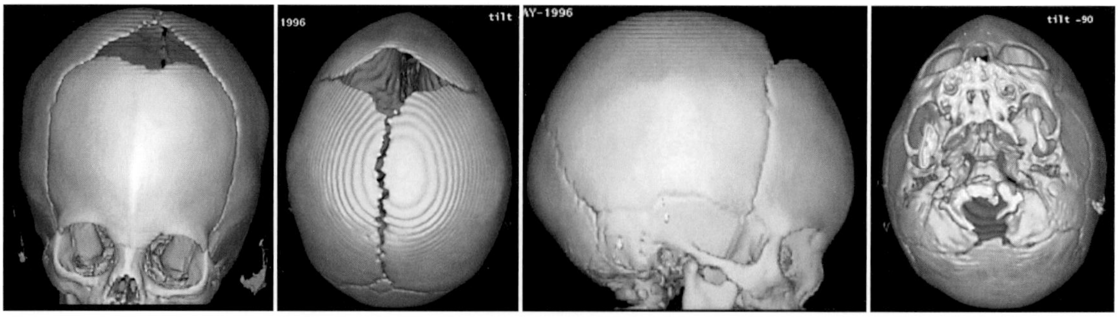

Fig. 7. AP, oblique, lateral, and axial views using 3-D CT scan imaging confirming metopic craniosynostosis in patient 2.

prompted us to perform similar testing on patient 2 which revealed a frameshift mutation in exon 6 of the *GLI3* gene (c.1018delA), resulting in a premature protein termination (p.Ser340ValfsX7). Parental studies are unavailable [20].

GLI3 Pathogenesis and Mutation Spectrum

The *GLI3* gene encodes a protein that is a zinc finger bi-functional transcription factor, having both a transcriptional repressor and activation effect. It is a downstream mediator of the Sonic hedgehog (SHH) signal-transduction pathway. This pathway is essential for early development as it plays a role in cell growth, cell specialization, and the patterning of structures such as the brain and limbs. Mutations in the *GLI3* gene have been found in patients with Pallister Hall syndrome (PHS), with variable clinical features including hypothalamic hamartoma, central and postaxial polydactyly, bifid epiglottis/laryngeal cleft, imperforate anus, and renal abnormalities; Greig cephalopolysyndactyly syndrome; postaxial polydactyly type A1; preaxial polydactyly type IV; and in one patient with acrocallosal syndrome, generally characterized by hallux duplication, postaxial polydactyly, absence of the corpus callosum, and developmental delay/mental retardation [22]. In addition, deletions including the *GLI3* gene have been identified in patients with overlapping features of GCPS and ACLS [3].

Genotype-phenotype correlations for *GLI3* mutations have been fairly well established [23]. Truncating mutations in the middle third of the gene are found in patients with Pallister-Hall syndrome. They generate a constitutive gain of function of the *GLI3* repressor protein that is likely to be independent of SHH controlled post-translational regulation. The remaining entities – GCPS, postaxial polydactyly type A1, and preaxial polydactyly type IV – are associated with *GLI3* mutations in the first and last third of the gene, resulting in haploinsufficiency. Postaxial polydactyly type A1 (OMIM #174200) is classically defined as having a well formed extra digit that articulates with the 5th finger or with an extra metacarpal. In addition, some individuals have broad thumbs. Preaxial polydactyly type IV (OMIM #174700) has postaxial polydactyly of the hand with more severe preaxial and postaxial polydactyly of the foot. Furthermore, the thumb may show a mild degree of duplication and there may be syndactyly of the 3rd and 4th fingers [24]. Radhakrishna et al. [24] have used the term *GLI3* morphopathy to lump these remaining entities, as the border of the phenotypic characterizations amongst the diagnoses is somewhat blurred. Johnston et al. [23] have also suggested that, 'many patients who present with features in the GCPS spectrum may not have manifestations amenable to phenotype diagnoses because of variable severity and nonspecific clinical features of GCPS' further stating that 'relaxed clinical criteria would be most useful in selecting patients for molecular analysis'.

With these 2 new cases in mind, it is noteworthy that Hootnick and Holmes in 1972 reported a father with polysyndactyly and his son with trigonocephaly, polysyndactyly and agenesis of the corpus callosum [27]. Thereafter this family was considered to have GCPS by Gorlin et al. [25]. Subsequently, in 1996, Guzzetta et al. [28] described a patient with trigonocephaly, polysyndactyly, and agenesis of the corpus callosum postulating a diagnosis of GCPS or Carpenter syndrome (now known to be caused by mutations in the *RAB23* gene). Though Fryns et al. [26] later suggested ACLS be considered as another diagnostic possibility for this patient, Gorlin et al. [25] comment that this would be an atypical case, in light of the fact that severe mental retardation is an almost universal finding in ACLS patients. Furthermore, they state, 'Since the child in the report of Guzzetta et al. also had trigonocephaly, it could be argued that this is a distinct, yet pathogenetically related condition'. Thus, it appears feasible that the patients described by Hootnick and Holmes and Guzzetta et al. [27, 28], both with metopic suture synostosis, polysyndactyly and normal development, as well as our 2 patients with trigonocephaly, polysyndactyly, and normal intelligence, due to confirmed *GLI3* mutations [20], represent a distinctive clinical presentation within the *GLI3* GCPS spectrum, highlighting the phenotypic variability emphasized by Radhakrishna et al. and their concept of *GLI3* morphopathy [24]. This is also supported by the biology of *GLI3*.

Genetic Mouse Models for *GLI3* Disorders

Given the essential role of the SHH-GLI3 signaling in antero-posterior specification of limb and digit formation, even a slight disturbance in the *GLI3* expression pattern is expected to produce a certain degree of limb deformity. Studies of a genetic mouse model for GCPS, *extra-toes* (Xt^{J}), which carries a *Gli3* null allele, show that heterozygous ($Gli3^{+/-}$) mice display mild preaxial polydactyly, while homozygous ($Gli3^{-/-}$) mice present severe polydactyly marked by complete loss of digit identity [29]. The greater severity exhibited in homozygous null mice underscores the importance of the expression level of GLI3 protein. Based on phenotypic similarity with $Gli3^{+/-}$ mice, the patients described in this report are likely to express functional GLI3 protein at a reduced level. However, the biochemical fate of the mutant RNAs and proteins has yet to be determined for their translatability, stability and function.

The polydactyly in $Gli3^{-/-}$ mouse mutants has been postulated to involve *Shh*. *Shh* is normally expressed only in the zone of polarizing activity (ZPA) located in the posterior part of the limb bud to organize antero-posterior patterning of the limb. In the $Gli3^{-/-}$ mutant limb bud, *Shh* is ectopically expressed on the anterior side opposite the ZPA, inducing the mirror image duplication of the limb and thus explaining the polydactyly [30]. In addition to determining digit identity and numbers, *Gli3* is involved in digit separation by inducing apoptosis in the mesenchyme through downstream effectors, Msx2 and possibly BMP4 [31, 32]. It is also involved in induction or maintenance of cell death by limiting the number of cells expressing *Fgf8* [33]. *Gli3* normally functions to repress *Fgf8*. In $Gli3^{-/-}$ mice, *Fgf8* is upregulated in the apical ectodermal ridge two-fold, with a reduction in apoptosis in the interdigital ridges, explaining the syndactyly.

Upregulation of *Fgf8* was seen in the anterior neural ridge, the isthmus, and the facial primordia in $Gli3^{-/-}$ mutant embryos [33]. FGF8 not only inhibits apoptosis but also stimulates Runx2 expression and osteoblast differentiation [34], which may explain for premature ossification of a midline suture. In fact, increasing evidence points to an inhibitory role of Gli3 repressor (Gli3-R) in skeletal development and osteogenesis. In vitro analyses have shown that Gli3-R inhibits expression and activity of 2 essential osteogenic factors, BMP2 and Runx2, respectively [35, 36]. The combination of a decrease in cell apoptosis and an increase in osteogenic differentiation may explain the occurrence of metopic synostosis as a part of the wide spectrum of non-overlapping clinical features in GLI3 morphopathies, which likely is a result of loss of GLI3-R function.

Conclusion and Implications

In summary, our 2 unrelated patients, with a rare collection of findings including trigonocephaly and polysyndactyly due to mutations within the last third (exon 14) and first third (exon 6) of the *GLI3* gene respectively [20], in conjunction with the patient reported by Kini et al. [19] with a confirmed mutation, and those reported by Hootnick and Holmes [27] and Guzzetta et al. [28], in whom no molecular analysis was pursued, represent a previously unrecognized presentation within the GCPS/GLI3 spectrum. Furthermore, based on the findings in these patients we would suggest *GLI3* mutational analysis and/or deletion studies in those individuals with metopic suture fusion and extremity anomalies along the spectrum of preaxial polydactyly type IV or postaxial polydactyly type AI in order to provide appropriate medical management and genetic counseling. As mutations in *GLI3* are inherited in an autosomal dominant manner, any affected individual would therefore have a 50% chance of having an affected offspring. Detection of a pathogenic mutation would also provide affected families with the options of preimplantation and prenatal diagnosis, and allow for identification of other at risk family members who may not have any outward phenotypic manifestations due to reduced penetrance. If *GLI3* mutation analysis becomes commonplace in patients presenting with this constellation of findings, it is likely that a larger cohort will emerge, and will perhaps render Cohen's remorse in having added craniosynostosis to the list of clinical features associated with GCPS to be considered unfounded.

Acknowledgements

The authors would like to thank Laurie Lunny, Sarah MacDougall, Kristin D'Aco, M.D., Patricia Schultz, M.S.N., Rosa Casasanto, and Rosa Soto for their expert assistance in the preparation of this manuscript, as well as the families of the 2 children presented here for allowing us to share their medical information and photographs.

References

1 Lajeunie E, Le Merrer M, Marchac D, Renier D: Syndromal and nonsyndromal primary trigonocephaly: Analysis of a series of 237 patients. Am J Med Genet 1998;75:211–215.
2 Lajeunie E, Barcik U, Thorne J, El Ghouzzi V, Bourgeois M, Renier D: Craniosynostosis and fetal exposure to sodium valproate. J Neurosurg 2001;95:778–782.
3 Johnston J, Olivos-Glander I, Turner J, Aleck K, Bird L, et al: Clinical and molecular delineation of the Greig cephalopolysyndactyly contiguous gene deletion syndrome and its distinction from acrocallosal syndrome. Am J Med Genet 2003;123A:236–242.
4 Azimi C, Kennedy S, Chitayat D, Chakraborty P, Clarke J, Forrest C, Teebi A: Clinical and genetic aspects of trigonocephaly: a study of 25 cases. Am J Med Genet 2003;117A:127–135.
5 Frydman M, Kauschansky A, Elian E: Trigonocephaly: a new familial syndrome. Am J Med Genet 1984;18:55–59.
6 Opitz JM, Johnson RC, McCreadie SR, Smith DW: The C syndrome of multiple congenital anomolies. Birth Defects 1969;5:161–166.
7 Say B, Meyer J: Familial trigonocephaly associated with short stature and developmental delay. Am J Dis Child 1981; 135:711–712.
8 Hennekam R, Van Den Boogaard M: Autosomal dominant craniosynostosis of the sutura metopica. Clin Genet 1990;38: 374–377.
9 Tartaglia M, Bordoni V, Velardi F, Basile R, Saulle E, et al: Fibroblast growth factor receptor mutational screening in newborns affected to metopic synostosis. Child's Nerv Syst 1999;15:389–394.
10 Van der Meulen J, Van den Ouweland A, Hoogeboom J: Trigonocephaly in Muenke syndrome. Am J Med Genet 2006; 140A:2493–2494.
11 Cristofori G, Filippi G: Saethre-Chotzen syndrome with trigonocephaly. Am J Med Genet 1992;44:611–614.

12 Hunter A, Rudd N, Hoffman H: Trigonocephaly and associated minor anomalies in mother and son. J Med Genet 1976; 13:77–79.
13 Cohen M, MacLean R: Craniosynostosis – Diagnosis, Evaluation and Management, 2nd ed. (Oxford University Press, New York 2000).
14 Kress W, Petersen B, Collmann H, Grimm T: An unusual FGFR1 mutation (fibroblast growth factor receptor 1 mutation) in a girl with non-syndromic trigonocephaly. Cytogenet Cell Genet 2000;91:138–140.
15 Jehee F, Alonso L, Cavalcanti D, Kim C, Wall S, et al: Mutational screening of FGFR1, CER1, and CDON in a large cohort of trigonocephalic patients. Cleft Palate-Cranio J 2006;43:148–151.
16 Biesecker L: What can you learn from one gene: GLI3. J Med Genet 2004;43: 465.
17 Biesecker L: The Greig cephalopolysyndactyly syndrome. Orphanet J Rare Dis 2008;3:10.
18 Cohen M, MacLean R: Craniosynostosis – Diagnosis, Evaluation and Management (Raven Press, New York 1986).
19 Kini U, Hurst JA, Byren JC, Hall SA, Johnson D, Wilkie AOM: Etiological heterogeneity and clinical characteristics of metopic synostosis: evidence from a tertiary craniofacial unit. Am J Med Genet Part A 2010;152A:1383–1389.
20 McDonald-McGinn DM, Feret H, Nah H-D, Bartlett SP, Whitaker LA, Zackai EH: Metopic craniosynostosis due to mutations in *GLI3*: a novel association. Am J Med Genet Part A 2010;152A: 1654–1660.
21 Elanko N, Sibbring JS, Metcalfe KA, Clayton-Smith J, Donnai D, et al: A survey of *TWIST* for mutations in craniosynostosis reveals a variable length polyglycine tract in asymptomatic individuals. Hum Mut 2001;18:535–541.
22 Elson E, Perveen R, Donnai D, Wall S, Black C: De novo *GLI3* mutation in acrocallosal syndrome: broadening the phenotypic spectrum of *GLI3* defects and overlap with murine models. J Med Genet 2002;39:804–806.
23 Johnston J, Olivos-Glander I, Killoran C, Elson E, Turner J, et al: Molecular and clinical analyses of Greig cephalopolysyndactyly and Pallister-Hall syndromes: robust phenotype prediction from the type and position of *GLI3* mutations. Am J Hum Genet 2005;76:609–622.
24 Radhakrishna U, Bornholdt D, Scott H, Patel U, Rossier C, et al: The phenotypic spectrum of GLI3 morphopathies includes autosomal dominant preaxial polydactyly type-IV and postaxial polydactyly type-A/B: no phenotype prediction from the position of *GLI3* mutations. Am J Hum Genet 1999;65: 645–655.
25 Gorlin R, Cohen M, Hennekam R: Syndromes of the Head and Neck, 4th ed. (Oxford University Press, New York 2001).
26 Fryns J, Devriendt K, Legius E: Polysyndactyly and trigonocephaly with partial agenesis of corpus callosum: an example of the variable clinical spectrum of the acrocallosal syndrome? Clin Dysmorphol 1997;6:285–286.
27 Hootnick D, Holmes L: Familial polysyndactyly and craniofacial anomalies. Clin Genet 1972;3:128–134.
28 Guzzetta V, Lecora M, Rossi G, Berni Canani M, Andria G: Polysyndactyly and trigonocephaly with partial agenesis of corpus callosum. Clin Dysmorphol 1996;5: 179–182.
29 Hui C, Joyner A: A mouse model of Greig cephalopolysyndactyly syndrome: the *extra-toes^J* mutation contains an intragenic deletion of the *Gli3* gene. Nat Genet 1993;3:241–246.
30 Büscher D, Bosse B, Heymer J, Rüther U: Evidence for genetic control of Sonic hedgehog by *Gli3* in mouse limb development. Mech Dev 1997;62:175–182.
31 Lallemand Y, Bensoussan V, Cloment C, Robert B: Msx genes are important apoptosis effectors downstream of the Shh/Gli3 pathway in the limb. Dev Biol 2009;331:189–198.
32 Bastida M, Delgado M, Wang B, Fallon JF, Fernandez-Teran M, Ros M: Levels of Gli3 repressor correlate with *Bmp4* expression and apoptosis during limb development. Dev Dyn 2004;231:148–160.
33 Aoto K, Nishimura T, Eto K, Motoyama J: Mouse GLI3 regulates *Fgf8* expression and apoptosis in the developing neural tube, face, and limb bud. Dev Biol 2002; 251:320–332.
34 Zhou Y, Xu X, Chen L, Li C, Brodie S, Deng C: A Pro250Arg substitution in mouse Fgfr1 causes increased expression of Cbfa1 and premature fusion of calvarial sutures. Hum Mol Genet 2000;9: 2001–2008.
35 Garrett I, Chen D, Gutierrez G, Zhao M, Escobedo A, et al: Selective inhibitors of the osteoblast proteasome stimulate bone formation in vivo and in vitro. J Clin Invest 2003;111:1771–1782.
36 Ohba S, Kawaguchi H, Kugimiya F, Ogasawara T, Kawamura N, et al: Patched1 haploinsufficiency increases adult bone mass and modulates Gli3 repressor activity. Dev Cell 2008;14:689–699.

Donna M. McDonald-McGinn
Clinical Genetics Center, Children's Hospital of Philadelphia
34th Street and Civic Center Boulevard
Philadelphia, PA, 19104 (USA)
Tel. +1 215 590 2920, Fax +1 215 590 3298, E-mail mcginn@email.chop.edu

Muenke M, Kress W, Collmann H, Solomon BD (eds): Craniosynostoses: Molecular Genetics, Principles of Diagnosis, and Treatment.
Monogr Hum Genet. Basel, Karger, 2011, vol 19, pp 152–164

Craniosynostosis and Chromosomal Alterations

M.R. Passos-Bueno · R.D. Fanganiello · F.S. Jehee

Human Genome Center, Department of Genetics and Evolutionary Biology, University of São Paulo, São Paulo, Brazil

Abstract

A large number of patients with craniosynostosis and chromosomal rearrangements have been described in the last decades. Through a comparative analysis of these cases, we discuss in this chapter their relative frequency, heterogeneity, complexity of the rearrangement, type of synostosis involved and their contribution to the characterization of the etiology of the craniosynostosis. The use of chromosomal abnormalities in the identification of causative loci and genes in craniosynostosis and suture development has not been straightforward, particularly due to the small number of cases per chromosomal abnormality, incomplete penetrance of the malformation's clinical signs, and the type of chromosomal rearrangements. However, progress has been made in recent years, and several novel candidates have been discovered. For genetic counseling purposes, chromosomal analysis through routine cytogenetics or by higher resolution techniques, such as MLPA or array CGH, is indicated once *FGFR-*, *TWIST1-* or *EFNB1*-related syndromes are excluded.

Craniosynostosis is a major congenital malformation that affects the craniofacial complex. It has an estimated prevalence of approximately 1:2,000–3,000 births and is characterized by the premature closure of one or several cranial sutures. Its onset can be variable, ranging from the prenatal developmental period until early childhood [1, 2].

Craniosynostosis is quite heterogeneous both in terms of its clinical aspects as well as its molecular etiology. It comprises both isolated (non-syndromic) forms, with the sagittal suture being the most affected of the sutures, and syndromic forms, which may be accompanied by a constellation of other signs, such as calvaria, orbit and/or face deformities, developmental delay, limb abnormalities, and heart defects. The primary treatment is usually surgical in nature, with goals of skull shape correction, intracranial pressure alleviation, and of creating space for the brain to follow its appropriate growth program [3].

It has been predicted that the precocious differentiation of stem cells to osteoblasts at the sutures would be the primary mechanism leading to this phenomenon. However, this proposition seems to be overall very general and even oversimplified, and a much more complex, cellularly and molecularly elaborate process might be involved, as exemplified by the demonstration that deficiency of ephrin, which is a causative mechanism of craniosynostosis, disturbs the boundaries between cranial neural stem cells and other cells during the development of the skull [4, 5].

Premature ossification in craniosynostosis can be triggered by 3 major events: environmental factors, gene mutations or chromosomal aberrations.

Amongst common environmental factors that may cause anomalies including craniosynostosis are intrauterine head compression [6–10], maternal or neonatal hyperthyroidism [11–14] and fetal exposure to teratogenic substances such as diphenylhydantoin [15], retinoids [16], valproate [17–19], aminopterin [20], fluconazole [21] and cyclophosphamide [22].

Currently, mutations in 8 genes, namely *FGFR1*, *-2*, and *-3*, *TWIST1*, *EFNB1*, *MSX2*, *POR* and *RAB23*, are unmistakably associated with syndromic craniosynostosis [23, 24]. Except for the recessive nature of the *RAB23* mutations, mutations in all the other loci are associated with an autosomal dominant pattern of inheritance with high penetrance, though clinical expressivity of the disease can be widely variable.

With the exception of chromosomes 16 and 19, a wide set of chromosomal aberrations, mainly deletions and duplications, have been described in association with craniosynostosis, including deletions 2q, 3p, 7p, 9p, 11p and duplications 1q, 5q, 13q and 15q [25–33]. This mechanism contributes to explain approximately 16% of syndromic craniosynostosis.

Our current knowledge of the pathogenetic mechanisms of craniosynostosis and of normal suture biology is still limited, and is mainly based on the identification of genes and gene defects in a few autosomal dominant and recessive craniosynostosis syndromes. The identification of structural chromosomal abnormalities in patients and the refinement of the segments involved in these rearrangements afford an interesting opportunity both to identify genes related to craniosynostosis and to determine important loci for canonical cranial suture development and closure.

Chromosomal Alterations

A broad range of chromosomal alterations involving almost all chromosomes have been reported in patients with syndromic craniosynostosis (table 1). Except for a few chromosomal alterations, which include the deletions 9p24-p21 and 11q23-q25, most of these have been described in only 1 case or in a small number of subjects. The extensive and remarkable variety of chromosomal abnormalities illustrates the great genetic heterogeneity of this family of malformations, and raises the possibility that there might be genes in several distinct chromosomal regions implicated in the molecular cause of craniosynostosis.

Even though a diverse group of chromosomal rearrangements has been described, deletions are the most prevalent type, followed by duplications. With the use of robust, high resolution techniques, such as array-based comparative genomic hybridization (array CGH), it has been possible to show that these chromosomal aberrations can be very complex and can include deleted and duplicated segments in the same chromosomal region [34–36]. Although full trisomy of chromosome 9 does not lead to viable individuals, mosaicism of this chromosome has been reported in a few patients with craniosynostosis [37]. It is thus possible that some cases of craniosynostosis are due to mosaicism restricted to a minute subset of tissues, including cranial tissues, a mechanism that could in part explain the difficulties in dissecting the genetics of this group of disorders.

Although it is necessary to be cautious about the correlation between the loci or type of chromosomal alteration and the synostotic site, one or more sutures are found to be associated with specific types of chromosomal alterations. Fusion of the metopic suture appears to be the most prevalent type of craniosynostosis, both in connection to deletions (~60%) and to duplications (~50%). While sagittal and lambdoid suture synostoses seem to be more prevalent among duplications (~40%) than among deletions (~20%), the involvement of coronal suture is more prevalent among chromosomal deletions (~20%; table 1). Intriguingly, while the metopic is the most commonly involved suture among the chromosomopathies, it is the least commonly affected suture in the autosomal

Table 1. Chromosomal alterations in patients with syndromic craniosynostosis. The first article where the referred aberration was reported is cited.

Chromosome aberration	Suture involved, craniosynostosis type	References
del 1p36	metopic, sagittal and coronal	[34]
del 1q24.4-q31	not specified	[64]
del 1qter	metopic	[52]
del 1qter/dup 13qter	metopic	[65]
del 1qter/dup 15qter	metopic	[52]
del 2q24.3-q31	coronal and sagittal	[66]
del 2q32.2-q34	metopic	[67]
del 2q32.1-q33	metopic	[52]
del 3p25-pter	brachy-trigonocephaly	[26]
del 3p25/dup 6q21	acrocephalosyndactyly	[68]
del 3p25/dup 7q36	mid segment of lambdoid and left coronal	[36]
del 3q	metopic (Opitz C syndrome)	[69]
del 4q21.1-q22.1	not specified	[70]
del 4q34.3-qter/dup 4q32.3-q34.3	metopic	[71]
del 5p14-pter/dup 13q13-qter	not specified	[72]
del 6q22.2-q23.1	not specified	[73, 74]
del 7p	metopic, coronal	[75]
del 7p22/dup 2q3	not specified	[76]
del 7p21-pter	metopic, coronal	[77]
del 7p15-pter	Saethre-Chotzen syndrome	[78]
del 7p14-p15.1	coronal bilateral	[52]
del 7p13-pter	metopic, coronal	[79]
del 7p13-p15	metopic, coronal	[79]
del 7p11.2-p15.1	sagittal	[53]
del 7q11.22-q11.23	not specified	[80]
del 8q21-q22	not specified	[81]
del 8q13.3-q22.1	lambdoid	[82]
del 9p24-pter/dup 5q32-qter	sagittal	[83]
del 9p23	metopic	[84]
del 9p22-pter	metopic	[85]
del 9p22.3-pter/dup 4qter	metopic	[43]
del 9p22.3-p24.2	metopic	[43]
del 9p21.3-pter	metopic	[43]
del 9p12-p13.3	not specified	[86]
del 9q22.32-q22.33	trigonocephaly	[87]
del 9q34.3	metopic (Opitz C syndrome)	[88]
del 9qter/dup 17qter	metopic	[52]

Table 1. Continued

Chromosome aberration	Suture involved, craniosynostosis type	References
del 10p13-pter	trigonocephaly	[89]
del 10q26-qter	metopic	[90]
del 11 q24.1-qter	metopic, brachycephaly	[31]
del 11q24.1-qter/dup 4q31.3-qter	trigonocephaly	[31]
del 11q23.3-qter	metopic	[43]
del 11q23.1	trigonocephaly	[91]
del 12p12	sagittal	[92]
del 12q	metopic	[93]
del 13q	not specified	[94]
del 14q22.1-q23.2	lambdoid	[95]
del 15q15-q22.1	turribrachycephaly	[96]
del 15q15-q22.2	coronal, metopic and sagittal	[97]
del 17p11.2-p11.2	brachycephaly	[98]
del 17q23.1-q24.2	not specified	[99]
del 18p/dup 20p	not specified	[100]
del 22q11.2	coronal unilateral and bilateral	[101]
45,X	not specified	[102]
45,X	metopic	[52]
46,XXX, del 2q14-q21	not specified	[103]
47,XXY, del 15q11-q13	coronal	[104]
del Y	not specified	[105]
dup/del 1p36.3-pter	metopic and sagittal	[97]
dup 1q24-qter	trigonocephaly	[106]
dup 2q3/del 7p22	not specified	[81]
dup 3pter	metopic	[107]
dup 3p21-pter/del 18p11-pter	not specified	[108]
dup 3q	not specified	[109]
dup 3q23-qter/del 3p25-pter	metopic (Opitz C syndrome)	[110]
dup 4p16.1-p16.3/del 2q37.1-qter	cloverleaf skull	[111]
dup 5p	not specified	[112]
dup 5q11.2-5q14	not specified	[29]
dup 5q34-qter	sagittal and lambdoid	[61]
dup 5q33.1/del 10q26.3	metopic	[113]
dup 5q35.1/del 17p13.3	metopic	[113]
dup 6p21/del 2p25	not specified	[114]
dup 6q25-qter	turricephaly	[115]
dup 6q/del 10q	acrocephalosyndactyly	[116]

Table 1. Continued

Chromosome aberration	Suture involved, craniosynostosis type	References
dup 7p11.1-pter	lambdoid	[117]
dup 9p22.3-p24.3	metopic	[118]
dup 8p23q22	not specified	[119]
dup 13q22-qter	metopic	[120]
dup 13q22/tetrasomy 13q	metopic	[30]
dup 11q13.5-q21	trigonocephaly	[121]
dup 11q11-q13.3 mosaic	metopic, sagittal, lambdoid	[57]
dup 13q14-qter	trigonocephaly	[122]
dup 14q	not specified	[123]
dup 15q26.1-qter/del 13q34-qter	sagittal	[25]
dup 15q26-qter/del 2q37-qter	not specified	[124]
dup 15q25.1-qter/del 13q34-qter	sagittal	[125]
dup 17q24.2-qter	sagittal	[52]
dup 17q24-q25.1	not specified	[126]
dup 17q24-qter/del 2pter	metopic (Opitz C syndrome)	[127]
dup Xq22.3	metopic (FG syndrome)	[43]
dup Xp22.2	metopic and coronal bilateral	[52]
dup Xp21.2-pter	not specified	[128]
tetrasomy 15q25.3-qter	sagittal, metopic	[129]
trisomy 9 mosaic	coronal	[37]
trisomy 21	metopic	[130]
triploidy	not specified	[131]
ins(7;9)(p21.2;p21.2p24.2)	Saethre-Chotzen syndrome (cloverleaf skull)	[52]
t(1;18)(p31;q11)	not specified	[132]
t(1;19)(p10;q10)	not specified	[133]
t(2;7)(p24;p21),ins(7)(p21.3q21.3q22)dn	bilateral coronal	[134]
t(5;21)(q13;q22)	not specified	[135]
t(9;13)(q32;q22)	metopic	[136]
t(9;11)(q33;p15)	lambdoid, sagittal	[56]

dominant conditions caused by mutations in the *FGFR* genes or *TWIST*. Considering also the fact that the metopic suture is the only one entirely of neural crest origin, this further suggests that the signaling pathways leading to its closure might be distinct from those involved in the fusion of the coronal suture, which has a dual origin: neural crest and mesenchyme. The small amount of cases described with each chromosomal aberration has been one of the major limitations to establish the most relevant chromosomal regions that might harbor genes involved in suture biology; in addition, the complexity of the rearrangements and the incomplete penetrance of the craniosynostoses can interfere with the determination of the effect of genes in the phenotype.

Despite these difficulties, progress has been achieved in the identification of candidate regions and/or genes.

Craniosynostosis Syndromes Due to Chromosomal Deletions: 9p and 11q

Partial deletions of the short arm of chromosome 9 (9p24-p22, monosomy 9p syndrome) and of the long arm of chromosome 11 (11q23-qter, monosomy 11q syndrome) are the most common recurrent chromosomal alterations associated with syndromic craniosynostosis. Due to the relatively large number of studied cases of monosomy 9p and 11q, the associated phenotypes have been relatively well described. Although penetrance is not complete, even for patients with comparable deletions [38–41], efforts have been made to identify the critical region and gene(s) for craniosynostosis in these chromosomal areas.

The main clinical manifestations of monosomy 9p syndrome (MIM #158170) include dysmorphic craniofacial features (trigonocephaly, midface hypoplasia, upward-slanting palpebral fissures and a long philtrum), hypotonia and mental retardation [42]. At the molecular level, deletion 9p is heterogeneous and is associated with variable extents of the deletion. The critical region for a consensus phenotype has recently been reduced from a 4–6-Mb interval to a 300-kb interval on 9p22 which excludes *CER1*, a gene previously suggested as candidate for trigonocephaly [42–44]. As a few patients have been reported with trigonocephaly and a 9p deletion that does not overlap this smaller candidate region, it has been suggested that there might be another candidate region for craniosynostosis [45]. In half of the cases, the breakpoint occurs in a de novo fashion at 9p22. The remaining cases, which mainly occur at band 9p24, result from association with other unbalanced chromosome segments, as a consequence of de novo rearrangements, or segregation of parental unbalanced chromosomes in gametogenesis [46]. It is also important to note that not all deletions can be detected through conventional karyotype analysis and therefore a patient with clinical features compatible with monosomy 9p and normal karyotype should be tested for 9p deletion with higher resolution techniques, such as MLPA or array CGH [43].

Deletion 11q syndrome, frequently called Jacobsen syndrome (JBS; OMIM 147791) is a contiguous gene syndrome clinically characterized by dysmorphic craniofacial features (trigonocephaly, hypertelorism, ptosis, downslanting palpebral fissures, a broad nasal bridge with a short nose, a thin upper lip and low set, and malformed ears), anomalous genitalia, thrombocytopenia, developmental delay, congenital heart disease and short stature [38]. In most cases (~85%), the partial monosomy of 11q is the result of a terminal de novo deletion, with breakpoints usually occurring at or distal to 11q23.3. Alternatively, rearrangements involving other chromosomes sometimes present in a balanced form in a family, and may subsequently result in deletion 11q in one patient, which in these cases can be associated with additional complex imbalances. The minimum region for expression of the JBS phenotype spans about 14 Mb. Despite difficulties in establishing correlations between the location of the deletion and the phenotype, association of some regions and genes with certain phenotypes has been attempted. For craniosynostosis, the main focus of this article, the candidate region containing genes involved in suture development has been localized to a region bounded by D11S933 (124 Mb) and D11S912 (128 Mb). The *BARX2* gene maps within this critical region, and based on its expression pattern it was suggested as a possible candidate gene for the development of facial dysmorphism and/or craniosynostosis in JBS [38].

Chromosomal Rearrangements and Their Contribution to the Identification of Craniosynostotic Candidate Genes

Chromosomal rearrangements involving the 7p21 region represent the most successful contribution of using structural chromosome alterations for the identification of genes associated with craniosynostosis. In the first half of the 1990s, Saethre-Chotzen syndrome (SCS) had its locus mapped to 7p21 through a combination of results from chromosome rearrangement studies and data from linkage analysis [47–49]. The comparison of patients with different chromosomal rearrangements was crucially important in narrowing down the candidate region for SCS, at a time period in which sequencing of the human genome was still a distant goal. The mapping of the *TWIST1* gene, which encodes a basic helix-loop-helix transcription factor, to 7p22-p21 and the demonstration in 2 seminal papers that mutations in this gene cause SCS, led the authors to consider it to be the responsible locus for this disease [50, 51]. Indeed, subsequently, this finding was confirmed by several other reports and there are currently at least 97 different disease causing mutations in the *TWIST1* gene described among 153 patients worldwide, mostly with SCS phenotype [24].

Characterization of the breakpoints of some cytogenetically balanced rearrangements in SCS patients revealed that the coding region of the *TWIST1* gene is preserved and it is thus possible that the breakpoints disrupt an important regulatory sequence of *TWIST1* or alternatively, a second gene on 7p [24]. The possibility that there might be other loci at 7p that, when disrupted, cause craniosynostosis, has also been suggested by the description of patients with craniosynostosis and 7p deletions that do not encompass the 7p21 region [52, 53]. These genes, however, have not yet been identified.

Based on the study of patients with different sized deletions, duplications and/or triplications of 1p36 and with overlapping or diametrically divergent phenotypes, Gajecka et al. were able to narrow the candidate region that might contain a gene for suture development [34]. They suggested that the haploinsufficiency of matrix metalloproteinase 23 genes *(MMP23A* and *MMP23B)*, which have been previously reported as involved in bone remodeling and in bone matrix resorption [54], would be associated with large and late-closing anterior fontanelles, while triplication of the region containing these genes would lead to craniosynostosis. Subsequently, patients with deletions or duplication at 1p36 that do not corroborate this association have been reported, suggesting that overexpression of *MMP23A/B* genes is not sufficient to cause craniosynostosis [52, 55].

SOX6 (11p15), *TLR4* and *CALCA* (9q33) genes have been suggested as candidate genes for craniosynostosis based on the cloning of the breakpoints of a male infant with a de novo balanced translocation t(9;11)(q33;p15) and craniofacial dysostosis, which included craniosynostosis of the lambdoid and of the sagittal sutures. In addition, a missense mutation in *SOX6* was identified in 1 out of 104 patients with craniosynostosis screened for mutations in these genes [56]. These genes are interesting candidates for craniosynostosis, though further studies are necessary to clarify if they indeed play a role in craniosynostosis and in suture biology in general.

The *FGF3* and *FGF4* genes, mapped at 11q11-q12, are 2 other interesting loci that have been suggested as candidates for craniosynostosis, based on the analysis of 2 syndromic patients with 11q duplication and premature fusion of the metopic, sagittal and lambdoid sutures in 1 patient and trigonocephaly in the other [57]. The potential functional role of *FGF3* and *FGF4* genes in suture biology was further supported by the observation of upregulation of Fgf3 and Fgf4 in mice with craniofacial abnormalities similar to some human craniosynostosis syndromes [58].

CD96, a member of the immunoglobulin superfamily, has been pointed out as candidate for C (Opitz trigonocephaly) syndrome, which includes premature fusion of the metopic suture as part of the phenotype. The *TACTILE* gene, which codes for CD96, was disrupted at the 3q13.3 breakpoint in a balanced chromosomal translocation, t(3;18)(q13.13;q12.1) in a boy with C syndrome [59]. In addition, a de novo missense mutation in the *TACTILE* gene in a patient with the diagnosis of C-like syndrome further supports the importance of this gene in the etiology of this syndromic form of trigonocephaly [59].

Clinical description combined with cytogenetic and molecular analysis of chromosomal alterations has also contributed to corroborate molecular mechanisms associated with suture biology. For example, only 1 single mutation in the *MSX2* gene has been so far reported as causative for an autosomal dominant form of craniosynostosis, the Boston type [60]. Overdose of MSX2 due to trisomy of 5q34-q35 was suggested to cause craniosynostosis, a common clinical alteration in patients with 5q trisomy [35, 61].

Submicroscopic Rearrangements: An Important Cause of Craniosynostosis?

Chromosomal alterations account for about 16–20% of the syndromic craniosynostotic cases, while point or small mutations in 5 of the 8 known genes contribute to about 30% [23]. Recent work by our group using a combination of methods, including conventional karyotype, polymorphic microsatellite segregation analysis (PMSA) at 9p and 11q regions, subtelomeric multiplex ligation-dependent probe amplification (MLPA) and array CGH in 45 syndromic craniosynostotic subjects, led to the identification of chromosomal anomalies in 42.2% of patients. Considering that 27.8% (10/36) of the patients with normal conventional karyotype carried submicroscopic imbalances, these results imply that submicroscopic chromosomal alterations represent an important causative mechanism in syndromic craniosynostosis [52]. The most prevalent type of suture involved was again the metopic suture (57.8%), but coronal synostosis (17.8%), multiple synostosis (15.6%) and sagittal synostosis (8.9%) were also reported. Even though craniosynostosis consists of a prominent feature in this set of patients, these proportions may not be representative of syndromic craniosynostosis in general because our sample is biased towards metopic synostosis and severe cases, in which we indeed expect a higher frequency of chromosomal abnormalities. Although these findings should be verified in other cohorts of patients, they suggest that further submicroscopic chromosomal analyses should be done in individuals with these disorders and with normal conventional karyotype.

Most cases of single metopic synostosis described herein presented as typical trigonocephaly. However a few exceptions are noted, such as the 2 patients with deletion 9p and associated turricephaly and turriplagiocephaly [42]. It is of note that the chromosomal abnormality by itself seems not to determine whether metopic synostosis will lead to typical trigonocephaly or other forms of craniostenosis, as seen in the 2 brothers with the same chromosomal abnormality derived from a der(9)t(9;4)(p22.3;q34), where only one of them developed turricephaly [42]. Brachycephaly without coronal involvement was also seen in a few cases of metopic synostosis, however, in these instances, it is difficult to define whether the cranial shape is a primary abnormality or secondary to a positional effect due to hypotonia and severe developmental delay.

Conclusions

The numerous and heterogeneous chromosomal rearrangements so far described indicate the complexity of suture development, which must depend on a large number of genes distributed within the human genome. The analysis of these alterations with high resolution techniques is now leading to the identification of novel potential candidate genes for suture biology and to novel insights for diagnosis. The genes and the intracellular signaling circuitry involved in metopic suture closure might be different from those associated with coronal, sagittal or lambdoid suture closure. Considering that deletions and duplications can cause craniosynostosis, both haploinsufficiency and gain of function or dominant negative mechanisms may be associated with premature ossification of the sutures. The importance of some of these genes in skull development has also been shown by the identification of patients who instead of craniosynostosis present with wide sutures due to an inverse dosage of the chromosomal region or of the specific gene associated with craniosynostosis, as exemplified by the *TWIST1* gene [62]. This, however, is not a rule for all genes involved in craniosynostosis, as demonstrated by duplication of 9p, which is not associated with delayed ossification of the sutures [63]. Regarding the diagnostic approach for patients with complex or syndromic craniosynostosis, particularly concerning syndromic cases, once the most common Mendelian forms are excluded by clinical and molecular evaluation, i.e. the *FGFR*, *TWIST1* and *EFNB1* syndromes, chromosomal analysis by cytogenetics and/or high resolution techniques is indicated.

References

1 Cohen MM, MacLean RE (eds): Craniosynostosis: Diagnosis, Evaluation, and Management, 2nd ed. Oxford, Oxford University Press, 2000.
2 Rice DP (ed): Craniofacial Sutures: Development, Disease and Treatment. Front Oral Biol. Basel, Karger, 2008.
3 Gorlin RJ, Cohen MM Jr, Hennekam RCM: Syndromes of the Head and Neck, 4th ed. (Oxford Monographs on Medical Genetics. Vol. 42). Oxford, Oxford University Press, 2001.
4 Merrill AE, Bochukova EG, Brugger SM, Ishii M, Pilz DT, et al: Cell mixing at a neural crest-mesoderm boundary and deficient ephrin-Eph signaling in the pathogenesis of craniosynostosis. Hum Mol Genet 2006;15:1319–1328.
5 Twigg SR, Kan R, Babbs C, Bochukova EG, Robertson SP, et al: Mutations of ephrin-B1 *(EFNB1)*, a marker of tissue boundary formation, cause craniofrontonasal syndrome. Proc Natl Acad Sci USA 2004;101:8652–8657.
6 Graham JM Jr, Badura RJ, Smith DW: Coronal craniostenosis: fetal head constraint as one possible cause. Pediatrics 1980;65:995–999.
7 Graham JM Jr, deSaxe M, Smith DW: Sagittal craniostenosis: fetal head constraint as one possible cause. J Pediatr 1979;95:747–750.
8 Graham JM Jr, Smith DW: Metopic craniostenosis as a consequence of fetal head constraint: two interesting experiments of nature. Pediatrics 1980;65:1000–1002.
9 Higginbottom MC, Jones KL, James HE: Intrauterine constraint and craniosynostosis. Neurosurgery 1980;6:39–44.
10 Hunenko O, Karmacharya J, Ong G, Kirschner RE: Toward an understanding of nonsyndromic craniosynostosis: altered patterns of TGF-beta receptor and FGF receptor expression induced by intrauterine head constraint. Ann Plast Surg 2001;46:546–553, discussion 553–554.
11 Leonard CO, Ralston C, Carey JC, Morales L: Craniosynostosis and facial dysmorphism due to maternal Graves disease. Clin Res 1987;35:225A.
12 Johnsonbaugh RE, Bryan RN, Hierlwimmer R, Georges LP: Premature craniosynostosis: a common complication of juvenile thyrotoxicosis. J Pediatr 1978; 93:188–191.
13 Menking FW, Schmid WU, Ebel KD, Holthusen WH, Schmidt WW: Premature craniosynostosis associated with hyperthyroidism. Ann Radiol (Paris) 1972;15:279–284.
14 Menking M, Wiebel J, Schmid WU, Schmidt WT, Ebel KD, Ritter R: Premature craniosynostosis associated with hyperthyroidism in 4 children with reference to 5 further cases in the literature. Monatsschr Kinderheilkd 1972;120: 106–110.
15 Char F, Herty JB, Wilson RS, Dungen WT: Patterns of malformations in infants exposed to gestational anticonvulsants. Presentation at the Birth Defects Meeting, San Francisco, June 1978.
16 Happle R, Traupe H, Bounameaux Y, Fisch T: Teratogene Wirkung von Etretinat beim Menschen. Dtsch Med Wochenschr 1984;109:1476–1480.
17 Ardinger HH, Atkin JF, Blackston RD, Elsas LJ, Clarren SK, et al: Verification of the fetal valproate syndrome phenotype. Am J Med Genet 1988;29:171–185.
18 Assencio-Ferreira VJ, Abraham R, Veiga JC, Santos KC: [Metopic suture craniosynostosis: sodium valproate teratogenic effect. Case report]. Arq Neuropsiquiatr 2001;59:417–420.
19 Lajeunie E, Barcik U, Thorne JA, El Ghouzzi V, Bourgeois M, Renier D: Craniosynostosis and fetal exposure to sodium valproate. J Neurosurg 2001;95: 778–782.
20 Cohen MM Jr: Etiopathogenesis of craniosynostosis. Neurosurg Clin N Am 1991;2:507–513.

21 Aleck KA, Bartley DL: Multiple malformation syndrome following fluconazole use in pregnancy: report of an additional patient. Am J Med Genet 1997;72:253–256.
22 Enns GM, Roeder E, Chan RT, Ali-Khan Catts Z, Cox VA, Golabi M: Apparent cyclophosphamide (cytoxan) embryopathy: a distinct phenotype? Am J Med Genet 1999;86:237–241.
23 Scott RR, Miller WL: Genetic and clinical features of p450 oxidoreductase deficiency. Horm Res 2008;69:266–275.
24 Passos-Bueno MR, Sertié AL, Jehee FS, Fanganiello R, Yeh E: Genetics of craniosynostosis: genes, mutations and genotype-phenotype correlations; in Rice DP (ed): Craniofacial Sutures: Development, Disease and Treatment. Basel, Karger, 2008, pp 107–143.
25 Nagai T, Shimokawa O, Harada N, Sakazume S, Ohashi H, et al: Postnatal overgrowth by 15q-trisomy and intrauterine growth retardation by 15q-monosomy due to familial translocation t(13;15): dosage effect of *IGF1R*? Am J Med Genet 2002;113:173–177.
26 Schwyzer U, Binkert F, Caflisch U, Baumgartner B, Schinzel A: Terminal deletion of the short arm of chromosome 3, del(3pter-p25): a recognizable syndrome. Helv Paediatr Acta 1987;42:309–315.
27 Huret JL, Leonard C, Forestier B, Rethore MO, Lejeune J: Eleven new cases of del(9p) and features from 80 cases. J Med Genet 1988;25:741–749.
28 Ramer JC, Mowrey PN, Robins DB, Ligato S, Towfighi J, Ladda RL: Five children with del(2)(q31q33) and one individual with dup(2)(q31q33) from a single family: review of brain, cardiac, and limb malformations. Am J Med Genet 1990;37:392–400.
29 Breslau-Siderius EJ, Wijnen JT, Dauwerse JG, de Pater JM, Beemer FA, Khan PM: Paternal duplication of chromosome 5q11.2–5q14 in a male born with craniostenosis, ear tags, kidney dysplasia and several other anomalies. Hum Genet 1993;92:481–485.
30 Chu TW, Teebi AS, Gibson L, Breg WR, Yang-Feng TL: FISH diagnosis of partial trisomy 13 and tetrasomy 13 in a patient with severe trigonocephaly (C) phenotype. Am J Med Genet 1994;52:92–96.
31 Lewanda AF, Morsey S, Reid CS, Jabs EW: Two craniosynostotic patients with 11q deletions, and review of 48 cases. Am J Med Genet 1995;59:193–198.
32 Brewer C, Holloway S, Zawalnyski P, Schinzel A, FitzPatrick D: A chromosomal deletion map of human malformations. Am J Hum Genet 1998;63:1153–1159.
33 Garcia-Heras J, Corley N, Garcia MF, Kukolich MK, Smith KG, Day DW: De novo partial duplications 1p: report of two new cases and review. Am J Med Genet 1999;82:261–264.
34 Gajecka M, Yu W, Ballif BC, Glotzbach CD, Bailey KA, et al: Delineation of mechanisms and regions of dosage imbalance in complex rearrangements of 1p36 leads to a putative gene for regulation of cranial suture closure. Eur J Hum Genet 2005;13:139–149.
35 Kariminejad A, Kariminejad R, Tzschach A, Ullmann R, Ahmed A, et al: Craniosynostosis in a patient with 2q37.3 deletion 5q34 duplication: association of extra copy of *MSX2* with craniosynostosis. Am J Med Genet A 2009;149A:1544–1549.
36 Ben-Shachar S, Bidwa BM, Potocki L, Lalani SR: Coexistence of an unbalanced chromosomal rearrangement and spinal muscular atrophy in an infant with multiple congenital anomalies. Am J Med Genet A 2009;149A:515–518.
37 Kaminker CP, Dain L, Lamas MA, Sanchez JM: Mosaic trisomy 9 syndrome with unusual phenotype. Am J Med Genet 1985;22:237–241.
38 Mattina T, Perrotta CS, Grossfeld P: Jacobsen syndrome. Orphanet J Rare Dis 2009;4:9.
39 Veitia RA, Nunes M, Quintana-Murci L, Rappaport R, Thibaud E, et al: Swyer syndrome and 46,XY partial gonadal dysgenesis associated with 9p deletions in the absence of monosomy-9p syndrome. Am J Hum Genet 1998;63:901–905.
40 De Pater JM, Ippel PF, Bijlsma JB, Van Nieuwenhuizen O: Interstitial deletion 11q: case report and review of the literature. Genet Couns 1997;8:335–339.
41 Leegte B, Kerstjens-Frederikse WS, Deelstra K, Begeer JH, van Essen AJ: 11q–syndrome: three cases and a review of the literature. Genet Couns 1999;10:305–313.
42 Christ LA, Crowe CA, Micale MA, Conroy JM, Schwartz S: Chromosome breakage hotspots and delineation of the critical region for the 9p-deletion syndrome. Am J Hum Genet 1999;65:1387–1395.
43 Jehee FS, Johnson D, Alonso LG, Cavalcanti DP, de Sa Moreira E, et al: Molecular screening for microdeletions at 9p22-p24 and 11q23-q24 in a large cohort of patients with trigonocephaly. Clin Genet 2005;67:503–510.
44 Swinkels ME, Simons A, Smeets DF, Vissers LE, Veltman JA, et al: Clinical and cytogenetic characterization of 13 Dutch patients with deletion 9p syndrome: delineation of the critical region for a consensus phenotype. Am J Med Genet A 2008;146A:1430–1438.
45 Shimojima K, Yamamoto T: Investigation of the candidate region for trigonocephaly in a patient with monosomy 9p syndrome using array-CGH. Am J Med Genet A 2009;149A:1076–1080.
46 Su PH, Kuo PL, Chen SJ, Huang SC, Chen JY, Hung HM: Six cases of deletion 9p24 and trisomy 19q13.4 inherited from a familial balanced translocation. J Formos Med Assoc 2005;104:525–530.
47 Brueton LA, van Herwerden L, Chotai KA, Winter RM: The mapping of a gene for craniosynostosis: evidence for linkage of the Saethre-Chotzen syndrome to distal chromosome 7p. J Med Genet 1992;29:681–685.
48 Lewanda AF, Cohen MM Jr, Jackson CE, Taylor EW, Li X, et al: Genetic heterogeneity among craniosynostosis syndromes: mapping the Saethre-Chotzen syndrome locus between D7S513 and D7S516 and exclusion of Jackson-Weiss and Crouzon syndrome loci from 7p. Genomics 1994;19:115–119.
49 van Herwerden L, Rose CS, Reardon W, Brueton LA, Weissenbach J, et al: Evidence for locus heterogeneity in acrocephalosyndactyly: a refined localization for the Saethre-Chotzen syndrome locus on distal chromosome 7p – and exclusion of Jackson-Weiss syndrome from craniosynostosis loci on 7p and 5q. Am J Hum Genet 1994;54:669–674.
50 Howard TD, Paznekas WA, Green ED, Chiang LC, Ma N, et al: Mutations in *TWIST*, a basic helix-loop-helix transcription factor, in Saethre-Chotzen syndrome. Nat Genet 1997;15:36–41.
51 el Ghouzzi V, Le Merrer M, Perrin-Schmitt F, Lajeunie E, Benit P, et al: Mutations of the *TWIST* gene in the Saethre-Chotzen syndrome. Nat Genet 1997;15:42–46.

52 Jehee FS, Krepischi-Santos AC, Rocha KM, Cavalcanti DP, Kim CA, et al: High frequency of submicroscopic chromosomal imbalances in patients with syndromic craniosynostosis detected by a combined approach of microsatellite segregation analysis, multiplex ligation-dependent probe amplification and array-based comparative genome hybridisation. J Med Genet 2008;45:447–450.
53 Zneimer SM, Cotter PD, Stewart SD: Telomere-telomere (end to end) fusion of chromosomes 7 and 22 with an interstitial deletion of chromosome 7p11.2→p15.1: phenotypic consequences and possible mechanisms. Clin Genet 2000;58:129–133.
54 Clancy BM, Johnson JD, Lambert AJ, Rezvankhah S, Wong A, et al: A gene expression profile for endochondral bone formation: oligonucleotide microarrays establish novel connections between known genes and BMP-2-induced bone formation in mouse quadriceps. Bone 2003;33:46–63.
55 D'Angelo CS, Kohl I, Varela MC, de Castro CI, Kim CA, et al: Extending the phenotype of monosomy 1p36 syndrome and mapping of a critical region for obesity and hyperphagia. Am J Med Genet A 2010;152A:102–110.
56 Tagariello A, Heller R, Greven A, Kalscheuer VM, Molter T, et al: Balanced translocation in a patient with craniosynostosis disrupts the *SOX6* gene and an evolutionarily conserved non-transcribed region. J Med Genet 2006;43:534–540.
57 Jehee FS, Bertola DR, Yelavarthi KK, Krepischi-Santos AC, Kim C, et al: An 11q11-q13.3 duplication, including *FGF3* and *FGF4* genes, in a patient with syndromic multiple craniosynostoses. Am J Med Genet A 2007;143A:1912–1918.
58 Carlton MB, Colledge WH, Evans MJ: Crouzon-like craniofacial dysmorphology in the mouse is caused by an insertional mutation at the *Fgf3/Fgf4* locus. Dev Dyn 1998;212:242–249.
59 Kaname T, Yanagi K, Chinen Y, Makita Y, Okamoto N, et al: Mutations in CD96, a member of the immunoglobulin superfamily, cause a form of the C (Opitz trigonocephaly) syndrome. Am J Hum Genet 2007;81:835–841.
60 Jabs EW, Muller U, Li X, Ma L, Luo W, et al: A mutation in the homeodomain of the human *MSX2* gene in a family affected with autosomal dominant craniosynostosis. Cell 1993;75:443–450.
61 Shiihara T, Kato M, Kimura T, Hayasaka K, Yamamori S, Ogata T: Craniosynostosis with extra copy of *MSX2* in a patient with partial 5q-trisomy. Am J Med Genet A 2004;128A:214–216.
62 Stankiewicz P, Thiele H, Baldermann C, Kruger A, Giannakudis I, et al: Phenotypic findings due to trisomy 7p15.3-pter including the *TWIST* locus. Am J Med Genet 2001;103:56–62.
63 Zou YS, Huang XL, Ito M, Newton S, Milunsky JM: Further delineation of the critical region for the 9p-duplication syndrome. Am J Med Genet A 2009; 149A:272–276.
64 Falk RE, Crandall BF, Sparkes RS, et al: Profound growth failure and minor congenital anomalies in a child with a small chromosome deletion: 46,XX,del(1)(pter→q24::q31→qter). Clin Res 1977;25: 176A.
65 De Vries BB, Knight SJ, Homfray T, Smithson SF, Flint J, Winter RM: Submicroscopic subtelomeric 1qter deletions: a recognisable phenotype? J Med Genet 2001;38:175–178.
66 Nixon J, Oldridge M, Wilkie AO, Smith K: Interstitial deletion of 2q associated with craniosynostosis, ocular coloboma, and limb abnormalities: cytogenetic and molecular investigation. Am J Med Genet 1997;70:324–327.
67 Van Buggenhout G, Van Ravenswaaij-Arts C, Mc Maas N, Thoelen R, Vogels A, et al: The del(2)(q32.2q33) deletion syndrome defined by clinical and molecular characterization of four patients. Eur J Med Genet 2005;48:276–289.
68 Tipton RE, Berns JS, Johnson WE, Wilroy RS Jr, Summitt RL: Duplication 6q syndrome. Am J Med Genet 1979;3:325–330.
69 Sargent C, Burn J, Baraitser M, Pembrey ME: Trigonocephaly and the Opitz C syndrome. J Med Genet 1985;22:39–45.
70 Fagan K, Gill A: A new interstitial deletion of 4q (q21.1::q22.1). J Med Genet 1989;26:644–647.
71 Van Buggenhout G, Maas NM, Fryns JP, Vermeesch JR: A dysmorphic boy with 4qter deletion and 4q32.3-34.3 duplication: clinical, cytogenetic, and molecular findings. Am J Med Genet A 2004;131:186–189.
72 Coco R, Penchaszadeh VB: Inherited parital duplication deficiency of chromosome 15 (p12;q22). J Genet Hum 1978;26:203–210.
73 Park P, Graham JM Jr, Berg SZ, Wurster-Hill DH: A de novo interstitial deletion of chromosome 6 (q22.2q23.1). Clin Genet 1988;33:65–68.
74 Chotai KA, Brueton LA, van Herwerden L, Garrett C, Hinkel GK, et al: Six cases of 7p deletion: clinical, cytogenetic, and molecular studies. Am J Med Genet 1994;51:270–276.
75 Gong BT, Norwood TH, Hoehn H, McPherson E, Hall JG, Hickman R: Chromosome 7 short arm deletion and craniosynostosis. A 7p-syndrome. Hum Genet 1976;35:117–123.
76 Fryns JP, Haspeslagh M, Agneessens A, van den Berghe H: De novo partial 2q3 trisomy/distal 7p22 monosomy in a malformed newborn with 7p deletion phenotype and craniosynostosis. Ann Genet 1985;28:45–48.
77 Schömig-Spingler M, Schmid M, Brosi W, Grimm T: Chromosome 7 short arm deletion, 7p21→pter. Hum Genet 1986; 74:323–325.
78 Touliatou V, Mavrou A, Kolialexi A, Kanavakis E, Kitsiou-Tzeli S: Saethre-Chotzen syndrome with severe developmental delay associated with deletion of chromosomic region 7p15→pter. Genet Couns 2007;18:295–301.
79 Hinkel GK, Tolkendorf E, Bergan J: [7p-deletion syndrome]. Monatsschr Kinderheilkd 1988;136:824–827.
80 Morimoto M, An B, Ogami A, Shin N, Sugino Y, et al: Infantile spasms in a patient with Williams syndrome and craniosynostosis. Epilepsia 2003;44: 1459–1462.
81 Donahue ML, Ryan RM: Interstitial deletion of 8q21→22 associated with minor anomalies, congenital heart defect, and Dandy-Walker variant. Am J Med Genet 1995;56:97–100.
82 Fryburg JS, Golden WL: Interstitial deletion of 8q13.3→22.1 associated with craniosynostosis. Am J Med Genet 1993;45:638–641.
83 Schimmenti LA, Higgins RR, Mendelsohn NJ, Casey TM, Steinberger J, et al: Monosomy 9p24→pter and trisomy 5q31→qter: case report and review of two cases. Am J Med Genet 1995;57:52–56.

84 Wagstaff J, Hemann M: A familial 'balanced' 3;9 translocation with cryptic 8q insertion leading to deletion and duplication of 9p23 loci in siblings. Am J Hum Genet 1995;56:302–309.
85 Alfi OS, Donnell GN, Allderdice PW, Derencsenyi A: The 9p– syndrome. Ann Genet 1976;19:11–16.
86 Eshel G, Lahat E, Reish O, Barr J: Neurodevelopmental and behavioral abnormalities associated with deletion of chromosome 9p. J Child Neurol 2002;17:50–51.
87 Redon R, Baujat G, Sanlaville D, Le Merrer M, Vekemans M: Interstitial 9q22.3 microdeletion: clinical and molecular characterisation of a newly recognised overgrowth syndrome. Eur J Hum Genet 2006;14:759–767.
88 Yatsenko SA, Cheung SW, Scott DA, Nowaczyk MJ, Tarnopolsky M, et al: Deletion 9q34.3 syndrome: genotype-phenotype correlations and an extended deletion in a patient with features of Opitz C trigonocephaly. J Med Genet 2005;42:328–335.
89 Francke U, Mahan GM, Dixson BK, Jones OW: 10p–: a new autosomal deletion syndrome? Birth Defects Orig Artic Ser 1975;11:207–212.
90 Lukusa T, Smeets E, Vermeesch JR, Fryns JP: Small terminal 10q26 deletion in a male patient with Noonan-like stigmata: diagnosis by cytogenetic and FISH analysis. Genet Couns 2002;13:417–425.
91 Bresson JL, Noir A: [Partial monosomy 11q. A new case]. Ann Genet 1977;20:63–66.
92 Orye E, Craen M: Short arm deletion of chromosome 12: report of two new cases. Humangenetik 1975;28:335–342.
93 Masuno M, Asano J, Yasuda K, Kondo T, Orii T: Balanced complex rearrangement involving chromosomes 8, 9, and 12 in a normal mother, derivative chromosome 9 with recombinant chromosome 12 in her daughter with minor anomalies. Am J Med Genet 1993;45:65–67.
94 Orbeli DJ, Lurie IW, Goroshenko JL: The syndrome associated with the partial D-monosomy: case report and review. Humangenetik 1971;13:296–308.
95 Lemyre E, Lemieux N, Décarie JC, Lambert M: Del(14)(q22.1q23.2) in a patient with anophthalmia and pituitary hypoplasia. Am J Med Genet 1998;77:162–165.
96 Shur N, Cowan J, Wheeler PG: Craniosynostosis and congenital heart anomalies associated with a maternal deletion of 15q15-22.1. Am J Med Genet A 2003;120A:542–546.
97 Hiraki Y, Fujita H, Yamamori S, Ohashi H, Eguchi M, et al: Mild craniosynostosis with 1p36.3 trisomy and 1p36.3 deletion syndrome caused by familial translocation t(Y;1). Am J Med Genet A 2006;140:1773–1777.
98 Stratton RF, Dobyns WB, Greenberg F, DeSana JB, Moore C, et al: Interstitial deletion of (17)(p11.2p11.2): report of six additional patients with a new chromosome deletion syndrome. Am J Med Genet 1986;24:421–432.
99 Thomas JA, Manchester DK, Prescott KE, Milner R, McGavran L, Cohen MM Jr: Hunter-McAlpine craniosynostosis phenotype associated with skeletal anomalies and interstitial deletion of chromosome 17q. Am J Med Genet 1996;62:372–375.
100 Cantu ES, Khan TA, Pai GS: Fluorescence in situ hybridization (FISH) of a whole-arm translocation involving chromosomes 18 and 20 with alpha-satellite DNA probes: detection of a centromeric DNA break? Am J Med Genet 1992;44:340–344.
101 McDonald-McGinn DM, Gripp KW, Kirschner RE, Maisenbacher MK, Hustead V, et al: Craniosynostosis: another feature of the 22q11.2 deletion syndrome. Am J Med Genet A 2005;136A:358–362.
102 Heinrichs C, Elmer C, Derasse M, Perlmutter N, Vamos E: Craniosynostosis in the Ullrich-Turner syndrome. Am J Med Genet 1991;40:252.
103 Lucas J, Faivre J, Le Mee F, Hubert S, Pluquailec K, Picard F: [De novo interstitial deletion of the long arm of chromosome 2: 46,XXX,del(2)(q14q21), associated with premature craniosynostosis]. Ann Genet 1987;30:33–38.
104 Carvalho DR, Trad CS, Pina-Neto JM: Atypical presentation of Prader-Willi syndrome with Klinefelter (XXY karyotype) and craniosynostosis. Arq Neuropsiquiatr 2006;64:303–305.
105 Fryns JP: Structural abnormalities of the Y-chromosome and craniosynostosis. Clin Genet 1992;42:100–101.
106 Gagnon JA, Richer CL, Lemieux N, Gauthier-Chouinard M: [De novo appearance of a partial trisomy 1q in mosaic due to a 1;9 translocation]. Ann Genet 1984;27:33–37.
107 McGaughran J, Aftimos S, Oei P: Trisomy of 3pter in a patient with apparent C (trigonocephaly) syndrome. Am J Med Genet 2000;94:311–315.
108 Buchinger G, Wettstein A, Metze H: Familial chromosome translocation t(3;18)(p21;p11). J Med Genet 1981;18:119–123.
109 Wilson GN, Dasouki M, Barr M Jr: Further delineation of the dup(3q) syndrome. Am J Med Genet 1985;22:117–123.
110 Preus M, Vekemans M, Kaplan P: Diagnosis of chromosome 3 duplication q23→qter, deletion p25→pter in a patient with the C (trigonocephaly) syndrome. Am J Med Genet 1986;23:935–943.
111 de Brasi D, Perone L, di Micco P, Andria G, Sebastio G, et al: Cloverleaf skull anomaly and de novo trisomy 4p. J Med Genet 1999;36:422–424.
112 Opitz JM, Patau K: A partial trisomy 5p syndrome. Birth Defects Orig Artic Ser 1975;11:191–200.
113 Wang JC, Steinraths M, Dang L, Lomax B, Eydoux P, et al: Craniosynostosis associated with distal 5q-trisomy: further evidence that extra copy of *MSX2* gene leads to craniosynostosis. Am J Med Genet A 2007;143A:2931–2936.
114 Bernheim A, Berger R, Vaugier G, Thieffry JC, Matet Y: Partial trisomy 6p. Hum Genet 1979;48:13–16.
115 Schmid W, D'Apuzzo V, Rossi E: Trisomy 6q25 to 6qter in a severely retarded 7-year-old boy with turricephaly, bow-shaped mouth, hypogenitalism and club feet. Hum Genet 1979;46:279–284.
116 Robertson KP, Thurmon TF, Tracy MC: Acrocephalosyndactyly and partial trisomy 6. Birth Defects Orig Artic Ser 1975;11:267–271.
117 Odell JM, Siebert JR, Bradley C, Salk D: Duplication 7p in a family with t(7;11): association with anomalies of the anterior cranial base. Am J Med Genet 1987;27:687–692.
118 Seghezzi L, Maraschio P, Bozzola M, Maserati E, Tupler R, et al: Ring chromosome 9 with a 9p22.3-p24.3 duplication. Eur J Pediatr 1999;158:791–793.
119 Sujansky E, Smith AC, Peakman DC, McConnell TS, Baca P, Robinson A: Familial pericentric inversion of chromosome 8. Am J Med Genet 1981;10:229–235.
120 Phadke SR, Patil SJ: Partial trisomy 13 with features similar to C syndrome. Indian Pediatr 2004;41:614–617.

121 Yelavarthi KK, Zunich J: Familial interstitial duplication of 11q; partial trisomy (11)(q13.5q21). Am J Med Genet A 2004;126A:423–426.
122 Hornstein L, Soukup S: A recognizable phenotype in a child with partial duplication 13q in a family with t(10q;13q). Clin Genet 1981;19:81–86.
123 Genest P, Genest FB, Gagnon-Blais D: [Unusual chromosomal rearrangement. An autosomal telomeric translocation on a multicentury satellited Y (Yqs) chromosome]. Ann Genet 1983;26:86–90.
124 Van Allen MI, Siegel-Bartelt J, Feigenbaum A, Teshima IE: Craniosynostosis associated with partial duplication of 15q and deletion of 2q. Am J Med Genet 1992;43:688–692.
125 Zollino M, Tiziano F, Di Stefano C, Neri G: Partial duplication of the long arm of chromosome 15: confirmation of a causative role in craniosynostosis and definition of a 15q25-qter trisomy syndrome. Am J Med Genet 1999;87:391–394.
126 Babovic-Vuksanovic D, Westman JA, Jalal SM, Lindor NM: Clinical characteristics associated with dup17(q24q25.1) in a mosaic mother and two non-mosaic daughters. Clin Dysmorphol 1998;7: 171–176.
127 Czako M, Riegel M, Morava E, Bajnóczky K, Kosztolányi G: Opitz "C" trigonocephaly-like syndrome in a patient with terminal deletion of 2p and partial duplication of 17q. Am J Med Genet A 2004;131:310–312.
128 Gustashaw KM, Zurcher V, Dickerman LH, Stallard R, Willard HF: Partial X chromosome trisomy with functional disomy of Xp due to failure of X inactivation. Am J Med Genet 1994;53:39–45.
129 Hu J, McPherson E, Surti U, Hasegawa SL, Gunawardena S, Gollin SM: Tetrasomy 15q25.3→qter resulting from an analphoid supernumerary marker chromosome in a patient with multiple anomalies and bilateral Wilms tumors. Am J Med Genet 2002;113:82–88.
130 Demyer W, Palmer C: Closed metopic suture with trigonocephaly in Down's syndrome. Neurology 1965;15:756–760.
131 Saadi AA, Juliar JF, Harm J, Brough AJ, Perrin EV, Chen H: Triploidy syndrome. A report on two live-born (69, XXY) and one still-born (69, XXX) infants. Clin Genet 1976;9:43–50.
132 Ward J, Vieto E, Lee D, Arosemena G: Acrocephalopolysyndactyly, pentalogy of Fallot, and hypoacusis in a patient with a de novo reciprocal translocation involving the short arm of chromosome 1 and the long arm of chromosome 18: 46,XX,t(1;18)(p31;q11). J Med Genet 1993;30:438–439.
133 Vazquez-Cardenas A, Vasquez-Velasquez AI, Barros-Núñez P, Mantilla-Capacho J, Rocchi M, Rivera H: Familial whole-arm translocations (1;19), (9;13), and (12;21): a review of 101 constitutional exchanges. J Appl Genet 2007;48: 261–268.
134 Schluth-Bolard C, Till M, Labalme A, Rey C, Banquart E, et al: *TWIST* microdeletion identified by array CGH in a patient presenting Saethre-Chotzen phenotype and a complex rearrangement involving chromosomes 2 and 7. Eur J Med Genet 2008;51:156–164.
135 Hordnes K, Engebretsen LF, Knudtzon J: De novo balanced 5;21 translocation in a child with acrobrachycephaly, ventriculomegaly, pulmonary stenosis, ectopic anus and mental retardation. Clin Genet 1995;48:321–323.
136 Fryns JP, Hendrickx G: Malformative syndrome with trigonocephaly, shallow orbits, ptosis, growth and mental retardation. De novo autosomal reciprocal t(9;13)(q32;q22) in a male patient. Ann Genet 1996;39:51–53.

Maria Rita Passos-Bueno
Department of Genetics and Evolutionary Biology
University of São Paulo
Rua do Matão, 277, São Paulo, SP, 05088-900 (Brazil)
Tel. +55 11 309 19910, Fax +55 11 309 17419, E-Mail passos@ib.usp.br

Muenke M, Kress W, Collmann H, Solomon BD (eds): Craniosynostoses: Molecular Genetics, Principles of Diagnosis, and Treatment.
Monogr Hum Genet. Basel, Karger, 2011, vol 19, pp 165–176

Nonsyndromic Craniosynostoses

H. Collmann[a] · B.D. Solomon[b] · T. Schweitzer[a] · W. Kress[c] · M. Muenke[b]

[a]Section of Pediatric Neurosurgery, Julius-Maximilians University, Würzburg, Germany; [b]Medical Genetics Branch, National Human Genome Research Institute, National Institutes of Health, Bethesda, Md., USA; [c]Institute of Human Genetics, Julius-Maximilians University, Würzburg, Germany

Abstract

The subtypes of nonsyndromic ('isolated') craniosynostosis are denominated according to the predominant deformity resulting from premature fusion of one of the major cranial sutures: scaphocephaly, trigonocephaly, anterior plagiocephaly, brachycephaly, posterior plagiocephaly, and oxycephaly. In most cases the underlying causes remain unknown although there is some overlap with syndromic craniosynostosis suggesting heterogeneous etiologies. In contrast to the oversimplified nomenclature, isolated craniosynostosis may involve two or more sutures at the same time or may progress with increasing age, thus indicating that the basic nature of craniosynostosis is a failure of growth regulation of the skull rather than a malformation.

The term nonsyndromic ('isolated') craniosynostosis implies that the diagnosis can only be established after excluding concurrent abnormalities apart from the skull that indicate the presence of a syndrome, but also after excluding secondary (metabolic, toxic, etc.) forms of craniosynostosis. Large epidemiological studies demonstrate that nonsyndromic craniosynostosis is much more common than the syndromic forms, accounting for up to 90% of all patients with craniosynostosis [1]. In practice it can be quite challenging in both the clinical and the research setting to distinguish syndromic from nonsyndromic craniosynostosis. This diagnostic dilemma is impressively illustrated by the way in which Muenke syndrome had been recognized, as initially it had been classified as hereditary isolated coronal synostosis until associated abnormalities of the inner ear and the brain, as well as subtle anomalies of the extremities, were appreciated [2, 3]. Likewise, a considerable proportion of individuals with a putative isolated metopic synostosis actually have syndromic craniosynostoses [4].

While a genetic cause for patients with syndromic craniosynostosis still remains unknown in over half of cases, an understanding of the basis of nonsyndromic craniosynostoses appears even more elusive [5]. Data from twin studies support evidence for a multifactorial etiology likely involving multiple interacting genes and environmental factors [6, 7], which corresponds with the lack of familial cases. Thus, as the etiology (including both the genetic and environmental bases) of isolated craniosynostosis is still obscure, any individual assignment of a patient to this largest subgroup remains somewhat preliminary.

As will be described in this chapter, much of the work regarding the genetics of nonsyndromic craniosynostosis has been based upon findings in patients with syndromic craniosynostosis. Looking to the future, it is critical to note that as new genomic technologies become available, it will likely become possible to unravel the complex causes of nonsyndromic craniosynostosis after involvement of known loci has been ruled-out (see also Chapter 15). Recently, techniques coupling high-throughput sequencing with statistical genomic analyses has revealed genetic causes of a number of conditions [8, 9]. This approach underscores the role of the clinician even as technology races forward: the use of large-scale genomic analysis for the discovery of new genetic etiologies hinges on careful patient phenotyping. It must also be stated, however, that making the leap from classical Mendelian to more complex conditions (such as nonsyndromic craniosynostosis) may be challenging even with the availability of the most rigorous and thorough research methodologies [10]. Research designs depending on large numbers of affected patients, such as the type involving genome wide association studies (GWAS), provide another line of inquiry, though the cost and necessary numbers of participants can be prohibitive. Ultimately, it will be valuable to link more traditional family based-studies involving patients affected by many types of craniosynostosis with newer genomic techniques in order to inform our overall understanding of nonsyndromic craniosynostosis [11, 12].

Since the basic morphological studies were performed by Rudolf Virchow, monosutural craniosynostoses have been classified according to 'Virchow's law', which describes the synostotic head shape as a result of restricted growth perpendicular to and compensatory overgrowth along the fused suture (see Chapter 1). Therefore, it became customary to use the head shapes caused by monosutural fusion as synonyms for the underlying sutural fusion.

Scaphocephaly

This deformity, resulting from premature sagittal suture fusion with prenatal onset, convincingly illustrates 'Virchow's law'. In addition to the dolichocephalic head shape, typical features comprise a bulging forehead and occiput, a shift of the vertex (the most cranial point of the head) to the bregma site, and underdeveloped parietal eminences. As a consequence of sutural fusion, the fontanelle may assume a triangular shape with its base at the fused suture (fig. 1d). Sometimes the fontanelle closes through a Wormian bone. As sutural fusion is a dynamic process the resulting deformity may vary depending on the site at which sutural fusion starts. Virchow already differentiated between 3 subgroups of scaphocephaly (fig. 1 a–c). The most common is 'sphenocephaly', in which the forehead width exceeds the interparietal diameter. This shape can be attributed to sutural fusion starting at the posterior half. 'Leptocephaly' refers to an equal narrowing of the head, attributable to simultaneous fusion of the whole suture. The least common type, 'clinocephaly', refers to a medial retrocoronal depression of the vault and is probably due to a fusion starting at the mid-portion of the suture. While these subgroups seem to be irrelevant in terms of function, the sphenocephalic and clinocephalic deformities are highly specific, hence diagnostic of sagittal synostosis. As a peculiar feature, mild hypertelorism has been noted in several patients with scaphocephaly who were examined in Würzburg [unpublished data]. The significance of scaphocephaly in terms of function has not yet been precisely defined. In routine measurements elevated intracranial pressure has been reported in 14% [13] and 23% [14] of individuals, respectively. In a small proportion of patients, severe intracranial hypertension causing papilledema and optic nerve damage may occur [15]. This is probably attributable to the fact that sutural fusion may sometimes proceed to involve the coronal and the lambdoid sutures as well [16]. On neuroimaging, intracranial structures do not

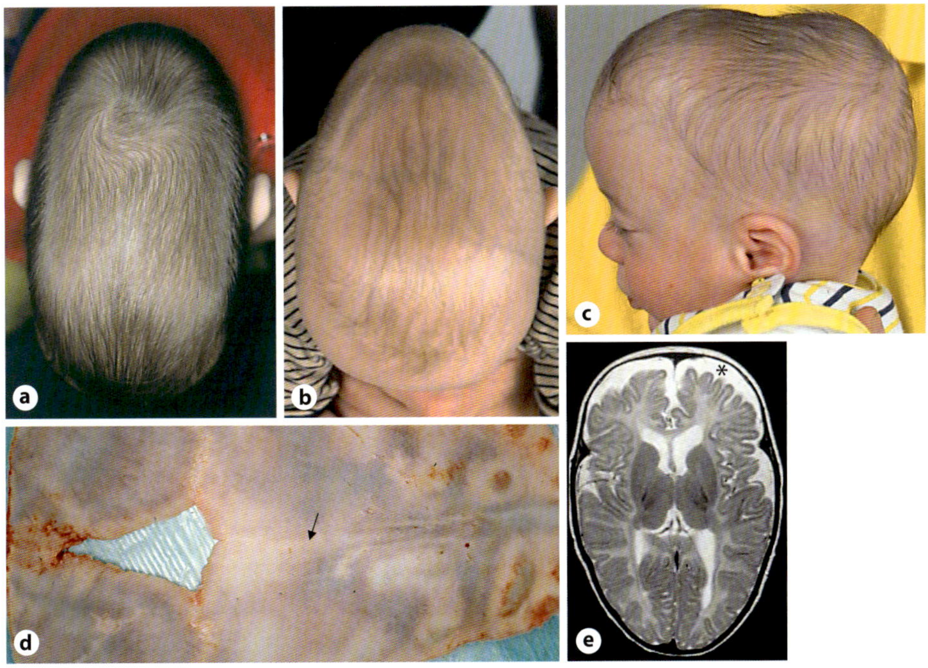

Fig. 1. Isolated scaphocephaly. Different deformities according to Virchow: leptocephaly (**a**), sphenocephaly (**b**), clinocephaly (**c**). Inner surface of a surgical specimen shows typical delta-shaped fontanelle with its base towards the closed sagittal suture (**d** arrow). Magnetic resonance image shows enlarged frontal subarachnoid space (**e**, asterisk).

seem to be significantly altered unless they are deformed. Dilation of the frontal subarachnoid space is a common phenomenon, which is probably due to accommodation of the cerebrospinal fluid by the bulging forehead (fig. 1e) [17]. Recent findings suggest that the mere deformation of the immature brain within the deformed skull may have a slight influence on neurodevelopment [18].

Isolated scaphocephaly is the most common type of craniosynostosis of all, accounting for roughly 50% of individuals referred to craniofacial centers. There is a male preponderance of 80%, and only 5% of patients have affected parents or siblings [6, 19]. An association with prematurity has also been posited [20]. In the vast majority of cases a genetic cause has not yet been identified. Seto et al. [21] found a *TWIST1* mutation in one of 83 scaphocephalic individuals, though other cohorts have not replicated this observation [22, 23]. While Seto et al. suggested a causative relationship, Kress et al. in a similar case believed this to be a non-disease-causing polymorphism [24]. McGillivray et al. [25] suspect a major role of the *FGFR2* gene in sagittal suture closure. Anderson et al. [23] tested for somatic mutations of the *FGFR* and *TWIST* genes in the sutural tissue of 8 individuals with single suture craniosynostosis. None of the tissue samples exhibited any mutations of the genes in question. In a clinical setting, it is important that some patients with Crouzon syndrome have a phenotype that at least postnatally resembles isolated scaphocephaly. Simple scaphocephaly may also be confused with some other rare syndromes (see Chapter 11) and some types of metabolic craniosynostosis. For instance, at the Würzburg

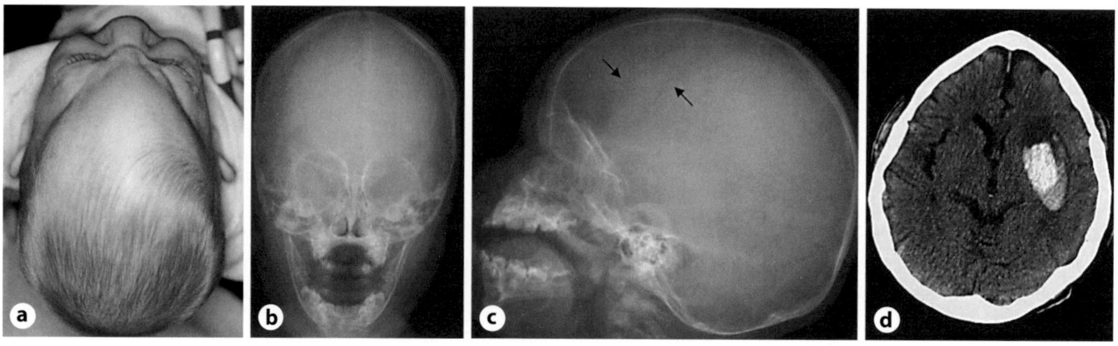

Fig. 2. Isolated trigonocephaly. Typical forehead deformity (**a**), reduced interorbital distance (**b**), hypoplastic frontal squama causing anterior shift of the coronal suture (**c**, arrows), incidental finding of untreated trigonocephaly in an 80-year-old man with intracerebral hemorrhage (**d**).

center this was the case in several patients with hypophosphatasia.

Few studies address the spontaneous evolution of untreated isolated scaphocephaly. In a longitudinal study involving 28 untreated patients, Barritt et al. found progression of dolichocephalic deformity in 15, which however was of clinical significance in only one patient [26]. In the remaining patients, the deformity either slightly improved or remained unchanged. In our own cohort, 21 individuals studied radiologically showed a medically insignificant deterioration of scaphocephalic deformity [unpublished data].

Trigonocephaly

Although specific for monosutural metopic synostosis, this deformity cannot be explained by applying 'Virchow's law'. This raises suspicion that the underlying pathogenic mechanism differs from that of other types of monosutural synostosis. In fact, the metopic suture derives from the neural crest mesenchyme (see Chapter 3). In mice, the metopic suture is the only one which continues to fuse over the animals' entire lifetime. In humans, it differs from the other major cranial sutures in that physiological fusion usually occurs as early as the end of the first year. This is important to realize if the diagnosis of premature sutural fusion should be established. In most cases the unique cranial deformity allows for a diagnosis to be easily made in the first clinical encounter (fig. 2a). During surgery or on neuroimaging it becomes obvious that the frontal squama is actually hypoplastic (fig. 2b, c). Typical features of isolated frontal suture synostosis include a keel-shaped forehead with a midline bony crest, absent frontal eminences, deficient lateral supraorbital ridges, hypotelorism due to a narrow ethmoid bone (fig. 2b), and prominent epicanthal folds. The compensatory increase of the parietal width contributes to the triangular head shape. Cranial deformity may vary in severity, and in its mildest form, premature frontal synostosis may consist of a metopic ridge only.

The estimated prevalence of typical trigonocephaly is about 1:15,000 [27]. Though the majority of cases appear to occur in a nonsyndromic context, this is an example where differentiation between syndromic and nonsyndromic craniosynostosis can be challenging. In fact, a multitude of different syndromes, chromosomal aberrations, or toxic fetopathies – e.g., exposure to valproic acid – may be associated with typical trigonocephaly [4, 27, 28, 29], many of which may not yet have been identified (see Chapter 15). In contrast to syndromic craniosynostosis with trigonocephaly, the nonsyndromic form tends to have a good prognosis [4, 30]. Intriguingly, an increasing incidence of trigonocephaly (as well as other types of nonsyndromic craniosynostosis to a lesser degree) has recently been reported, the cause of which is unknown [31, 32]. As in scaphocephaly, there is a distinct male preponderance, and approximately 5–6% of cases are familial [6, 27]. The etiologic heterogeneity likely accounts for a reported 10 to 30% rate of neurodevelopmental delay [4, 33]. Conclusive data about the impact of trigonocephalic deformity on the developing brain are lacking, although a few centers reported a favourable effect of surgery on mental development [33]. Likewise, data about the spontaneous evolution of untreated trigonocephaly are scarce and conflicting. Slight improvement has been sufficiently documented in a single case [34], whereas data from another study are less convincing [35]. The center in Würzburg is aware of 4 distinct cases of untreated isolated trigonocephaly in adulthood, which appeared to remain unchanged since early childhood (fig. 2d). Progressive plurisutural synostosis is a rare complication in isolated trigonocephaly, a single case being detected in a well documented study group of 128 trigonocephalic patients in Würzburg. As in certain other types of nonsyndromic craniosynostosis, insights from syndromic craniosynostosis have not allowed the identification of causal factors for nonsyndromic trigonocephaly, though some recurrent genomic imbalances detectable by microarray analysis were suggestive as causative for at least a subset of cases [36, 37, see also Chapter 13].

Anterior Plagiocephaly

The complex deformity resulting from unilateral coronal synostosis is best visualized by means of 3-dimensionally reformatted computed tomography, although in clinical practice this particular radiological technique is actually rarely required. The abnormal cranial shape is readily inferred by applying Virchow's law. In essence, restricted growth perpendicular to and overgrowth along the fused suture results in a 2-fold bending of the midsagittal plane: towards the affected side in an anterior-posterior direction and to the other side in the vertical direction (fig. 3). Typical craniofacial features include retrusion of the ipsilateral forehead and the supraorbital rim resulting in a reduced distance between outer canthus and tragus – a phenomenon most notable at the sides of glasses. The forehead retrusion is compensated by contralateral frontal bossing. Craniofacial scoliosis with its convexity towards the affected side and deviation of the nasal septum and the chin to the opposite side is an important diagnostic feature. Depression of the ipsilateral petrous bone and glenoid fossa results in a depressed plane of dental occlusion. An ovoid deformity of the ipsilateral orbit and the elevation of the ipsilateral lesser sphenoid wing contribute to the typical 'harlequin eye' appearance in X-rays (see Chapter 18). Strabismus is a frequent feature deserving particular attention as it carries the risk of amblyopia. Ophthalmologic findings would be consistent with superior oblique paresis, but the actual cause appears to be asymmetric insertion of the muscles in asymmetrically distorted orbits [38]. Currently, other functional consequences have not been verified.

Few data exist about the incidence of isolated unilateral coronal synostosis. Reported values are no longer valid since many cases formerly considered to be isolated forms of craniosynostosis actually represent patients with conditions such as Muenke or Saethre-Chotzen syndrome. At the craniofacial center of Würzburg, after exclusion of *FGFR1–2* related syndromes, molecular analysis of 111 cases of anterior plagiocephaly resulted in classification into 81 isolated cases, 7 individuals with Muenke syndrome, and 23 cases of Saethre-Chotzen syndrome. Another study involving a separate cohort of patients with 'isolated unilateral craniosynostosis' showed that over ten percent of patients harbored mutations associated with forms

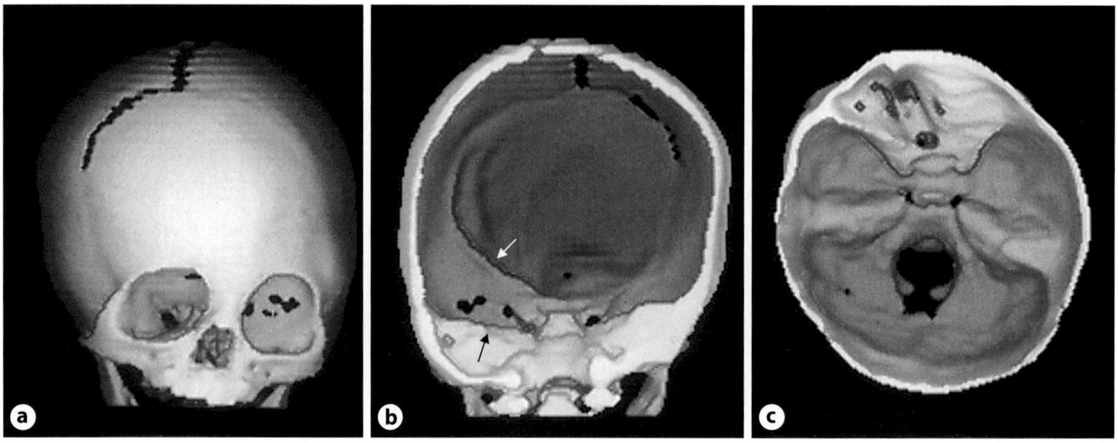

Fig. 3. Left-sided unicoronal synostosis. Note the deformities of the orbits and the deviation of the facial midline to the opposite side (**a**), the elevated left lesser sphenoid wing (**b**, white arrow) and the depressed ipsilateral petrous bone (**b**, black arrow), severe scoliosis of the cranial base (**c**).

of syndromic craniosynostosis, with mutations identified in *FGFR2*, *FGFR3*, and *TWIST1* [39]. These data suggest that molecular analysis may be warranted in at least this type of patient. Isolated unilateral coronal synostosis showed a distinct female preponderance of 77 percent in 81 individuals studied in Würzburg [unpublished data]. Little information is available about the spontaneous evolution of untreated isolated anterior plagiocephaly. While some authors have reported a slight improvement of deformity, others even noted progressive deformity. The Würzburg cohort includes two sufficiently documented cases showing insignificant improvement of the deformity.

Brachycephaly

While the term originally referred to an increased cephalic index only (see Chapter 17) it is now used by clinicians to denote bilateral coronal synostosis (fig. 4). Apart from shortening and widening of the skull, the height of the skull is commonly increased, which is why the term 'turricephaly' has been used as a synonym. The typical facial aspect includes a high and broad, often protruding forehead, widely separated frontal eminences, and recessed supraorbital ridges. Hypertelorism is common, while midfacial growth is fairly normal in the isolated form. Shortening of the anterior cranial fossa is the predominant feature at the cranial base. The lesser wing of the sphenoid bone and its process is elevated on both sides, and the orbits are laterally elevated and assume an ovoid shape, which result in the typical bilateral 'harlequin eye'.

The true prevalence of isolated brachycephaly is surprisingly low. This is obviously due to the fact that the majority of cases actually occur in a syndromic context, in particular Muenke and Saethre-Chotzen syndromes. In our cohort, after excluding Crouzon, Pfeiffer and Apert syndromes, molecular analysis of 125 brachycephalic individuals actually demonstrated the presence of Muenke syndrome in 44 patients and a Saethre-Chotzen syndrome in another 49 patients, while only 32 patients could finally be verified as having isolated forms by exclusion of mutations in the above genes (without question, currently unidentified 'syndromic' loci may also be causative).

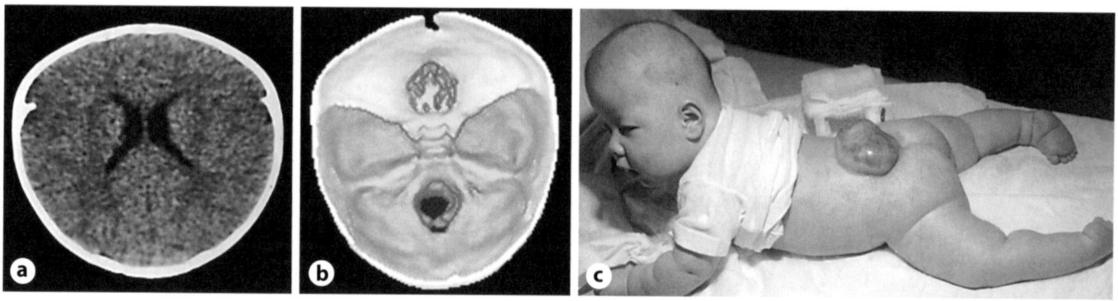

Fig. 4. Isolated brachycephaly. Computed tomography shows the typical head shape (**a**) and the broad, but shortened anterior cranial fossa (**b**). Coronal synostosis is sometimes associated with myelomeningocele, as seen in this baby (**c**).

Males and females were equally represented among patients with the isolated form. For the same reason, reports on the impact of bicoronal synostosis on brain function have to be critically examined. More recent studies performed on genetically tested patients actually suggested some interference with mental development, yet these findings need to be further verified [40]. None of the above-mentioned 32 patients with nonsyndromic bicoronal synostosis presented with papilledema at any point before surgery or during follow-up.

As a peculiar phenomenon, uni- or bicoronal synostosis has been found to be associated with neural tube defects. Four cases (2 unicoronal and 2 bicoronal synostoses) have been verified at our institution during a 20-year period (fig. 4c), but additional cases are reported in the literature [41]. As this coincidental finding involves the coronal suture exclusively, a random phenomenon appears unlikely. However, the etiology of this association remains obscure.

Posterior Plagiocephaly

Synostotic posterior plagiocephaly is caused by unilateral lambdoid synostosis. In this rare type of isolated craniosynostosis, the cranial deformity can also be inferred by applying Virchow's law: sutural growth restriction results in ipsilateral flattening of the occiput, while compensatory overgrowth along the fused suture leads to depression of the ipsilateral petrous bone and auricle and a characteristic bulging of the contralateral parietal region (fig. 5a–c). Another typical, yet not invariably present sign is a bony crest above the ipsilateral mastoid process (fig. 5a, b). Because of the reduced size of the posterior fossa on the affected side, the ipsilateral cerebellar tonsil usually herniates into the foramen magnum (fig. 5c). As the opposite tonsil remains normal, neurological sequelae typical for Chiari I malformation seem unlikely. Synostotic posterior plagiocephaly has often been confused with deformity resulting from positional molding, which is of little if any functional significance. Differential diagnosis is therefore important and will be addressed in Chapter 17. Positional deformation has been estimated to be approximately one hundred times more frequent than the synostotic form [42]. Unilateral lambdoid synostosis is believed to account for roughly 1–3% of all craniosynostoses [42, 43]. In the cohort of 1100 individuals examined at Würzburg, the proportion was even less, as only 6 cases (0.5%) of true unilateral lambdoid synostosis were identified. Genetic analysis shows that mutations in the known 'hotspots' of the *FGFR1–3*

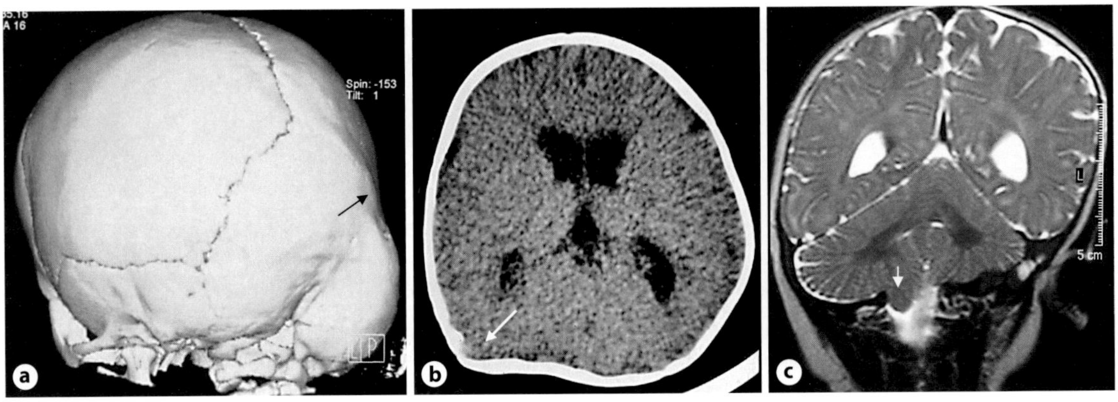

Fig. 5. Right-sided unilateral lambdoid synostosis. 3-dimensional computed tomography shows ridging of the closed suture (**a**, **b**, arrows), MR imaging shows contralateral parietal bulging and ectopia of the ipsilateral cerebellar tonsil (**c**, arrow).

genes do not appear to play a role in at least non-syndromic plagiocephaly [44].

Bisutural Synostosis

Various combinations are possible and have been reported [45]. For example, sagittal synostosis may be combined with frontal, uni- and bicoronal or lambdoid synostosis. Likewise, coronal and frontal suture synostosis may co-occur. However, the present authors are not aware of a single case of combined coronal and lambdoid suture fusion.

The co-existence of sagittal and metopic suture synostosis is a rare event and results in scaphocephaly with less striking trigonocephaly. Only 2 individuals with this particular subtype of isolated craniosynostosis have been identified in the Würzburg cohort of 1100 patients. Prenatal frontal suture fusion combined with bicoronal synostosis is likewise a rare subtype represented by 3 cases in the Würzburg cohort. This combination causes a typical turricephalic deformity with a narrow forehead which however lacks the prominent midline keel of isolated monosutural frontal synostosis (fig. 6a). A quite similar deformity may be observed in patients with Saethre-Chotzen syndrome and 'metopic synostosis' (see Chapter 9, fig. 4). Reliable data as to the functional significance of this subtype are lacking.

Sagittal suture synostosis combined with coronal synostosis is much more common, accounting for about 2% (24/1100 individuals) of the Würzburg series. In this cohort there was a distinct male preponderance of 83%. In nearly half of the cases, scaphocephaly was combined with typical anterior plagiocephaly, indicating unilateral involvement of the coronal suture although bilateral coronal synostosis was ultimately confirmed in some of these cases (fig. 6b). From this observation one may speculate that some of these cases actually represent a transient stage within progressive multisutural synostosis, especially as sutural fusion in scaphocephaly may actually proceed to pansynostosis [16].

The combined sagittal and lambdoid suture fusion results in a peculiar deformity referred to as the 'Mercedes-Benz pattern' [46], because prominent bony crests along the fused lambdoid suture and the posterior part of the sagittal suture resemble the emblem of this car company (fig. 6c, d).

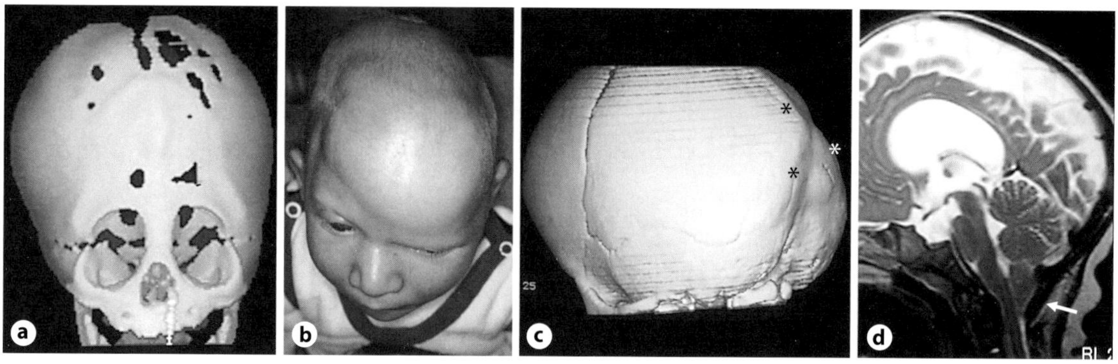

Fig. 6. Bisutural synostosis. Computed tomography of combined bicoronal and metopic synostosis (**a**), infant with sagittal and right-sided unicoronal synostosis (**b**), sagittal and bilambdoid synostosis (**c**, **d**) – note the ridging of the fused sagittal and lambdoid sutures giving the appearance of the Mercedes-Benz emblem (**c**, asterisks), note the ectopic cerebellar tonsils (**d**, arrow).

Typical features include brachyturricephaly, a bulging forehead, biparietal narrowing, and an occipital midline concavity.

This type of craniosynostosis has been described several decades previously [47] and accounts for about 1% of all craniosynostosis cases [48], a value consistent with the numbers observed in Würzburg (14 cases in a total series of 1100). Once again, there is a male preponderance (10:4). Usually both sides of the lambdoid suture are involved, but unilateral fusion has also been observed. Early fusion of the lambdoid suture results in poor growth expansion of the posterior fossa. As a consequence the cerebellar tonsils are pushed down into the cervical spinal canal ('Chiari I malformation'), thereby potentially causing hydrocephalus, brain stem dysfunction, and hydrosyringomyelia (for details, see Chapter 18). As of yet, no theory as to the etiology of this type of craniosynostosis has been set forth. Molecular testing did not reveal any mutations in the common genes related to syndromic craniosynostosis [49]. A possible relationship to dosage of the *MSX2* gene, as suggested by Shiihara [50], remains to be verified.

Oxycephaly

The term refers to multisutural craniosynostosis (pansynostosis), although historically it has also been used as a synonym for brachycephaly [51]. Strictly speaking, the diagnosis of oxycephaly should be confined to postnatal progressive closure of all major cranial sutures, since prenatal onset of multisutural fusion causes Kleeblatt deformity. As all major sutures of the vault are involved to a similar degree, major cranial deformity is not to be expected, and may even sometimes be totally absent (fig. 7). Often the most striking feature is a bregmatic bump giving the appearance of a sugar loaf or a 'chapeau de clown', from which the term 'oxycephaly' (pointed head) has been derived. Subnormal head circumference is also a common feature which may cause confusion with microcephaly due to reduced brain bulk growth ('micrencephaly'), particularly because the latter condition is often associated with secondary pansynostosis. In most cases of true oxycephaly, multisutural fusion causes intracranial hypertension, putting the optic nerve at significant risk, which is important, as clinical complaints are usually

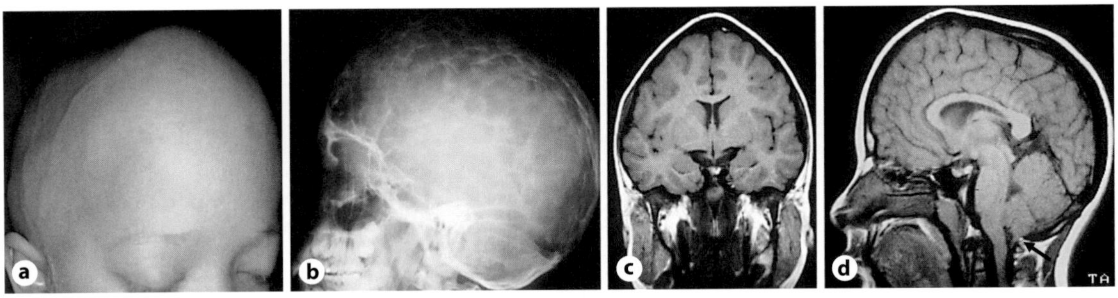

Fig. 7. Oxycephaly. Typical bregmatic bump is clearly seen on a patient with a shaved skull (**a**), absent sutures and copper beaten pattern on plain radiograph (**b**), typical deformity and an appearance of intracranial crowding on magnetic resonance images (**c**, **d**), mild descent of cerebellar tonsils (**d**, arrow).

lacking. Ophthalmologic signs usually become apparent only after the first year of life [51]. In up to 75% of affected individuals the deficient expansion of the posterior fossa results in a Chiari I malformation as described above (fig. 7d, also fig. 5 in Chapter 18). Oxycephaly is a fairly rare type of isolated craniosynostosis in Central Europe, accounting for only 2% of the total cohort studied in Würzburg, while it is observed at a rate of 40% or even higher in Mediterranean countries, particularly in the northern part of Africa [51, 52]. At this point, the question of etiology remains unanswered. Renier et al. speculated on a metabolic disorder related to the rachitic spectrum, but could not substantiate this assumption [51]. Conversely, the existence of affected families in consanguineous regions suggests an autosomal recessive inheritance.

Acknowledgements

This work was in part supported by the Division of Intramural Research, National Human Genome Research Institute, National Institutes of Health, Department of Health and Human Services, United States of America.

References

1 Boulet SL, Rasmussen SA, Honein MA: A population-based study of craniosynostosis in metropolitan Atlanta, 1989–2003. Am J Med Genet A 2008; 146A:984–991.
2 Bellus GA, Gaudenz K, Zackai EH, Clarke LA, Szabo J, Francomano CA, Muenke M: Identical mutations in three different fibroblast growth factor receptor genes in autosomal dominant craniosynostosis syndromes. Nat Genet 1996; 14:174–176.
3 Muenke M, Gripp KW, McDonald-McGinn DM, Gaudenz K, Whitaker LA, et al: A unique point mutation in the fibroblast growth factor receptor 3 gene *(FGFR3)* defines a new craniosynostosis syndrome. Am J Hum Genet 1997;60: 555–564.
4 Collmann H, Sörensen N, Krauß J: Consensus trigonocephaly. Childs Nerv Syst 1996;12:664–668.
5 Passos-Bueno MR, Serti Eacute AE, Jehee FS, Fanganiello R, Yeh E: Genetics of craniosynostosis: genes, syndromes, mutations and genotype-phenotype correlations. Front Oral Biol 2008;12:107–143.
6 Lajeunie E, Crimmins DW, Arnaud E, Renier D: Genetic considerations in nonsyndromic midline craniosynostoses: a study of twins and their families. J Neurosurg 2005;103:353–356.
7 van Aalst JA, Schultz G, Eppley BL: Craniosynostosis anomalies in twins. J Craniofac Surg 2005;16:696–699.
8 Ng SB, Buckingham KJ, Lee C, Bigham AW, Tabor HK, et al: Exome sequencing identifies the cause of a mendelian disorder. Nat Genet 2010;42:30–35.

9 Roach JC, Glusman G, Smit AF, Huff CD, Hubley R, et al: Analysis of genetic inheritance in a family quartet by whole-genome sequencing. Science 2010;328:636–639.
10 Baranzini SE, Mudge J, van Velkinburgh JC, Khankhanian P, Khrebtukova I, et al: Genome, epigenome and RNA sequences of monozygotic twins discordant for multiple sclerosis. Nature 2010;464:1351–1356.
11 Stein CM, Elston RC: Finding genes underlying human disease. Clin Genet 2009;75:101–106.
12 Lasky-Su J, Won S, Mick E, Anney RJ, Franke B, et al: On genome-wide association studies for family-based designs: an integrative analysis approach combining ascertained family samples with unselected controls. Am J Hum Genet 2010;86:573–580.
13 Renier D, Sainte-Rose C, Marchac D: Intracranial pressure in craniostenoses, in Marchac D (ed): Craniofacial Surgery: Proc 1st Int Congr Int Soc Cranio-Maxillo-Facial surgery, Cannes-La Napoule 1985, pp 110–113 (Springer, Berlin 1987).
14 Thompson DN, Malcolm GP, Jones BM, Harkness WJ, Hayward RD: Intracranial pressure in single-suture craniosynostosis. Pediatr Neurosurg 1995;22:235–240.
15 Florisson JM, van Veelen ML, Bannink N, van Adrichem LN, van der Meulen JJ, Bartels MC, Mathijssen IM: Papilledema in isolated single-suture craniosynostosis: prevalence and predictive factors. J Craniofac Surg 2010;21:20–24.
16 Reddy K, Hoffman H, Armstrong D: Delayed and progressive multisutural CS. Neurosurgery 1990;26:442–448.
17 Collmann H, Sörensen N, Krauss J: Hydrocephalus in craniosynostosis: a review. Childs Nerv Syst 2005;21:902–912.
18 Kapp-Simon KA, Speltz ML, Cunningham ML, Patel PK, Tomita T: Neurodevelopment of children with single suture craniosynostosis: a review. Childs Nerv Syst 2007;23:269–281.
19 Lajeunie E, Le Merrer M, Bonaïti-Pellie C, Marchac D, Renier D: Genetic study of scaphocephaly. Am J Med Genet 1996;62:282–285.
20 Butzelaar L, Breugem CC, Hanlo P, Mink van der Molen AB: Is isolated sagittal synostosis an isolated condition? J Craniofac Surg 2009;20:399–401.
21 Seto ML, Hing AV, Chang J, Hu M, Kapp-Simon KA, et al: Isolated sagittal and coronal craniosynostosis associated with TWIST box mutations. Am J Med Genet A 2007;143:678–686.
22 Zeiger JS, Beaty TH, Hetmanski JB, Wang H, Scott AF, et al: Genetic and environmental risk factors for sagittal craniosynostosis. J Craniofac Surg 2002;13:602–606.
23 Anderson PJ, Cox TC, Roscioli T, Elakis G, Smithers L, David DJ, Powell B: Somatic *FGFR* and *TWIST* mutations are not a common cause of isolated nonsyndromic single suture craniosynostosis. J Craniofac Surg 2007;18:312–314.
24 Kress W, Schropp C, Lieb G, Petersen B, Büsse-Ratzka M, et al: Saethre-Chotzen syndrome caused by *TWIST1* gene mutations: functional differentiation from Muenke coronal synostosis syndrome. Eur J Hum Genet 2006;14:39–48.
25 McGillivray G, Savarirayan R, Cox TC, Stojkoski C, McNeil R, et al: Familial scaphocephaly syndrome caused by a novel mutation in the FGFR2 tyrosine kinase domain. J Med Genet 2005;42:656–662.
26 Barritt J, Brooksbank M, Simpson D: Scaphocephaly: aesthetic and psychosocial considerations. Dev Med Child Neurol 1981;23:183–191.
27 Lajeunie E, Le Merrer M, Marchac D, Renier D: Syndromal and nonsyndromal primary trigonocephaly: analysis of a series of 237 patients. Am J Med Genet 1998;75:211–215.
28 Lajeunie E, Barcik U, Thorne JA, El Ghouzzi V, Bourgeois M, Renier D: Craniosynostosis and fetal exposure to sodium valproate. J Neurosurg 2001;95:778–782.
29 Kini U, Hurst JA, Byren JC, Wall SA, Johnson D, Wilkie AO: Etiological heterogeneity and clinical characteristics of metopic synostosis: evidence from a tertiary craniofacial unit. Am J Med Genet A 2010;152A:1383–1389.
30 Azimi C, Kennedy SJ, Chitayat D, Chakraborty P, Clarke JT, Forrest C, Teebi AS: Clinical and genetic aspects of trigonocephaly: a study of 25 cases. Am J Med Genet A 2003;117A:127–135.
31 van der Meulen J, van der Hulst R, van Adrichem L, Arnaud E, Chin-Shong D, et al: The increase of metopic synostosis: a pan-European observation. J Craniofac Surg 2009;20:283–286.
32 Di Rocco F, Arnaud E, Renier D: Evolution in the frequency of nonsyndromic craniosynostosis. J Neurosurg Pediatr 2009;4:21–25.
33 Bottero L, Lajeunie E, Arnaud E, Marchac D, Renier D: Functional outcome after surgery for trigonocephaly. Plast Reconstr Surg 1998;102:952–958.
34 Ousterhout DK, Peterson-Falzone SJ: Long-term follow-up on a case of untreated trigonocephaly. Cleft Palate J 1980;27:72–75.
35 Dominguez R, Sang K, Bender T, Girdany B: Uncomplicated trigonocephaly. Radiology 1981;140:681–688.
36 Jehee FS, Johnson D, Alonso LG, Cavalcanti DP, de Sá Moreira E, et al: Molecular screening for microdeletions at 9p22–p24 and 11q23–q24 in a large cohort of patients with trigonocephaly. Clin Genet 2005;67:503–510.
37 Jehee FS, Alonso LG, Cavalcanti DP, Kim C, Wall SA, et al: Mutational screening of *FGFR1*, *CER1*, and *CDON* in a large cohort of trigonocephalic patients. Cleft Palate Craniofac J 2006;43:148–151.
38 Gosain AK, Steele MA, McCarthy JG, Thorne CH: A prospective study of the relationship between strabismus and head posture in patients with frontal plagiocephaly. Plast Reconstr Surg 1996;97:881–891.
39 Mulliken JB, Gripp KW, Stolle CA, Steinberger D, Müller U: Molecular analysis of patients with synostotic frontal plagiocephaly (unilateral coronal synostosis). Plast Reconstr Surg 2004;113:1899–1909.
40 Arnaud E, Meneses P, Lajeunie E, Thorne JA, Marchac D, Renier D: Postoperative mental and morphological outcome for nonsyndromic brachycephaly. Plast Reconstr Surg 2002;110:6–12.
41 Martínez-Lage JF, Poza M, Lluch T: Craniosynostosis in neural tube defects: a theory on its pathogenesis. Surg Neurol 1996;46:465–469.
42 Mulliken JB, Vander Woude DL, Hansen M, LaBrie RA, Scott RM: Analysis of posterior plagiocephaly: deformational versus synostotic. Plast Reconstr Surg 1999;103:371–380.
43 Renier D, Lajeunie E, Arnaud, E, Marchac D: Management of craniosynostoses. Childs Nerv Syst 2000;16:645–658.
44 Dhamcharee V, Boles RG: *FGFR* mutations and plagiocephaly. J Craniofac Surg 2008;19:290–291.

45 Greene AK, Mulliken JB, Proctor MR, Meara JG, Rogers GF: Phenotypically unusual combined craniosynostoses: presentation and management. Plast Reconstr Surg 2008;122:853–862.
46 Moore MH, Abbott AH, Netherway DJ, Menard R, Hanieh A: Bilambdoid and posterior sagittal synostosis: the Mercedes Benz syndrome. J Craniofac Surg 1998;9:417–422.
47 Neuhäuser G, Kaveggia EG, Opitz JM: Studies of malformation syndromes of man XXXIX: a craniosynostosis-craniofacial dysostosis syndrome with mental retardation and other malformations: 'craniofacial dyssynostosis'. Eur J Pediatr 1976;123:15–28.
48 Rhodes JL, Kolar JC, Fearon JA: Mercedes Benz pattern craniosynostosis. Plast Reconstr Surg 2010;125:299–304.
49 Hing AV, Click ES, Holder U, Seto ML, Vessey K, et al: Bilateral lambdoid and sagittal synostosis (BLSS): a unique craniosynostosis syndrome or predictable craniofacial phenotype? Am J Med Genet A 2009;149A:1024–1032.
50 Shiihara T, Kato M, Kimura T, Hayasaka K, Yamamori S, Ogata T: Craniosynostosis with extra copy of *MSX2* in a patient with partial 5q trisomy. Am J Med Genet Part A 2004;128A:214–216.
51 Renier D, Cinalli G, Lajeunie E, Arnaud E, Marchac D: Oxycéphalie, une craniosténose sévère. A propos d'une série de 129 cas. Arch Pédiatr 1997;4:722–729.
52 Acquaviva R, Tamic PM, Lebascle J, Kerdoudi H, Berrada A: Les craniosténoses en milieu marocain. A propos de 140 observations. Neurochirurgie (Paris) 1966;12:561–566.

Hartmut Collmann
Department of Pedriatric Neurosurgery
Julius-Maximilian's University
Josef-Schneider-Str. 2, 97074 Würzburg (Germany)
Tel. +49 931 201 24809, Fax +49 931 201 24540, E-Mail collmann.h@nch.uni-wuerzburg.de

Muenke M, Kress W, Collmann H, Solomon BD (eds): Craniosynostoses: Molecular Genetics, Principles of Diagnosis, and Treatment.
Monogr Hum Genet. Basel, Karger, 2011, vol 19, pp 177–183

Molecular Genetic Testing of Patients with Craniosynostosis

U. Hehr

Center for and Department of Human Genetics, University of Regensburg, Regensburg, Germany

Abstract

Craniosynostosis is an etiologically heterogeneous condition and includes isolated and syndromal forms, which may result from exogenous as well as genetic factors. Genetic testing of patients with craniosynostosis is today an integral part of the routine diagnostic workup and allows identifying causal genetic alterations in up to 45% of unselected patient cohorts. Test results may provide important information on the expected further clinical course and long-term prognosis of the individual patient and may directly influence further therapy decisions. Furthermore, identification of causal genetic alterations allows individual genetic counseling of the affected families on the mode of inheritance, the recurrence risk for further pregnancies and related aspects including potential options of prenatal genetic diagnosis. In contrast to the preceding chapters, this article will focus on the practical approaches of molecular genetic testing in craniosynostosis patients during direct medical care: Which genetic regions should be tested in which patients? How to proceed? The most frequent clinical situations will be addressed and appropriate workup will be suggested according to current knowledge, but also considering the limited resources available in many health care systems as well as potential implications of the anticipated test results for further medical care.

Genetic testing today is an integral part of the diagnostic workup of patients with suspected genetic disorders. Like many other conditions, craniosynostosis is etiologically heterogeneous and may develop as part of a more complex genetic or non-genetic disease, occur as isolated craniosynostosis caused by exogenous factors and/or genetic alterations or, due to current limited insights or ignorance, be classified as 'idiopathic'. Applying current genetic testing strategies, a causal genetic alteration today can be identified for up to 45% of unselected cohorts of craniosynostosis patients [1–3].

Identification of the causal mutation(s) solves the differential diagnosis for the individual patient by defining the underlying genetic cause and distinct clinical condition. It allows a more precise prediction of the expected clinical course and accurate genetic counseling for the affected family regarding the recurrence risk for further relatives as well as related aspects including potential options for prenatal genetic testing in subsequent pregnancies or even preimplantation genetic diagnosis. Furthermore, results of genetic testing in craniosynostosis patients may directly influence recommended surveillance intervals and therapy decisions (e.g. [4]).

First Step: Clinical Evaluation

Genetic testing of craniosynostosis patients should always be based on individual clinical presentation and clearly benefits from an interdisciplinary setting including evaluation by at least both a trained craniosurgeon and clinical dysmorphologist (see Chapters 17 and 18).

Important clinical and anamnestic information to be considered includes:

- Involved cranial sutures and resulting head shape
- Associated craniofacial abnormalities/dysmorphism
- Brain malformations and/or anomalies
- Extracranial malformations/abnormalities, e.g. limb malformations
- Positive family history for craniosynostosis, cranial surgery and/or abnormal head shape, skeletal or seizure disorders, developmental delay or other potentially genetic conditions, suggesting an underlying Mendelian trait.

A positive family history for and/or the presence of additional extracranial malformations and/or profound delay of motor/mental development should prompt simultaneous evaluation by a trained dysmorphologist to exclude the presence of craniosynostosis as part of a more complex chromosomal or monogenic disorder (see Chapters 11 and 13). Conventional karyotyping and/or array comparative genomic hybridization (CGH) may be warranted for these patients as first line genetic testing to search for genomic imbalances. Depending upon the overall clinical presentation, additional testing of other genes may be necessary (see Chapter 17). Some craniosynostosis syndromes (e.g. Apert syndrome or craniofrontonasal syndrome) can directly be diagnosed based on a distinct combination of clinical features, and the diagnosis can then be confirmed by straightforward and cost-efficient syndrome-specific genetic testing.

Second Step: Genetic Workup of Craniosynostosis

In the absence of an obvious syndrome-specific overall appearance and extracranial malformations genetic testing should be planned based on the involved sutures and the resulting craniofacial morphology (fig. 1). Based on their own experience in the diagnostic workup Wilkie et al. [2] proposed a straightforward genetic approach for the molecular genetic testing of craniosynostosis patients to identify the underlying genetic alteration, which since then has been successfully adopted by our group as well as others.

Brachycephaly and Anterior Plagiocephaly Resulting from Predominant Coronal Craniosynostosis

The common 'syndromic' forms of uni- or bilateral coronal synostosis show autosomal dominant inheritance. These include the clinical entities Apert syndrome, Crouzon syndrome, Jackson-Weiss syndrome (JWS), Muenke syndrome, Pfeiffer syndrome and Saethre-Chotzen syndrome (SCS) and are clinically characterized by a congenital and progressive brachycephaly. Synostosis frequently is asymmetric and may affect additional sutures, with the most severe end of the spectrum presenting as cloverleaf skull. Patients may show additional skeletal anomalies, in particular affecting the hands and feet and/or a distinct facial gestalt including proptosis, midface hypoplasia or a beaked nose (for detailed clinical descriptions see individual preceding chapters). This overall clinical appearance may directly lead to the clinical diagnosis of Apert, classic Pfeiffer or craniofrontonasal syndrome (CFNS).

Considering the known clinical variability and phenotypic overlap, all other patients with predominantly coronal craniosynostosis may be subdivided for the genetic workup into patient cohorts with the most severe manifestation, such as clover leaf skull/plagiocephaly (severe Crouzon or Pfeiffer syndrome) and a uniform patient cohort

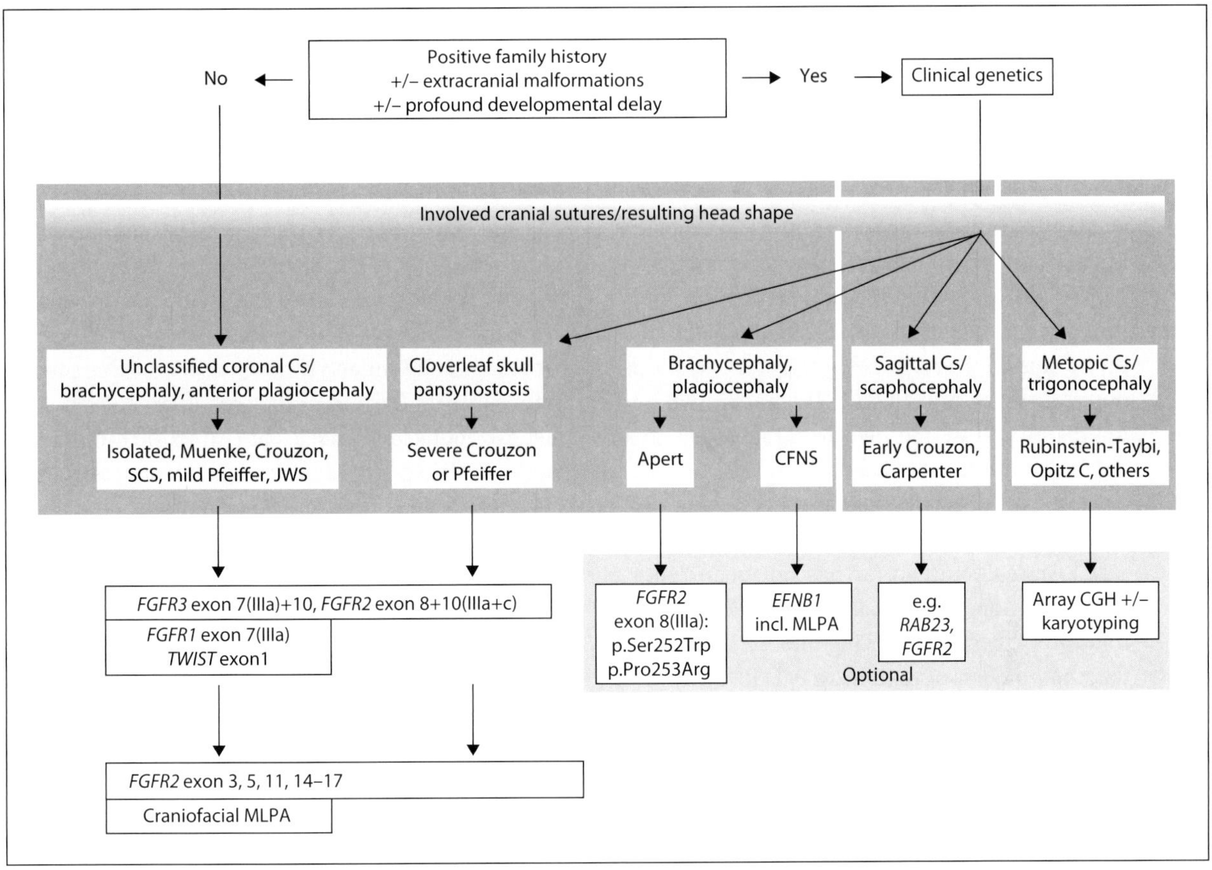

Fig. 1. Suggested genetic workup of craniosynostosis based on clinical findings and family history. CFNS, craniofrontonasal syndrome; Cs, craniosynostosis; JWS, Jackson-Weiss syndrome; SCS, Saethre-Chotzen syndrome.

including all milder forms of predominant coronal craniosynostosis with or without additional clinical features (isolated coronal craniosynostosis, Crouzon or Pfeiffer syndrome, Muenke syndrome, SCS, JWS).

Patients with the characteristic Apert phenotype should receive confirmatory testing for the 2 common mutations associated with this condition, p.Ser252Trp and p.Pro253Arg in exon 8 (IIIa) of the *FGFR2* gene, which together account for more than 98% of cases. Anecdotally, Apert patients without characteristic sequence alterations but with typical clinical features resulting from an exon deletion of, or Alu insertions into, exon 10 (IIIc) of *FGFR2* have been reported, but testing currently may only be available on a research basis [5].

Female patients with the characteristic combination of coronal craniosynostosis, severe hypertelorism, a bifid nose, and longitudinal ridging of the nails, suggestive of CFNS, should first be tested for sequence variants and exon deletions of the *EFNB1* gene.

For all other patients with predominant uni- or bilateral coronal synostosis first line genetic testing should start with testing for the Muenke mutation in *FGFR3* exon 7 (IIIa), followed by sequence analysis of *FGFR2* exons 8 and 10 (IIIa and IIIc), *FGFR3* exon 10 (Crouzon syndrome with acanthosis), and for milder forms in addition *FGFR1* exon 7 (IIIa) as well as *TWIST* exon 1. If negative, second line genetic testing in addition should encompass sequence analysis of *FGFR2* exons 3, 5, 11 and 14–17, as well as for milder craniosynostosis application of a craniofacial multiplex ligation-dependent probe amplification (MLPA) to detect deletions or duplications within the *TWIST* and *EFNB1* coding regions. Mutation detection rates vary greatly, depending on the clinical characterization and inclusion criteria for the tested patient cohort and for mixed patient cohorts may reach 25% [2].

Cloverleaf skull so far has not been reported in association with *FGFR1*, *TWIST* or *EFNB1* mutations; hence screening should only include the known hotspot regions in *FGFR2* and *FGFR3*. Genetic workup of syndromic cloverleaf skull in patients with rhizomelic short limb dwarfism is discussed in more detail under the section prenatal testing.

Microscopically visible and submicroscopic chromosomal imbalances appear to be a rare cause of coronal craniosynostosis, but array CGH may be indicated as first or third line genetic testing, particularly in the presence of additional abnormalities, e.g. profound developmental delay [3].

Scaphocephaly Resulting from Sagittal Craniosynostosis

The most common form of isolated craniosynostosis affects the midline sagittal (and metopic) sutures, is usually not the result of an underlying *FGFR* or *TWIST* mutation, and is only occasionally due to microscopic or submicroscopic chromosomal imbalances [2, 3]. Therefore further genetic workup should primarily be based on individual clinical presentation. Some patients with Crouzon syndrome initially present with sagittal craniosynostosis, only later followed by synostosis of the coronal suture(s). Therefore, sequence analysis of selected exons of *FGFR2* may be considered in young patients with the combination of sagittal craniosynostosis and a Crouzonoid facial gestalt [6].

Recently Jenkins et al. [7] identified the genetic basis of the very rare autosomal recessively inherited Carpenter syndrome, which in addition to predominant synostosis of midline sutures (sagittal and metopic) includes the characteristic combination of obesity and postaxial polydactyly and/or soft-tissue syndactyly. Most if not all characteristic patients harbor homozygous or compound heterozygous predicted loss-of-function mutations of the *RAB23* gene (MIM 606144) located on chromosome 6p11.2. The nonsense mutation p.L145X appears to be a predominant founder mutation in patients of Northern European origin (25/34 alleles from 15 independent families reported in [7]). Patients with characteristic phenotype but negative for p.L145X, should be tested by direct sequencing of the entire *RAB23* coding region.

Trigonocephaly Resulting from Metopic Craniosynostosis

Genetic alterations identified in patients with trigonocephaly predominantly are chromosomal imbalances, which may be identified in up to 30% of patients with metopic craniosynostosis [3]. Hence first line genetic testing should include array CGH and/or conventional karyotyping. If negative and/or in the presence of additional extracranial abnormalities, further evaluation by a clinical dysmorphologist is indicated in order to exclude distinct monogenic disorders like Opitz trigonocephaly syndrome (syn. C syndrome; OMIM 211750) [8].

Genetic Testing of Patients with Craniosynostosis as Part of Other Genetic Syndromes

Craniosynostosis in addition has been associated with a wide variety of rare syndromes with or without associated genetic alterations (see Chapters 11, 13, 17). Further diagnostic workup should regard the overall phenotypic presentation and family history, e.g. X-linked inheritance with a more pronounced phenotype in females may prompt direct genetic testing of *EFNB1*. In the presence of associated features affecting connective tissue, e.g. arterial aneurysms or dissections, joint laxity or scoliosis testing of *TGFBR1* and *TGFBR2* may be considered. The characteristic combination of craniosynostosis with obesity and polydactyly may prompt testing of *RAB23*.

Choosing the Laboratory
Genetic testing of craniosynostosis patients should be preferentially referred to genetic laboratories that meet specific quality standards (i.e., CLIA, ISO DIN) and which have expertise in the evaluation of test results for genes associated with craniosynostosis. Regularly updated lists of genetic laboratories offering genetic testing are available in databases such as:
http://www.ncbi.nlm.nih.gov/sites/GeneTests/lab?db = GeneTests
http://www.hgqn.org/
http://www.eurogentest.org/

These lists also provide links to the laboratory homepage with further information on sample requirements, shipping and handling recommendations, as well as download of information and consent forms. Informed consent of the patients or the legal custodian should be obtained prior to any genetic testing and a copy of the signed consent form should be included with shipment of the sample. Many laboratories additionally offer clinical advice on the most efficient testing strategy considering the available clinical and anamnestic data of the patient and may assist referring clinicians with further questions including cost coverage.

Third Step: Interpretation of Test Results and Genetic Counseling

Reports of genetic testing results regularly include detailed information on the method of testing applied (e.g. sequencing, MLPA) and the covered genetic regions (e.g. only particular exons or entire coding region analyzed). As a general rule, negative results of any diagnostic genetic testing do not exclude other genetic causal alterations not covered with the performed analysis; hence do not rule out an underlying genetic disorder with an increased recurrence risk for further relatives.

In general, conventional karyotyping will identify microscopically visible numerical or structural chromosomal anomalies (e.g. trisomy 21 or chromosomal translocations), but will not detect intragenic sequence alterations.

'Molecular genetic karyotyping' or array CGH will pick up microscopic and in addition submicroscopic chromosomal imbalances, e.g. duplications or deletions of chromosomal segments, but will not detect balanced chromosomal rearrangements without gain or loss of chromosomal material (balanced translocations) or intragenic point mutations.

MLPA (MRC Holland) is designed for individual clinical situations and contains probes to identify deletion or duplication of one or several exons, e.g. in the genes associated with craniofacial disorders *TWIST*, *EFNB1* and selected exons of the *FGFR* genes. The individual MLPAs will not detect chromosomal rearrangements or intragenic sequence alterations.

Sequence analysis will detect smaller sequence alterations within the amplified PCR products of the analyzed gene, but will neither identify larger chromosomal rearrangements, heterozygous deletions or duplications nor any mutations outside the tested coding regions. Most recent technologies like next generation sequencing currently collect sequence data from more than 80% of the entire genome of the individual patient; feasible costs are within reach now, and major current problems like sequence coverage, reassembly and analysis of the obtained vast amount of sequence information and variants identified are expected to be solved within the next few years.

Genetic Counseling and Estimation of the Recurrence Risk

Results of any genetic testing should be communicated to the patient and/or his/her family in a genetic counseling session. For difficult situations, particularly regarding prospective prenatal or predictive testing, additional genetic counseling prior to any genetic test is strongly recommended and in some countries mandatory. The main aspects of the counseling session should be documented, including written consent of the patient and/or his/her guardian with the intended genetic analysis.

For relatives of patients with identified genetic alteration(s) and hence clinical condition, the recurrence risk is given according to the underlying Mendelian trait. If a mutation for an autosomal dominant inherited condition is identified for the first patient of a family, clinical evaluation and/or genetic testing of both parents should be offered considering the known data on penetrance and clinical variability for the underlying disorder and genetic alteration. It is not a rare situation, that one parent of a child, e.g. with an *FGFR*-associated coronal synostosis, in fact presents with mild clinical signs such as brachycephaly or broad thumbs not previously considered as manifestation of a monogenic craniosynostosis syndrome.

For siblings of a seemingly sporadic 'non-syndromic' craniosynostosis patient without evidence for a craniosynostosis minor manifestation in one parent and without identified mutation, an overall empiric recurrence risk of 1% has been suggested, or 3% in the case of sporadic coronal craniosynostosis [9]. If a mutation has been identified in the index case, but excluded for both parents (a so called de novo mutation), the recurrence risk for further siblings depends on the probability of germ line mosaicism for the individual gene. For example, for prospective siblings of patients with presumed de novo mutation in one of the *FGFR* genes, a slightly increased but low recurrence risk below 1% has been reported due to mosaicism exclusively in the paternal germ cells [2] (see Chapter 6).

Prenatally Suspected Craniosynostosis

Prenatal detection of a fetal malformation or abnormality is always a challenge for both the expectant parents as well as the involved health care professionals. This situation requires rapid differential diagnosis and identification of the underlying clinical condition in order to reach an informed decision based on precise data on the expected clinical course, treatment options and long-term outcome of the individual child.

Prenatally suspected craniosynostosis should always prompt detailed sonographic evaluation of the fetus by an expert in prenatal medicine in order to search for associated malformations/anomalies (see Chapter 16). For example, a cloverleaf skull due to fusion of several cranial sutures and associated severe micromelia and narrow thorax suggest thanatophoric dysplasia, a perinatally lethal condition. Prenatal detection of the milder allelic disorder achondroplasia in association with craniosynostosis has also been reported [10]. Both conditions today can be rapidly confirmed by sequence analysis of selected exons of the *FGFR3* gene in 99% of characteristic cases within a few days. Genetic workup of prenatally identified isolated craniosynostosis during the 2nd and 3rd trimester should follow the stepwise recommended analysis depending upon affected cranial sutures and head shape (fig. 1).

Prenatal Diagnosis in Families with Positive Family History for Craniosynostosis

Some families with a positive family history for craniosynostosis may request prenatal or preimplantation genetic diagnosis. In general, precise exclusion of the recurrence risk for an ongoing pregnancy will only be possible if a causal mutation has been identified in this family prior to the intended prenatal testing. We here recommend genetic counseling of the family prior to any prenatal testing, which in addition to the recurrence risk should also cover the ethical issues of reduced penetrance and inter- and intrafamilial variability for the individual clinical condition.

If a mutation has not been identified in the family so far, genetic testing of an index proband of this family with characteristic clinical signs may be arranged to identify the underlying genetic cause. However, if no mutation can be identified in an index proband with or without negative family history, predictive testing of an ongoing pregnancy without sonographic fetal abnormalities to clarify the empiric recurrence risk is not recommended considering the etiological heterogeneity of craniosynostosis.

References

1 Morriss-Kay GM, Wilkie AO: Growth of the normal skull vault and its alteration in craniosynostosis: insights from human genetics and experimental studies. J Anat 2005;207:637–653.

2 Wilkie AO, Bochukova EG, Hansen RM, Taylor IB, Rannan-Eliya SV, et al: Clinical dividends from the molecular genetic diagnosis of craniosynostosis. Am J Med Genet A 2007;143A:1941–1949.

3 Jehee FS, Krepischi-Santos AC, Rocha KM, Cavalcanti DP, Kim CA, et al: High frequency of submicroscopic chromosomal imbalances in patients with syndromic craniosynostosis detected by a combined approach of microsatellite segregation analysis, multiplex ligation-dependent probe amplification and array-based comparative genome hybridisation. J Med Genet 2008;45:447–450.

4 Woods RH, Ul-Haq E, Wilkie AO, Jayamohan J, Richards PG, et al: Reoperation for intracranial hypertension in *TWIST1*-confirmed Saethre-Chotzen syndrome: a 15-year review. Plast Reconstr Surg 2009;123:1801–1810.

5 Bochukova EG, Roscioli T, Hedges DJ, Taylor IB, Johnson D, et al: Rare mutations of *FGFR2* causing Apert syndrome: identification of the first partial gene deletion, and an Alu element insertion from a new subfamily. Hum Mutat 2009;30:204–211.

6 McGillivray G, Savarirayan R, Cox TC, Stojkoski C, McNeil R, et al: Familial scaphocephaly syndrome caused by a novel mutation in the FGFR2 tyrosine kinase domain. J Med Genet 2005;42: 656–662.

7 Jenkins D, Seelow D, Jehee FS, Perlyn CA, Alonso LG, et al: *RAB23* mutations in Carpenter syndrome imply an unexpected role for hedgehog signaling in cranial-suture development and obesity. Am J Hum Genet 2007;80:1162–1170.

8 Kaname T, Yanagi K, Chinen Y, Makita Y, Okamoto N, et al: Mutations in CD96, a member of the immunoglobulin superfamily, cause a form of the C (Opitz trigonocephaly) syndrome. Am J Hum Genet 2007;81:835–841.

9 Harper PS: Practical Genetic Counselling, 6th ed. Oxford, Oxford University Press, 2004.

10 Karadimas C, Trouvas D, Haritatos G, Makatsoris C, Dedoulis E, et al: Prenatal diagnosis of achondroplasia presenting with multiple-suture synostosis: a novel association. Prenat Diagn 2006;26:258–261.

PD Dr. med. Ute Hehr
Zentrum und Institut für Humangenetik, Universität Regensburg
Universitätsklinikum D3, Franz-Josef-Strauss-Allee 11
93053 Regensburg (Germany)
Tel. +49 941 944 5410, Fax +49 941 944 5402, E-Mail ute.hehr@humangenetik-regensburg.de

Muenke M, Kress W, Collmann H, Solomon BD (eds): Craniosynostoses: Molecular Genetics, Principles of Diagnosis, and Treatment.
Monogr Hum Genet. Basel, Karger, 2011, vol 19, pp 184–198

Prenatal Sonographic Diagnosis of Craniosynostosis

T. Schramm

Prenatal Medicine Munich, Human Genetics and Obstetrics, Munich, Germany

Abstract
High-resolution and 3-dimensional ultrasound opens new possibilities for the examination of fetal bony structures. Prenatal ultrasound screening could potentially reveal most of the cases of craniosynostosis. Detailed expert examination allows for diagnosing most of syndromic and symptomatic cases. This study describes and discusses sonographic signs of craniosynostosis and typical findings in syndromic cases which are important for the indication of molecular genetic diagnosis.

The incidence of isolated craniosynostosis is reported to be 3 to 5 in 10,000. The incidence of syndromic craniosynostosis is significantly lower, estimated at 0.15 in 10,000 pregnancies [1]. Malformations of other organs, e.g. severe malformations of the heart (40 in 10,000 pregnancies) or spina bifida (5 in 10,000 pregnancies), that are potentially recognizable by prenatal ultrasound typically demonstrate a similar or higher incidence.

Despite the relatively high incidence, there are no data on the validity of prenatal ultrasound screening for craniosynostosis. Reports on the use of ultrasound as an important tool in the hands of an expert mainly deal with syndromic craniosynostosis, as in cases of Apert syndrome or Pfeiffer syndrome, both of which are associated with additional malformations.

Ultrasound Examination of the Normal Fetal Skull

For routine ultrasound examinations, two-dimensional (2D) ultrasound is used.

Detailed examination by experts in specialized centers is performed using both 2D- and three-dimensional (3D) ultrasound. With 3D ultrasound, it is possible to acquire volumes of 2D images that can be subsequently analyzed off-line. Clearly, this latter modality allows the display of three-dimensional images of the surface of an embryo or fetus. By eliminating soft tissue echoes and prominently emphasizing highly echogenic structures, bony structures can be demonstrated as appearing on an X-ray or spiral CT. Furthermore, multiplanar and tomographic displays of 2D-images are possible.

The vault of the skull, with its curvilinear bones and the sutures and fontanelles, is an important structure that is specifically assessed more accurately by 3D rendering than by 2D ultrasound [2, 3].

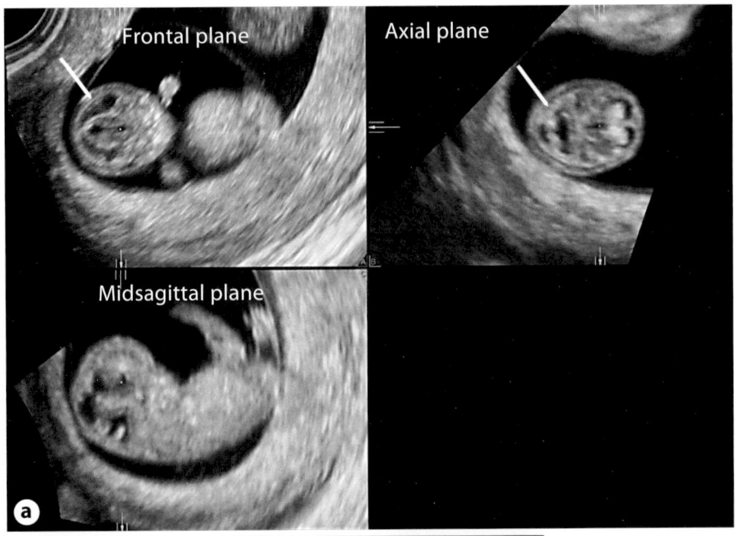

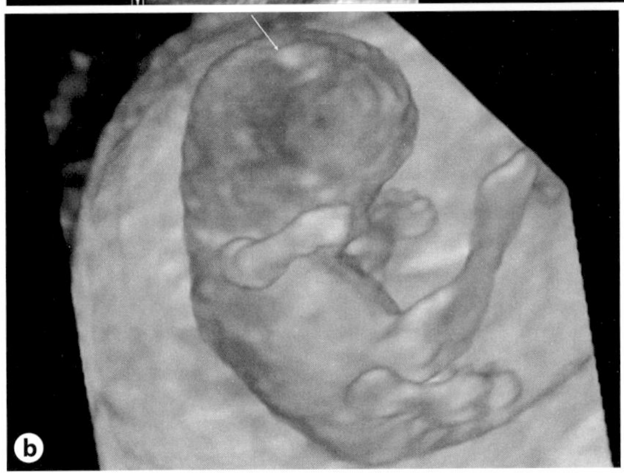

Fig. 1. **a** Embryo at 9 weeks 4 days (crown-rump-length 29 mm) in triplanar 2D display. The point of intersection between the 3 planes lies in the third ventricle. **b** Same embryo in 3D surface rendering. The skull shows only some small calcifications as precursors of the later bones (arrows).

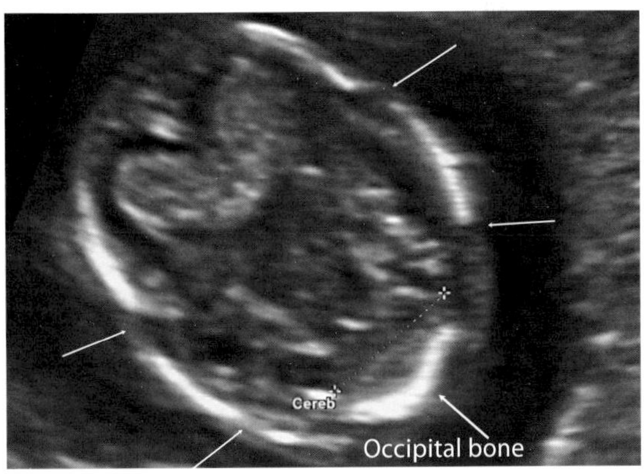

Fig. 2. Fetus at 12 weeks 4 days. Axial plane. Measurement of the hindbrain. Arrows indicate the coronal and lambdoid sutures and the occipital bone.

The bones of the fetal skull can be identified as hyperechogenic areas, which represent the ossification centers, as early as 9 weeks of gestation (note that gestational age is equivalent to menstrual age) (fig. 1). Early prenatal identification of sutures and fontanelles is possible from 12 to 13 weeks of gestation onwards using 2D- and 3D-ultrasound. The sutures are clearly seen as hypoechogenic spaces between the bones of the skull (figs. 2 and 3). With advancing gestational age, the sutures become narrower (figs. 4 and 5).

The growth of the skull, which depends on the growth of the brain, can be easily measured. The standard axial plane for measurement is the

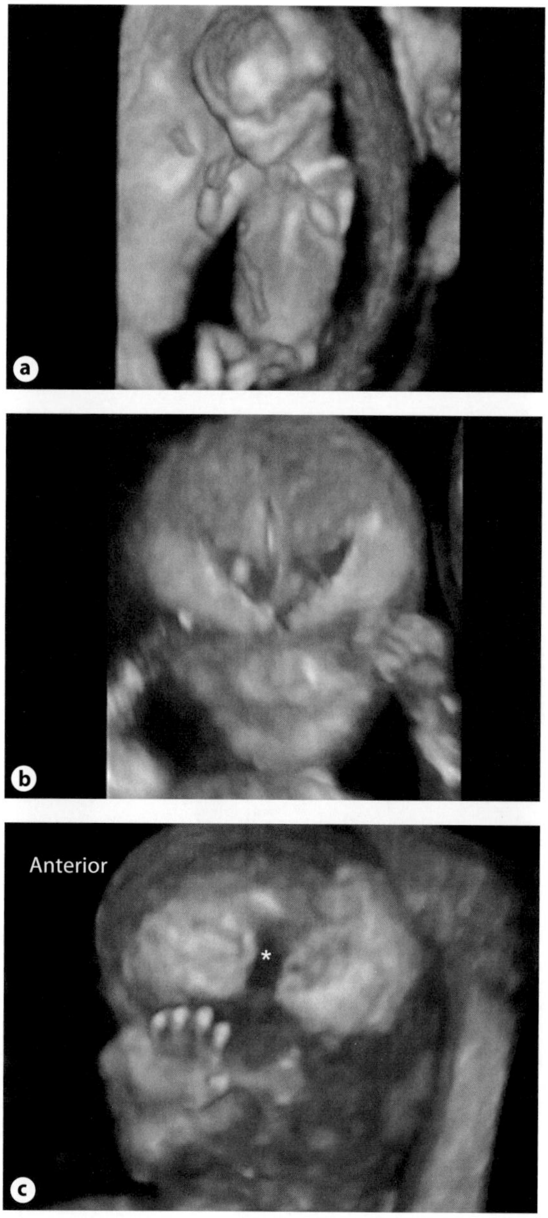

Fig. 3. **a** Whole fetus at 12 weeks 3 days. **b** Frontal view with frontal bones and metopic suture (11 weeks 4 days). **c** Lateral view with frontal bone, parietal bones and coronal suture (*).

occipitofrontal plane at the level of the thalami, the posterior horns of the lateral ventricles, and the cavum septi pellucidi (fig. 4). Biparietal and occipitofrontal diameters between 20 and 30 weeks of gestation normally show a ratio of 0.8 (0.73–0.85) [4].

Ultrasound in Craniosynostosis

In ultrasound screening, important signs of craniosynostosis are: loss of the hypoechogenic gap between the bones; irregular thickened inner sutural margin; in most cases, altered biometric parameters.

Figure 6a–c shows 2D images taken in a transthalamic axial plane of the fetal skull in cases of Apert syndrome, Muenke syndrome, and Pfeiffer syndrome, type 1 at 23 and 21 weeks. These fetuses demonstrate the typical signs of premature closure of the coronal suture. In some cases, a more or less discrete indentation of the sutures can be apparent, especially in fetuses with Pfeiffer syndrome [5]. The closure of the sutures leads to typical partial sonographic shadowing of the brain. When cloverleaf skull is present, major parts of the brain are not visible in axial standard views due to synostosis of all sutures except the metopic and squamosal sutures (fig. 6d). In trigonocephaly, where the metopic suture is closed, it will be impossible to see the midsagittal plane with the corpus callosum visible (fig. 6e).

Depending on the type of craniosynostosis, there may be brachycephaly in cases with craniosynostosis of the coronal sutures, or scaphocephaly when the sagittal suture is prematurely fused. Oxycephaly is difficult to assess prenatally, as there are no standard values for the craniocaudal size of the skull.

Using 3D ultrasound, it is possible to show an entire suture line in most cases. Closure of a part or of a whole suture can be demonstrated [6, 7]. In figure 7, a case with a complete synostosis of both coronal sutures and hydrocephalus internus

Caudal

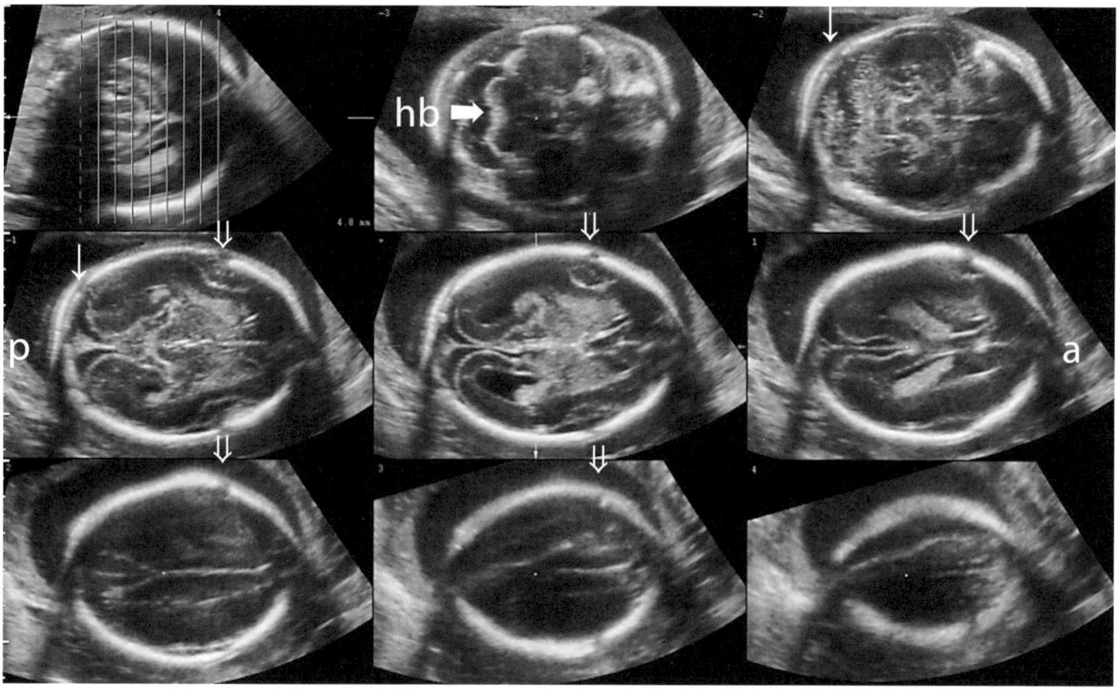

a Cranial

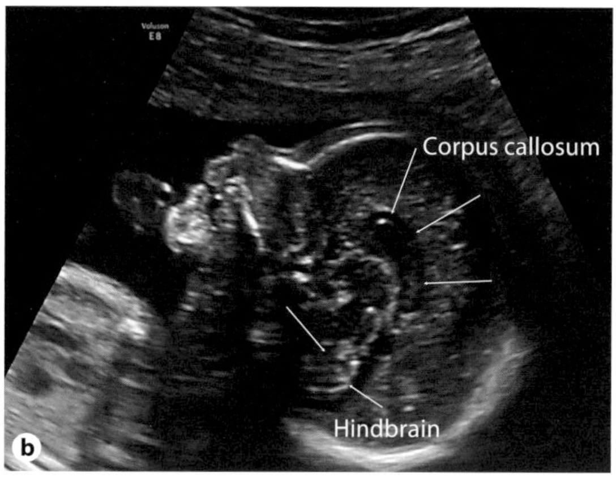

Fig. 4. Fetus at 21 weeks. **a** Axial sections in tomographic view (a = anterior, p = posterior, hb = hindbrain). Coronal and lambdoid sutures are visible as hyperechogenic gaps (coronal: open arrows; lambdoid: filled arrows). **b** Midsagittal section (arrows indicate the corpus callosum and the vermis of the hindbrain). As the metopic suture is open, the cerebral structures can be clearly identified (compare with fig. 6e).

is demonstrated. Figure 7b and c shows coronal synostosis in a case of Muenke syndrome at 21 weeks of gestation.

It is not precisely known when in pregnancy the closure of sutures occurs in cases of craniosynostosis. There is some evidence that the facial dysmorphism and the deformation of the skull may precede the osseous fusion by several weeks [8].

The most important issue of expert prenatal sonography is the differentiation and exact diagnosis of fetal malformations. The indication for

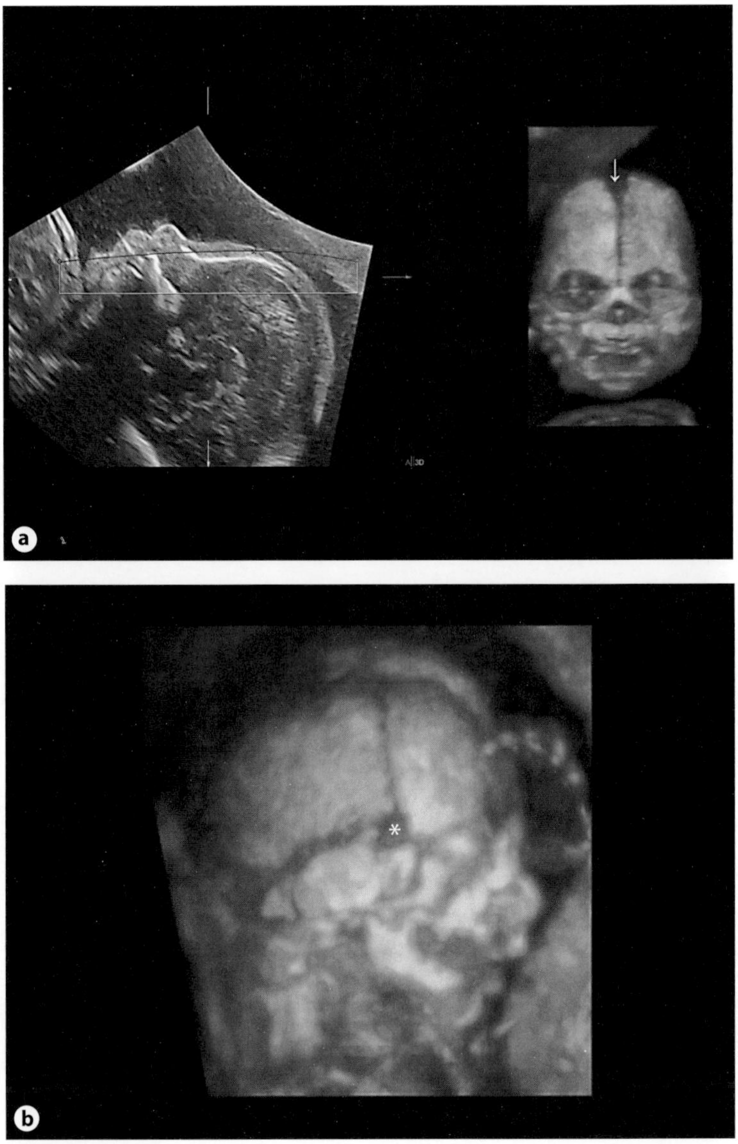

Fig. 5. Fetus at 21 weeks. 3D reconstruction of the sutures. **a** Metopic suture (arrow). On the left side is the 2D image. The black line indicates the point of view for the 3D-rendered image, which is a frontal view. **b** Lateral view with the coronal suture and the sphenoidal fontanelle (*).

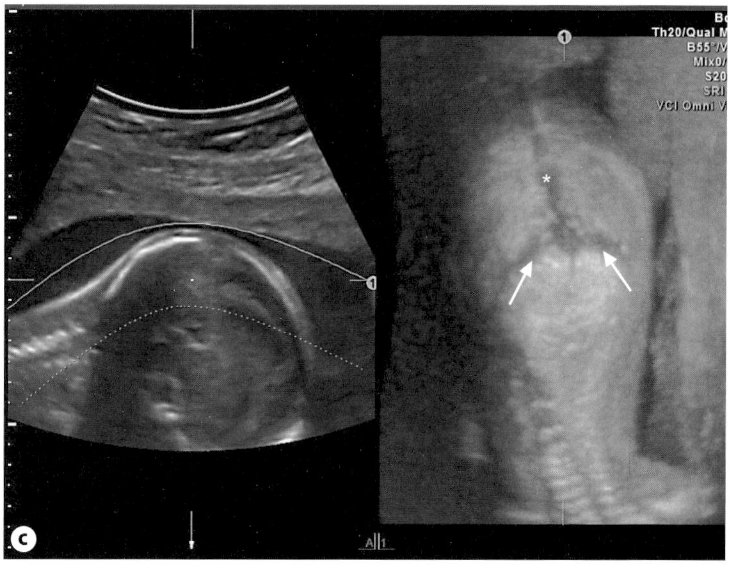

Fig. 5. **c** Sagittal suture (*) and lambdoid sutures (arrows). The solid white line indicates the perspective from the back of the fetus).

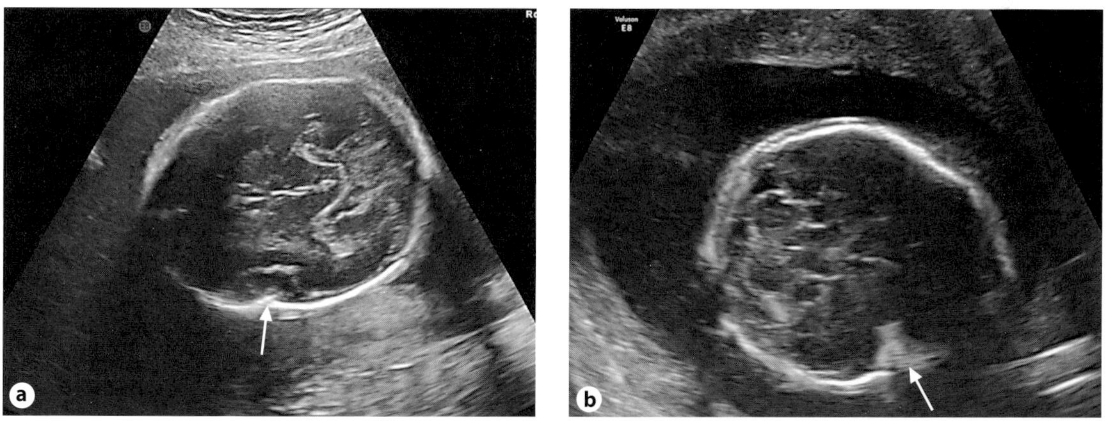

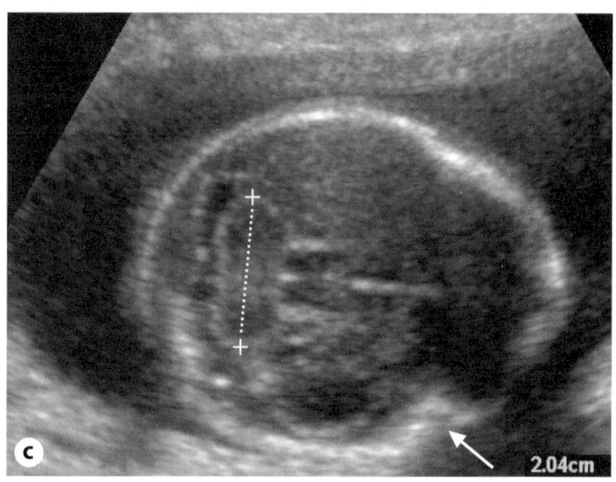

Fig. 6. 2D images of craniosynostosis. Note the thickening of the inner margin of the suture in every case (arrow) and the loss of the hypoechogenic gap between the bones. **a** Apert syndrome at 23 weeks. **b** Muenke syndrome at 21 weeks. **c** Pfeiffer syndrome type 1 at 21 weeks.

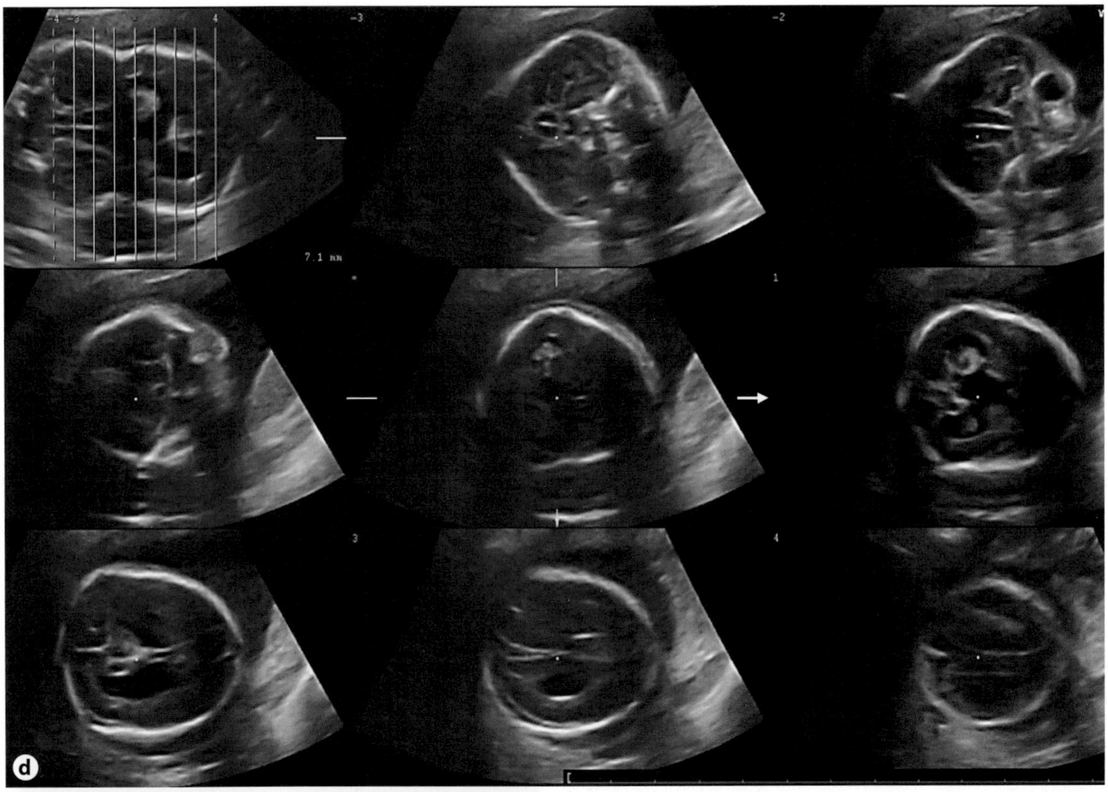

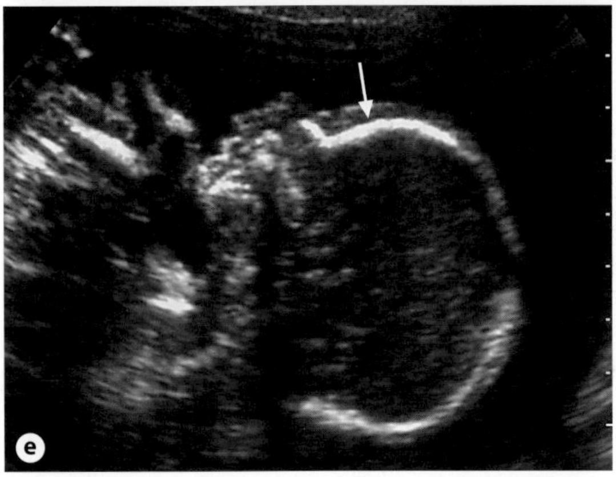

Fig. 6. d Cloverleaf skull in thanatophoric dysplasia type 2, 21 weeks (tomographic display of axial sections). **e** Trigonocephaly at 20 weeks, midsagittal section. There is acoustic shadowing behind the synostosis of the fused metopic suture (arrow).

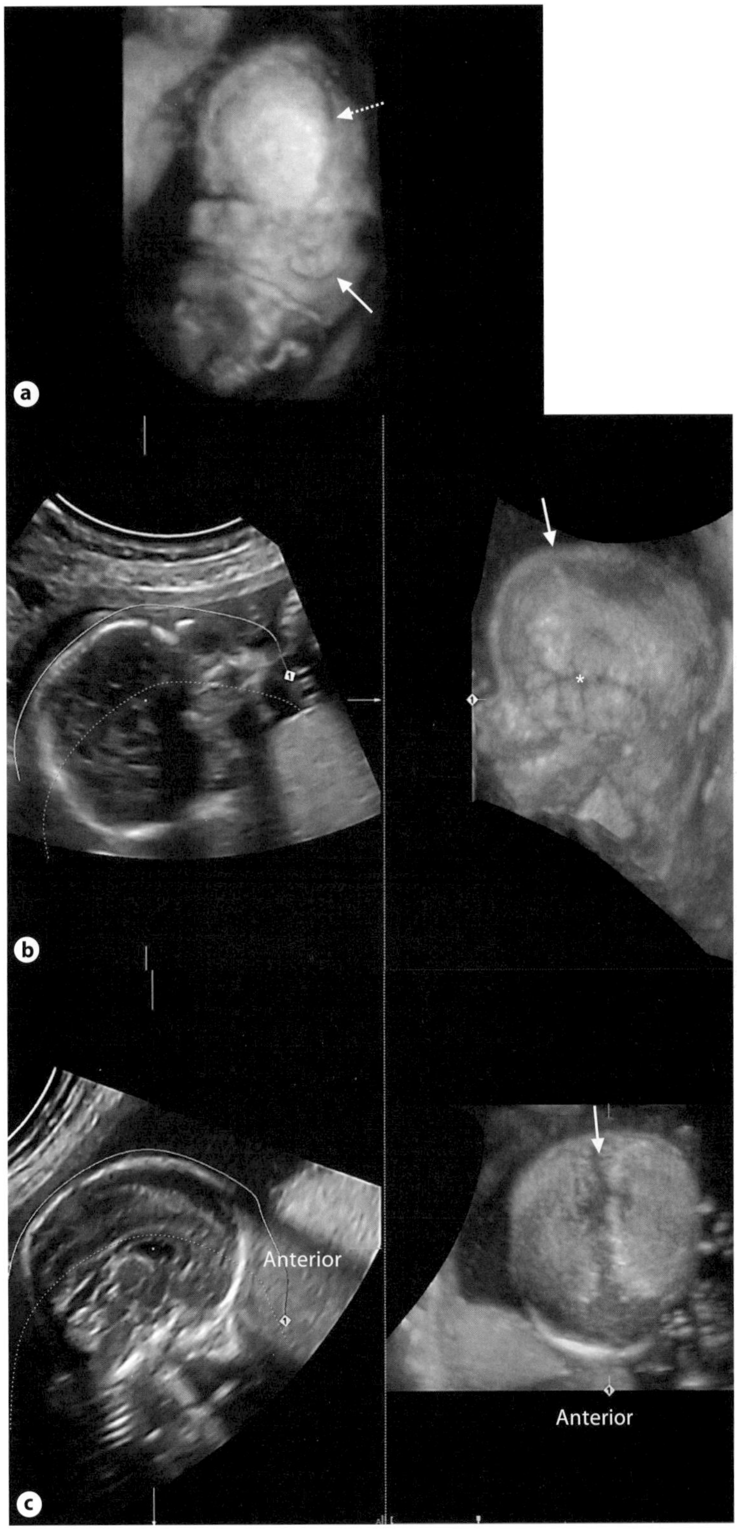

Fig. 7. 3D reconstruction of craniosynostosis. **a** Coronal synostosis (interrupted arrow) and hydrocephalus at 27 weeks (note the deeply located ear – arrow). Molecular genetic diagnosis did not reveal a distinct entity. **b** Muenke syndrome at 21 weeks (lateral view as indicated by the white line in the left part of the image). The coronal suture is closed (arrow). The sphenoidal fontanelle is indicated by an asterisk. **c** Same fetus from the top: normal sagittal suture (arrow). The coronal suture is not visible.

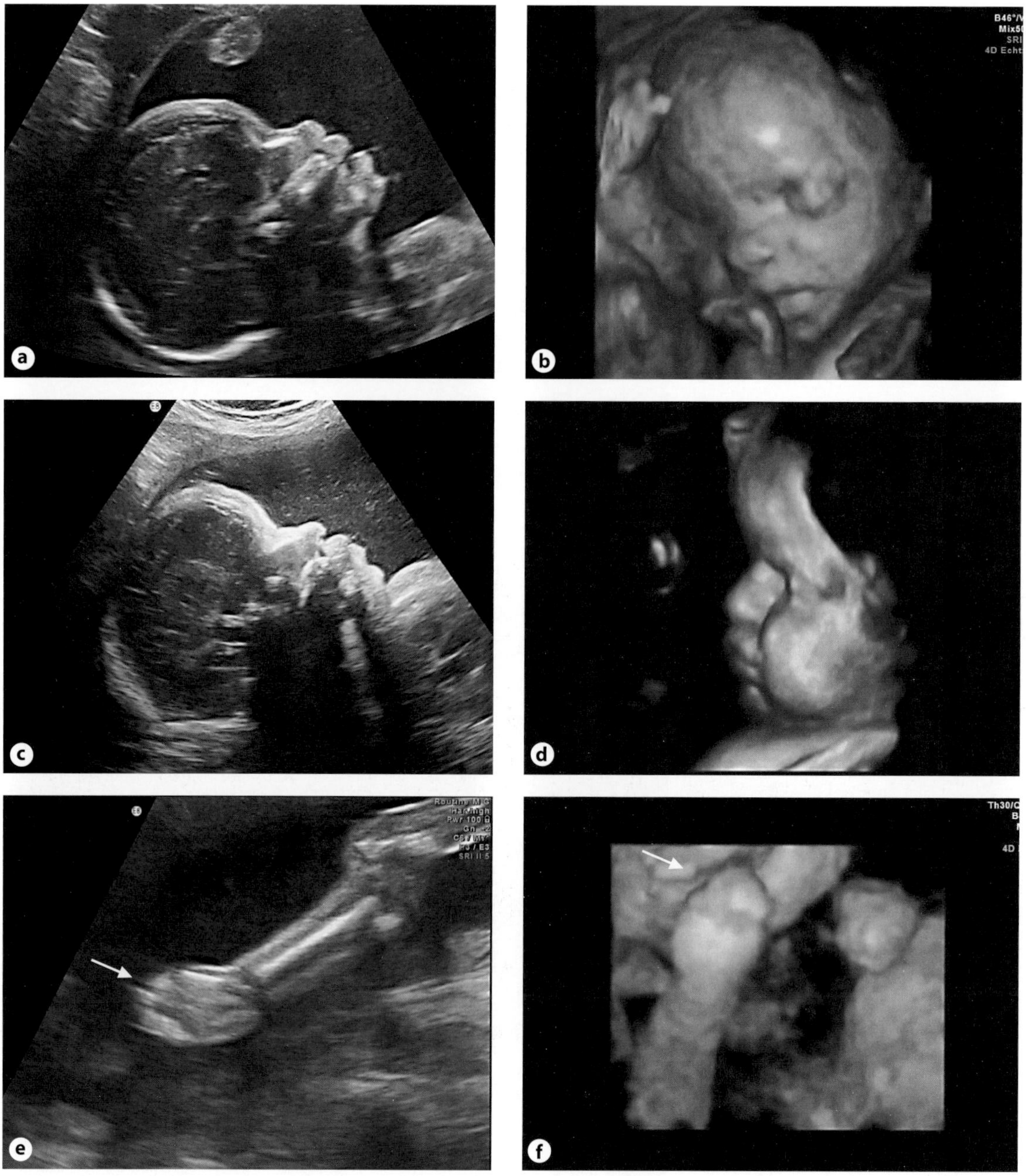

Fig. 8. Apert syndrome. **a** and **b** Face 2D and 3D at 23 weeks. The midfacial hypoplasia and frontal bossing are clearly visible. **c** and **d** Same fetus at 35 weeks. The appearance of the face is more dysmorphic than at 23 weeks. **e** and **f** 'Mitten'-hands at 21 weeks. The fingers are fused (arrows).

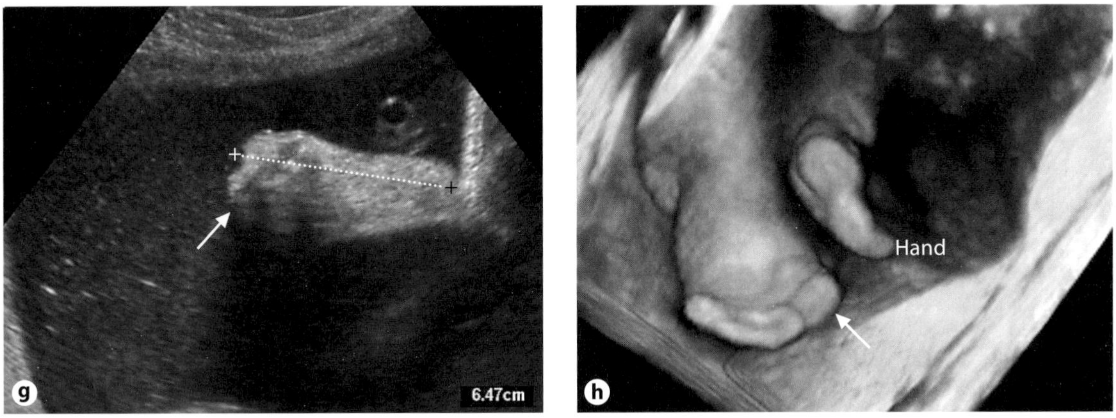

Fig. 8. g and **h** Cutaneous and osseous syndactyly of one foot in another fetus at 34 weeks. Note the fusion of the toes (arrows).

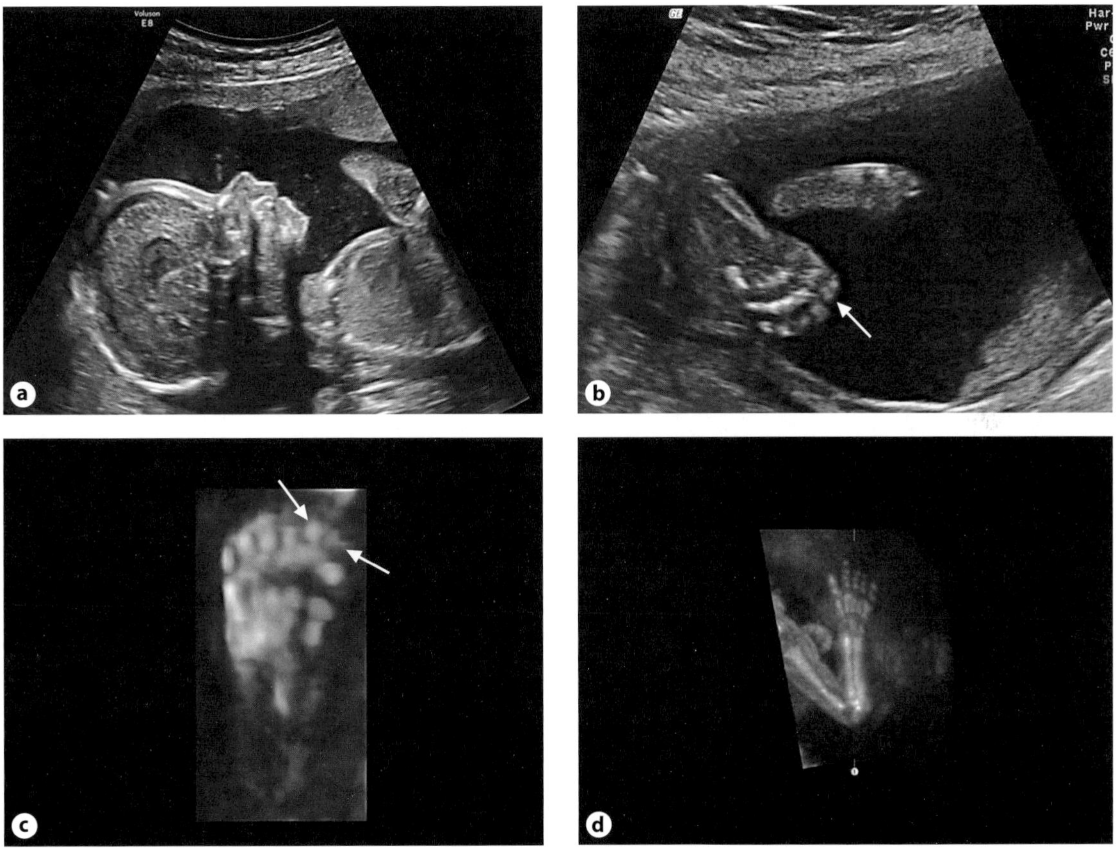

Fig. 9. Muenke syndrome at 21 weeks. **a** Typical face in 2D midsagittal section (note the short head and midfacial hypoplasia). **b** and **c** Foot with broad hallux, 2D and 3D. **d** Normal hand in 3D.

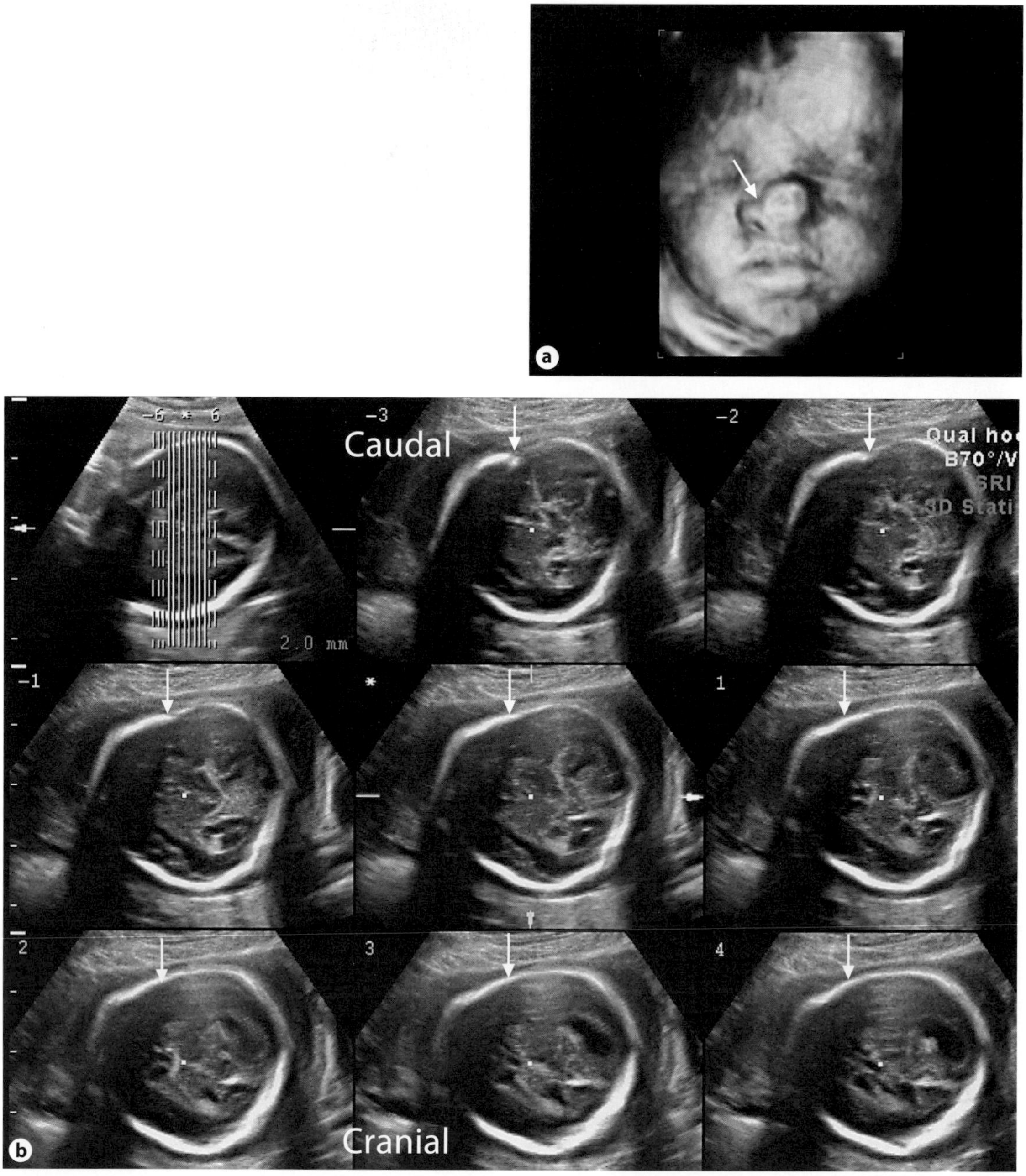

Fig. 10. Cerebro-oculo-nasal syndrome at 26 weeks. **a** 3D surface. Note the bifid nasal tip (arrow) and the rudimentary eyes. **b** Tomographic display of the skull with synostosis of the coronal suture (arrows). Note the short head.

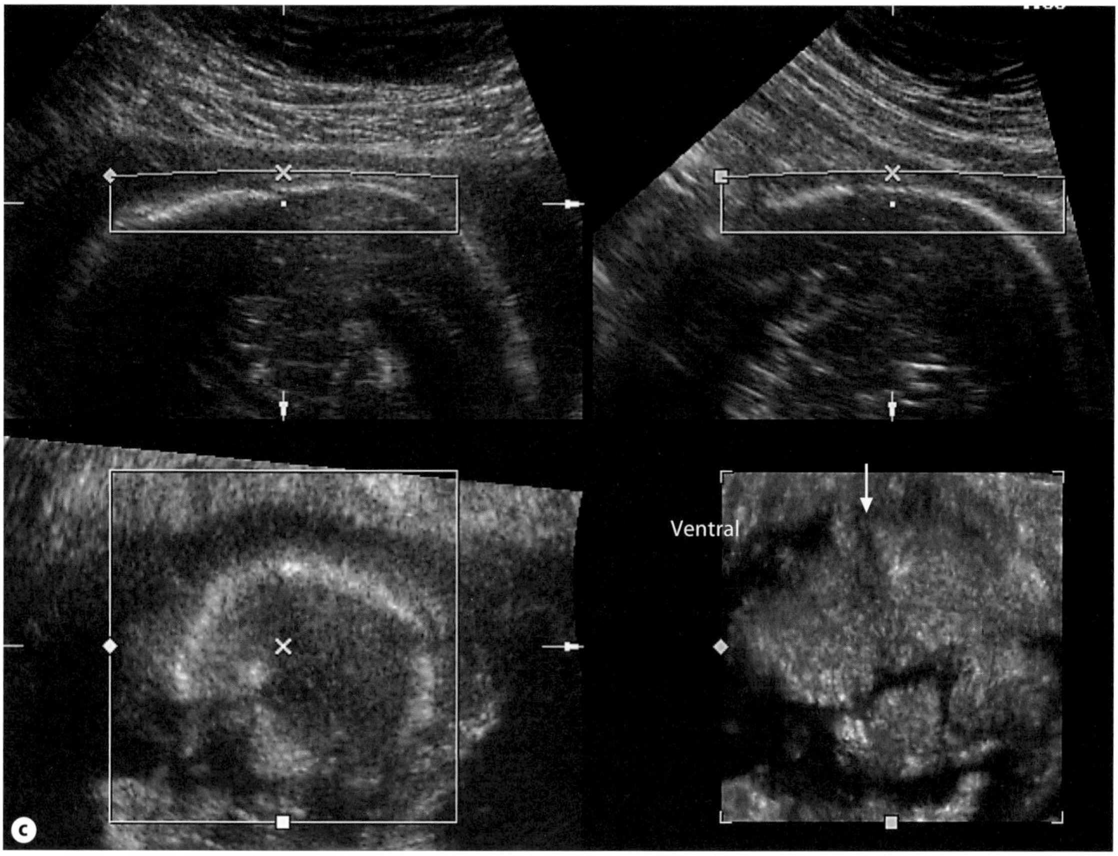

Fig. 10. **c** 3D reconstruction of the synostosis (arrow).

targeted genetic diagnostic testing and prenatal genetic counseling (regarding the prognosis, possible therapies, and the risk of recurrence, keeping in mind that these may be points to be discussed after birth) depend heavily on a precise description and interpretation of the anatomy. In craniosynostosis syndromes, a variety of facial dysmorphisms, limb abnormalities, and sometimes malformations of the brain can be seen. To a certain degree, the various features allow a sonographic differentiation between the syndromes.

The signs in cases of Apert syndrome are the most specific and well-recognized of the syndromic craniosynostoses. The head shows bilateral coronal craniosynostosis and an abnormal shape with acrobrachycephaly. The deformation of the face includes frontal bossing, a depressed nasal bridge, midface hypoplasia, as well as hypertelorism and exophthalmos. These findings may be subtle at 20 weeks gestation, and become more obvious late in pregnancy. Relatively specific signs include bilateral osseous and cutaneous syndactyly of the hands and feet (fig. 8). Possible malformations of the CNS reported in some studies on the prenatal diagnosis of Apert syndrome include ventriculomegaly and/or partial or complete agenesis of the corpus callosum [9].

In Pfeiffer syndrome, types 1 and 3, the aspect of the skull and face may be similar to that of cases of Apert syndrome, with the proptosis

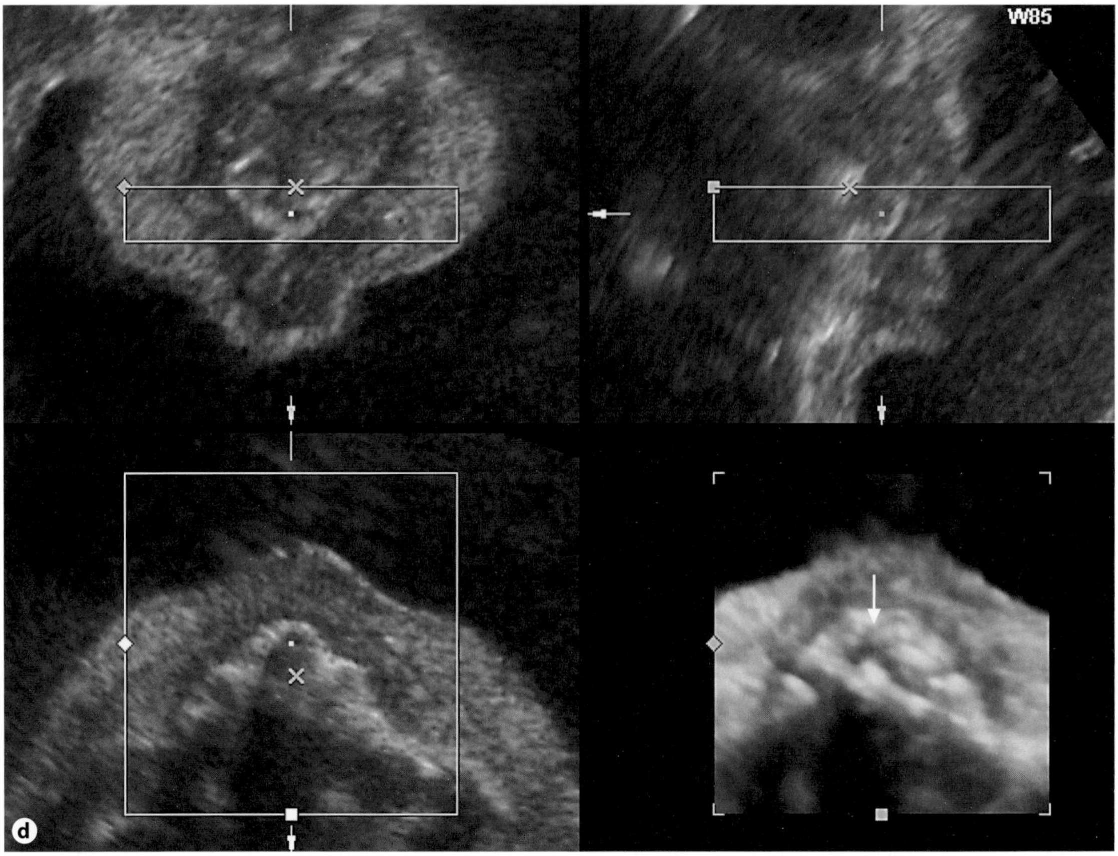

Fig. 10. d Maxilla from the bottom with single incisor (arrow). This is a multiplanar display with 3D reconstruction directly below.

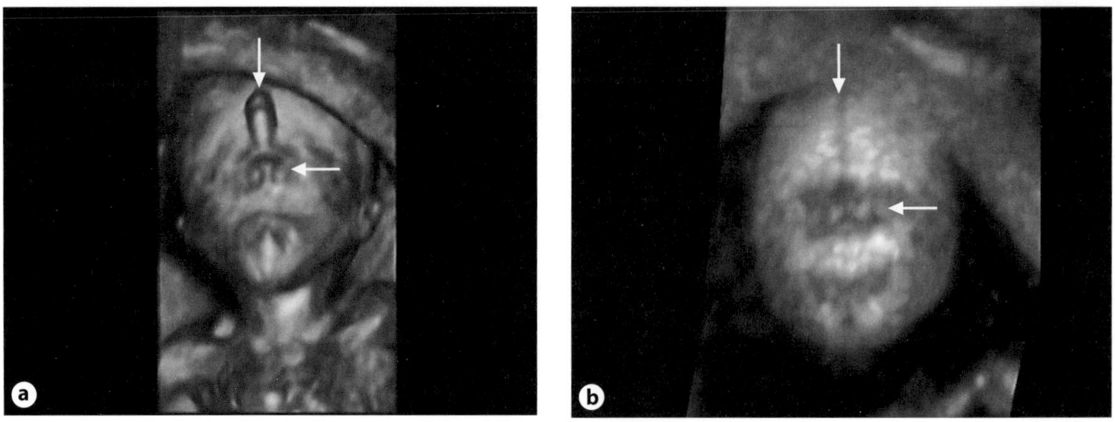

Fig. 11. Trisomy 13 at 15 weeks. Holoprosencephaly, cyclopia, proboscis, premature closure of the metopic suture. **a** and **b** show frontal views. **a** Surface reconstruction: proboscis (thin arrow), single orbit (thick arrow). **b** Skeletal reconstruction: the metopic suture is nearly closed (thin arrow), single orbit (thick arrow).

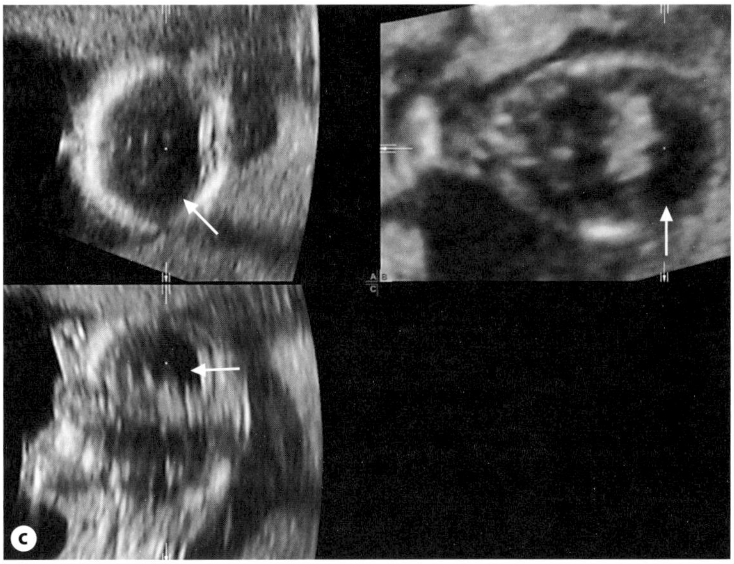

Fig. 11. **c** Multiplanar display of holoprosencephaly (arrows).

usually more pronounced in the former conditions. In Pfeiffer type 2, which is very rare, the craniosynostosis results in a cloverleaf skull deformity which is associated with hydrocephalus in most cases (fig. 6d). In cases of prenatal hindbrain herniation, visualization should be possible. Additionally, the abnormalities of the limbs are more subtle than in Apert syndrome. The hands and especially the feet show broad and medially deviated thumbs and halluces respectively. There may be a variable brachydactyly and discrete syndactyly [10].

In fetuses with Muenke syndrome, which most commonly includes coronal craniosynostosis, the limb abnormalities may be even more discrete, demonstrating only broad halluces and brachydactyly (fig. 9). Other symptoms as the fusion of the carpal and tarsal bones, thimble-like middle phalanges or epiphyseal coning are too discrete for sonographic visualization. Though there is little available in the medical literature, in this author's experience, similar findings may be found in cases of Jackson-Weiss syndrome or other craniosynostosis syndromes.

In addition to the craniosynostosis syndromes described above, there are a great variety of syndromes where craniosynostosis may occur as one manifestation of the broader condition. In OMIM, 114 entities with craniosynostosis are listed; in the Winter-Baraitser Dysmorphology Database, there are 205 entries [11, 12]. See Chapter 11 in this volume.

Differentiating the craniosynostosis syndromes from other phenotypically overlapping disorders does not tend to be difficult: micromelia is the most common finding in skeletal dysplasias, where the skull and face may look similar to the craniosynostosis syndromes, e.g. achondroplasia or thanatophoric dysplasia type 2 (TD 2) and other skeletal dysplasias. Anomalies of the ribs, hands and feet as well as of the spine allow the separation of these entities [13].

In some very rare diseases, the finding of craniosynostosis is helpful in establishing the diagnosis completely, such as in the example case of Cerebro-oculo-nasal syndrome. This very rare syndrome, which includes multiple congenital anomalies, is characterized by CNS anomalies such as hydrocephalus, ocular anomalies such as anophthalmia, typical alterations of the nose with a bifid nasal tip, asymmetric nares, microstomia, a single incisor, and altered bone growth of the skull (fig. 10).

In cases of holoprosencephaly, premature closure of the metopic suture is regularly determined prenatally. In holoprosencephaly, this finding is due to the frontal bones being derived from the neural crest. Disturbed migration of the neural crest cells leads to abnormally accelerated growth of the frontal bones and to impaired cleavage of the forebrain and midline defects of the face, such as cyclopia and facial clefts [14, 15] (fig. 11).

Conclusion

Craniosynostosis can be diagnosed by prenatal ultrasound. Expert examination allows the exact diagnosis of syndromic craniosynostosis and specific indications for molecular genetic diagnosis in most cases, especially those with Apert syndrome. Additional findings of the limbs may be discrete and overlapping with the other syndromic craniosynostoses.

References

1 Cohen MM, MacLean RE: Craniosynostosis: Diagnosis, Evaluation, and Management, 2nd ed. (Oxford University Press, New York 2000).
2 Ginath S, Debby A, Malinger G: Demonstration of cranial sutures and fontanelles at 15 to 16 weeks of gestation: a comparison between two-dimensional and three-dimensional ultrasonography. Prenat Diagn 2004;24:812–815.
3 Faro C, Benoit B, Wegrzyn P, Chaoui R, Nicolaides KH: Three-dimensional sonographic description of the fetal frontal bones and metopic suture. Ultrasound Obstet Gynecol 2005;26:618–621.
4 Snijders RJ, Nicolaides KH: Fetal biometry at 14–40 weeks' gestation. Ultrasound Obstet Gynecol 1994;4:34–48.
5 Nazzaro A, Della Monica M, Lonardo F, Di Blasi A, Baffico M, et al: Prenatal ultrasound diagnosis of a case of Pfeiffer syndrome without cloverleaf skull and review of the literature. Prenat Diagn 2004;24:918–922.
6 Benacerraf BR, Spiro R, Mitchell AG: Using three-dimensional ultrasound to detect craniosynostosis in a fetus with Pfeiffer syndrome. Ultrasound Obstet Gynecol 2000;16:391–394.
7 Esser T, Rogalla P, Bamberg C, Kalache KD: Application of the three-dimensional maximum mode in prenatal diagnosis of Apert syndrome. Am J Obstet Gynecol 2005;193:1743–1745.
8 Delahaye S, Bernard JP, Rénier D, Ville Y: Prenatal ultrasound diagnosis of fetal craniosynostosis. Ultrasound Obstet Gynecol 2003;21:347–353.
9 Quintero-Rivera F, Robson CD, Reiss RE, Levine D, Benson C, Mulliken JB, Kimonis VE: Apert syndrome: what prenatal radiographic findings should prompt its consideration? Prenat Diagn 2006;26: 966–972.
10 Blaumeiser B, Loquet P, Wuyts W, Nöthen MM: Prenatal diagnosis of Pfeiffer syndrome type II. Prenat Diagn 2004;24:644–646.
11 OMIM®- Online Mendelian Inheritance in Man. http://www.ncbi.nlm.nih.gov/omim [Accessed 23 May 2010].
12 Winter R, Baraitser M: Winter-Baraitser Dysmorphology Database, Version 1.0.19 (London medical databases Ltd, London, UK, 2007).
13 Schramm T, Gloning KP, Minderer S, Daumer-Haas C, Hörtnagel K, Nerlich A, Tutschek B: Prenatal sonographic diagnosis of skeletal dysplasias. Ultrasound Obstet Gynecol 2009;34:160–170.
14 Faro C, Wegrzyn P, Benoit B, Chaoui R, Nicolaides KH: Metopic suture in fetuses with holoprosencephaly at 11 + 0 to 13 + 6 weeks of gestation. Ultrasound Obstet Gynecol 2006;27:162–166.
15 Raam MS, Solomon BD, Shalev SA, Muenke M: Holoprosencephaly and craniosynostosis: A report of two siblings and review of the literature. Am J Med Genet C Semin Med Genet 2010; 154C:176–182.

Thomas Schramm
Praenatal-Medizin München
Lachnerstrasse 20
80639 München (Germany)
Tel. +49 89 1307440, Fax +49 89 13074499, E-Mail schramm@praenatal-medizin.de

Muenke M, Kress W, Collmann H, Solomon BD (eds): Craniosynostoses: Molecular Genetics, Principles of Diagnosis, and Treatment.
Monogr Hum Genet. Basel, Karger, 2011, vol 19, pp 199–215

Clinical Approach to Craniosynostosis

K.W. Gripp

Alfred I. duPont Hospital for Children, Wilmington, Del., USA

Abstract

Although abnormal skull shape is the typical presentation of craniosynostosis, it is more often due to deformational forces than to premature suture fusion. These mechanisms can usually be differentiated based on physical examination and review of the medical history. Premature suture fusion results in characteristic skull changes that vary with the affected suture, and imaging studies may confirm suspected synostosis. Craniectomy is the definitive treatment for craniosynostosis, and a single well-timed surgical procedure is sufficient in many patients with isolated synostosis. In contrast, craniosynostosis in combination with other congenital abnormalities implies more complex medical needs. Multiple congenital anomalies can have many different causes including teratogen exposure, single gene disorders, and chromosome abnormalities. A comprehensive dysmorphology evaluation, review of systems, and family history will inform the differential diagnosis, which in turn guides molecular genetic testing. When an underlying cause is identified, additional evaluation may focus on organ systems typically affected by the specific disorder, and the surgical approach may be modified based on the anticipated outcome. Family members benefit from the delineation of a specific cause because they can be counseled regarding the presence or absence of recurrence risk and its implications.

An abnormal head shape noted in infancy or early childhood often raises a concern for craniosynostosis. However, numerous other congenital anomalies or environmental influences can result in an abnormal head shape, and thus it is necessary to confirm the presence of craniosynostosis. A thorough clinical evaluation of patients with suspected or confirmed craniosynostosis will determine the most appropriate and cost-effective treatment approach.

Abnormal Head Shape in the Absence of Craniosynostosis

Skull asymmetry or a configuration significantly different from the expected rounded head shape may lead to a concern for craniosynostosis. However, such abnormalities are more often the result of environmental factors than of craniosynostosis. The most frequent cause of head shape irregularities is deformational plagiocephaly resulting from external molding forces on the malleable skull. These forces may occur in the intrauterine environment through crowding or abnormal birth position, or after birth by a nonvarying head position. The dolichocephalic head shape seen in many premature infants is an example of positional deformation, and although this elongated head shape resembles that seen

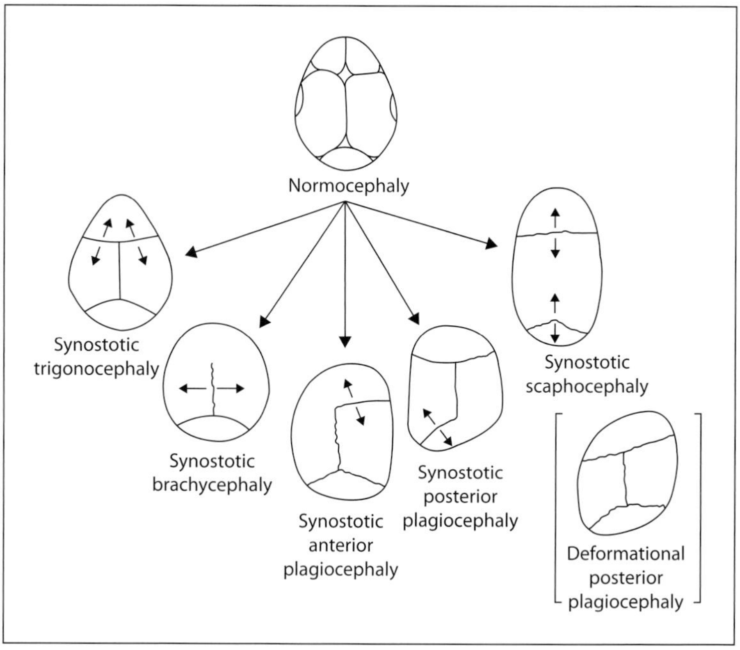

Fig. 1. Diagram of skull shapes resulting from synostosis or deformation. Drawing courtesy of M.M. Cohen, Jr.

with sagittal synostosis, these can easily be distinguished on clinical examination. It has been suggested that the supine sleeping position promoted for neonates in order to prevent sudden infant death resulted in increased posterior positional plagiocephaly [1]. Other risk factors for positional plagiocephaly include male sex and prematurity, but the most frequently identified contributing factor is congenital muscular torticollis resulting in a head rotational preference. Active head rotational preference can be measured, as delineated by Rogers et al. in 2009 [2], and typically shows a rotational preference to the flattened side. Positional plagiocephaly is characterized by unilateral flattening of the occiput, slight ipsilateral frontal protrusion, and anterior change in the ear position (figs. 1 and 2). These changes can be quantified by several different techniques [3, 4]. Congenital muscular torticollis is typically amenable to physical therapy. Other factors, such as ocular and vertebral abnormalities resulting in a head positional preference in oculoauriculovertebral defect spectrum or Goldenhar syndrome, need to be considered because physical therapy does not benefit these patients. Epibulbar dermoids, microtia, preauricular skin tags, and facial asymmetry with an underdeveloped mandible on the affected side suggest an underlying diagnosis of oculoauriculovertebral defect spectrum, and associated structural vertebral anomalies may occur along the entire spine. Cardiac and renal structural abnormalities are not uncommon in these individuals [5]. Regardless of its ultimate cause, the head shape resulting from deformational forces can be differentiated from that seen in craniosynostosis (figs. 1 and 2).

Abnormal Head Shape Due to Craniosynostosis

Premature fusion of one or more cranial sutures restricts normal head growth, leading to compensatory growth in dimensions not restricted by the

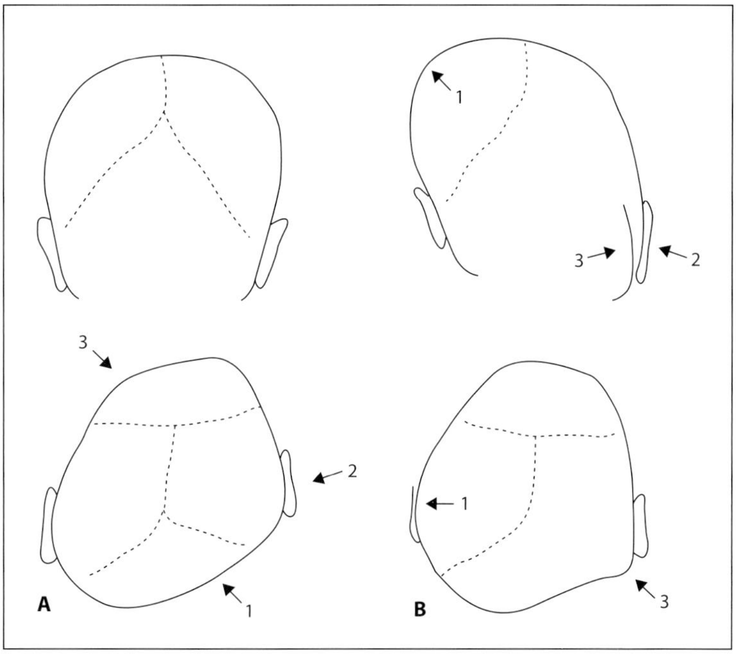

Fig. 2. Differential diagnosis of posterior plagiocephaly. **A** Positional deformity. 1, Occipital flattening; 2, anteriorly displaced auricle; 3, mild contralateral forehead retrusion. **B** Unilateral lambdoid synostosis. 1, Contralateral parietal bulging; 2, low-set ipsilateral ear; 3, bony crest above the mastoid process. Drawing courtesy of H. Collmann.

synostosis. Inspection of the abnormal head shape provides information about the suture or sutures affected by synostosis (figs. 1 and 2). Sagittal synostosis leads to an increase in the anteroposterior diameter of the skull, called dolichocephaly or scaphocephaly. Objective measurements of head length and width can be obtained using calipers, and measurements can be compared with age-matched standards [6]. Length is measured between the nasion and the ophistocranion, or alternatively at the most prominent area of the forehead and occiput to reflect the greatest anteroposterior dimension in patients with severe frontal bossing (fig. 3). Cranial width is measured between the most lateral points of the parietal bones (fig. 3). The ratio of head width to length is calculated using the formula for cephalic index, CI = head width × 100/head length. The typical CI ranges from 76% to 81%, and a CI <76% is considered dolichocephalic. Physical examination will reveal additional physical signs of sagittal synostosis including frontal bossing, a prominent occiput with flattened parietal eminences, and, rarely, palpable ridging of the fused suture. The location of the bregma, the intersection of the coronal with the sagittal suture, may be shifted posteriorly in close proximity to the vertex, the highest point of the skull. The fontanelle is triangular, rather than the typical rhomboid.

Synostosis of the coronal sutures may affect one or both sides, resulting in different head shapes. Unilateral coronal synostosis gives rise to an asymmetric skull with retrusion of the forehead, which is most obvious on the supraorbital rim of the affected side, and contralateral protrusion. This asymmetric skull is referred to as anterior plagiocephaly. It differs from deformational plagiocephaly by mild posterior flattening occurring ipsilateral to the forehead retrusion. Additionally, abnormal growth forces affect the midface, leading to facial scoliosis with nasal deviation to the contralateral side and a shortened

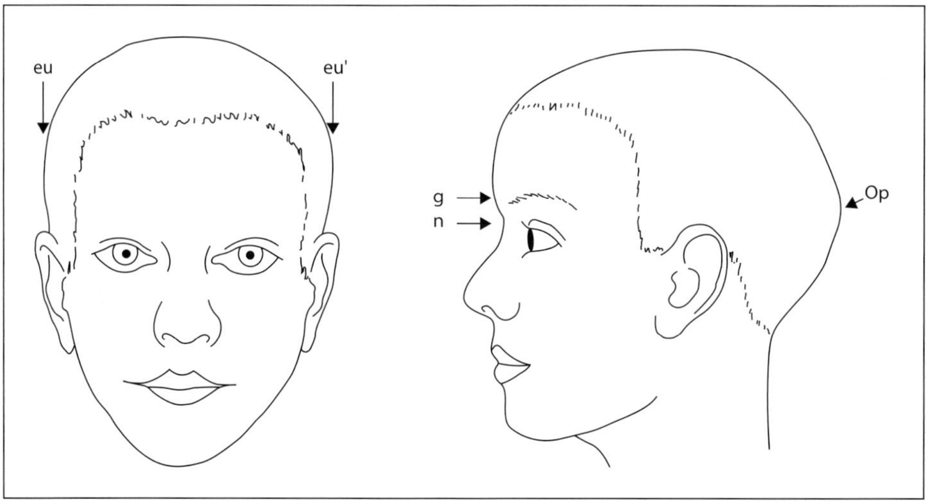

Fig. 3. Anatomical landmarks of the head. Eu, eurion (most lateral part of parietal bone); g, glabella; n, nasion; Op, ophistocranion (prominence of occiput). Head length: distance g–Op; head width: distance eu–eu'. The head circumference (occipitofrontal circumference, OFC) is measured so that the largest measurement is obtained, usually just above the glabella and horizontal to the ophistocranion. Drawing courtesy of H. Collmann.

distance between tragus and outer canthus on the affected side (fig. 4).

Bicoronal synostosis leads to a foreshortened anteroposterior diameter of the skull, termed brachycephaly (figs. 1, 3). A cephalic index >81% is characteristic for brachycephaly, but can also result from deformational forces or represent a normal variant. The restricted growth in the anteroposterior direction in bicoronal synostosis is compensated by upward growth with increased skull height, termed acrocephaly or turricephaly. Skull height can be measured with calipers from the nasion to the highest point of the head [6]. A more accurate approach may be to measure skull height on a radiograph, or to calculate it on digital images. Bicoronal synostosis causes forehead retrusion, easily recognized by the recessed supraorbital rims. Compensatory bulging of the temporal squama is common and most striking in syndromic brachycephaly.

Premature fusion of the metopic suture causes wedging of the forehead with prominence of the metopic region and increased parietal width (fig. 1), called trigonocephaly. Whereas mild trigonocephaly results only in a prominent metopic ridge, more severe cases demonstrate hypotelorism, upslanting palpebral fissures, and epicanthal folds.

In addition to the inspection of the skull shape, palpation of the sutures and fontanelles may reveal ridging of fused sutures or part of sutures. The fontanelles may be fused prematurely, or may be significantly enlarged. Persistent round ossification defects in the parietal bones, termed parietal foramina, and other irregular areas of delayed ossification can be identified by palpation of the skull.

Imaging Studies to Confirm Synostosis

In typical deformities and in the absence of functional or treatment consequences, there may be no need for routine radiographic confirmation of the synostosis. Radiographs of the skull may be

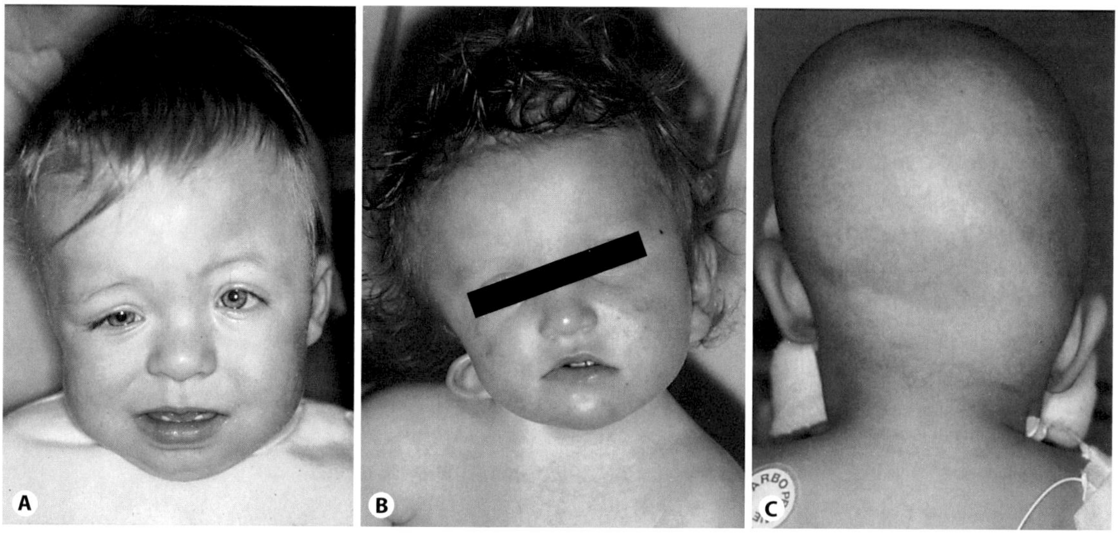

Fig. 4. Photographs of patients with left unicoronal synostosis (**A**), Goldenhar syndrome (**B**) and right lambdoidal synostosis (**C**). Courtesy of H. Collmann.

used to assess patency of sutures if craniosynostosis is suspected; however, early or partial synostosis may be missed on radiographs. More detailed information can be obtained through computed tomography (CT) studies, which allow precise visualization of each suture. Three-dimensional reconstruction of CT images can be digitally manipulated to provide the most detailed assessment (see Chapter 18 for a detailed discussion of these issues).

Underlying Etiology Varies by Affected Suture or Sutures

Craniosynostosis can occur as a sporadic and non-genetic abnormality, may be part of a malformation syndrome, or may have a genetic cause not resulting in additional malformations. Sagittal synostosis is the most common type, representing about half of all craniosynostoses in craniofacial centers. Sagittal synostosis is typically of non-genetic origin, but can occasionally occur in Crouzon syndrome. Coronal synostosis is the second most common form and may be an isolated finding or due to a genetic cause. Bicoronal synostosis is more likely than unicoronal to have an underlying genetic cause. The well-delineated craniosynostosis syndromes including Apert, Pfeiffer, Crouzon, Saethre-Chotzen, Muenke, and craniofrontonasal syndrome (CFNS) typically affect the coronal sutures. Pansynostosis, a term implying synostosis of all neurocranial sutures but often used for synostosis affecting the sagittal and the coronal sutures, is most characteristic for Crouzon syndrome. Severely restricted brain growth resulting in lack of expanding forces on the sutures may result in generalized secondary synostosis.

Typical trigonocephaly due to metopic synostosis is quite heterogeneous and has been reported after intrauterine valproic acid exposure, in numerous chromosome anomalies, and as an isolated finding. In Saethre-Chotzen syndrome, metopic synostosis is usually accompanied by fusion of the coronal sutures (see Chapter 9). Fusion of more than one suture results in complex skull-shape abnormalities. The most striking of these is Kleeblattschädel, or cloverleaf skull, with a trilobed configuration due to bulging of the cerebrum through the widely patent sagittal suture, or a very wide anterior fontanelle. Kleeblattschaedel is caused by fusion of multiple sutures during early fetal life. See specific chapters in this volume for more detailed discussion on many of the individual conditions.

Clinical Evaluation: Family History

A thorough family history is an important part of the complete clinical evaluation for a patient with craniosynostosis. Biological relatives, including siblings, parents, and grandparents, need to be considered, and additional relatives are included as needed. To identify familial cases, any history of craniofacial surgery, skull or facial abnormalities, and any other birth defects should be discussed. It is particularly important to inquire about multiple congenital abnormalities resulting in stillbirth or infant death, because this information may not be considered relevant by the family and may not be provided unless specifically asked. Multiple pregnancy losses or individuals with multiple congenital anomalies may suggest a chromosome abnormality. Although a balanced chromosomal rearrangement can be asymptomatic and transmitted from one generation to the next, it may also result in an unbalanced chromosome complement causing pregnancy loss or congenital anomalies.

If there are multiple relatives with craniosynostosis, the pedigree provides information about the inheritance pattern. Autosomal dominant inheritance will result in affected males and females in several generations. Findings in affected relatives provide information about the phenotypic variability of the condition and may differentiate between syndromes (table 1). Consanguinity between the proband's parents, particularly when siblings are affected, suggests an autosomal recessive condition (see Chapter 11). Affected females in the absence of affected males, or affected females born to fathers with mild hypertelorism only, can suggest CFNS, an unusual X-linked condition with more severe physical effects in females than in males [7, 8] (see Chapter 10). If the proband is the first affected individual in the family, the father's age should receive particular attention. Older fathers, often defined as at least age 34 years at the time of conception, increase the risk for a new mutation arising in the paternal germline. This mechanism has been documented for Apert syndrome, typically resulting from a de novo mutation in *FGFR2* [9].

Clinical Evaluation: Past Medical History

A review of the proband's past medical history should include the pregnancy and maternal medical conditions. Maternal hyperthyroidism as well as cigarette smoking during the pregnancy have been associated with craniosynostosis [10]. Rarely, prenatal exposure to diphenylhydantoin, aminopterin, methotrexate, fluconazole, or cyclophosphamide can cause craniosynostosis. Uterine abnormalities or multiple gestations may result in severe crowding and have been implicated in craniosynostosis, but this mechanism remains controversial. A brief review of organ systems may uncover differences in addition to the skull abnormality and can prompt further questions about the family history. Specific questions about developmental milestones are important in order to assess developmental delay or cognitive impairment. Previously performed imaging studies and chromosome analysis or molecular testing should be reviewed. It is particularly important to obtain documentation of all genetic study results as these can easily be misinterpreted or misunderstood (for a detailed discussion see Chapter 15).

Table 1. Brief overview of syndromic craniosynostoses, main physical findings, and causal genes

	Apert syndrome	Crouzon syndrome	Pfeiffer syndrome	Muenke syndrome	Saethre-Chotzen syndrome	Boston type	Cranio-frontonasal syndrome
Synostosis, skull findings	bicoronal, irregular with ossification defects	bicoronal; rarely pansynostosis or cloverleaf skull	bicoronal; cloverleaf skull in type 2	uni- or bicoronal synostosis; rarely macro-cephaly only	bi- or unicoronal, rarely metopic	bicoronal with turribrachy-cephaly; or pansynostosis with cloverleaf skull	uni- or bicoronal
Facial findings	hyper-telorism, down-slanting palpebral fissures; cleft palate	proptosis, hyper-telorism; beaked nose	proptosis, hyper-telorism, down-slanting palpebral fissures	mild facial findings, down-slanting palpebral fissures	ptosis, small ears with a prominent crus, facial asymmetry	fronto-orbital recession or rarely frontal bossing, no midfacial hypoplasia	hyper-telorism, broad nasal bridge and tip; rarely cleft lip
Hand and foot abnor-malities	severe syndactyly of hands and feet	none	broad and medially deviated thumbs and halluces; rarely symphal-angism	mild brachy-dactyly	hallux valgus, partial duplication of the first halluces, mild syndactyly of hands and feet; brachy-dactyly	short first metatarsals on radiograph	broad first toe, partial soft tissue syndactyly; longitudinal ridging of nails
Internal organs	cardiac and renal structural anomalies		tracheal sleeve in types 2 and 3	sensori-neural hearing loss			
Other	mental retardation common	none	multiple mal-formations in types 2 and 3	possible learning disabilities	mental retardation common with micro-deletion	variable expression in single large family	X-linked; more severe expression in females; unilateral breast hypoplasia
Gene mutations	*FGFR2* Ser252Trp or Pro253Arg	*FGFR2* mutations, multiple	*FGFR1* Pro252Arg; *FGFR2* mutations, multiple	*FGFR3* Pro250Arg	*TWIST* mutations; rarely complete gene deletion	*MSX2* Pro148His; rarely gene duplication or triplication	*EFNB1* mutations; rarely gene deletion

Clinical Evaluation: Physical Examination

A complete evaluation combines dysmorphology and general physical examinations. The general examination covers all organ systems and assesses any acute distress. In contrast, the dysmorphology examination identifies subtle abnormalities that may lack functional significance, but can suggest specific underlying diagnoses. Height, weight and head circumference measurements are placed on sex-specific growth curves and the centiles are noted. Occipitofrontal head circumference (OFC) is measured where the largest measurement is obtained, typically horizontal just above the glabella (fig. 3). A distorted skull shape can make it challenging to obtain this measurement. Palpation of the skull identifies the shape of the fontanelles, and their size can be measured. Fontanelles may be unusually wide and late closing, as typically seen in Apert syndrome, or close early in Crouzon syndrome, isolated pansynostosis, and scaphocephaly. Palpation of the skull identifies ridging of sutures, fontanelle location and size, and the presence of ossification defects including enlarged parietal foramina (see Chapters 2 and 9). The evaluation of the skull considers measurements, shape and information obtained by palpation. Hair texture may be wiry in CFNS, and the anterior hairline can be low in Saethre-Chotzen syndrome. A break in the continuity of the eyebrows is frequently seen in Apert syndrome [11].

The eyes appear asymmetric in unicoronal synostosis due to retrusion of the ipsilateral forehead and orbit. The palpebral fissure on the affected side becomes overly rounded, whereas the contralateral fissure appears narrow (fig. 4). Ptosis, defined as drooping of the upper eyelid resulting in a partially covered pupil, is common in Saethre-Chotzen syndrome and can occur in *FGFR2*-related syndromes. The distance between the inner and outer canthi and between the pupils is measured. Hypertelorism is defined as an increase in the interpupillary distance. In contrast, lateral displacement of the inner canthi without an increase in the interpupillary distance results in telecanthus (fig. 5). To assess palpebral fissure slant, imaginary lines intersecting the inner and outer canthi when the eyes are relaxed are compared with a horizontal line through the inner canthi. Upslanting or downslanting palpebral fissures can be noted upon visual inspection, and normative values for palpebral fissure inclination can be compared [6].

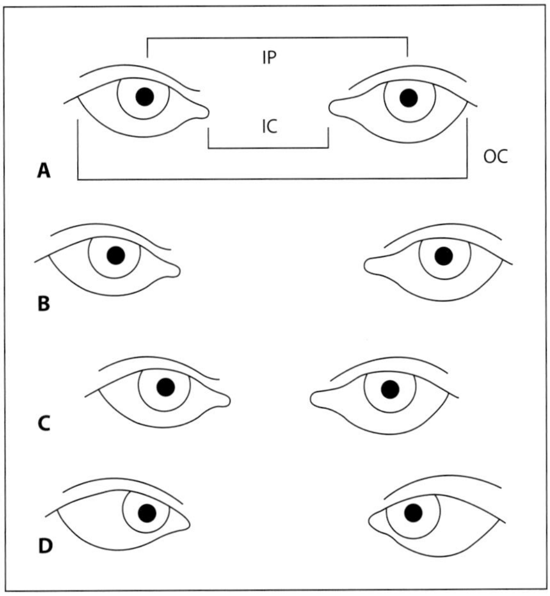

Fig. 5. Diagram depicting positional eye differences. **A** Normal eye position, with indication of landmarks used to obtain measurements. IP, Interpupillary distance; IC, inner canthal distance; OC, outer canthal distance. **B** Hypertelorism, characterized by increased IC, IP and OC distances. **C** Hypotelorism, characterized by decreased IC, IP and OC distances. **D** Telecanthus, characterized by lateral displacement of inner canthi resulting in increased IC distance, with normal IP and OC distance. Drawing courtesy of H. Collmann.

The position of the globe in the coronal plane, relative to the orbital rim, is referred to as orbital protrusion. Orbital protrusion can be measured with a clear plastic ruler. The head should be horizontal, with the facial profile in a vertical plane. The ruler is held against the lateral margin of the orbit, with the long axis parallel to the long axis of the globe. The distance between the lateral orbital rim and the maximum protrusion of the globe is measured in millimeters (fig. 6). Bicoronal synostosis causes symmetrical retrusion of the forehead and supraorbital rims, resulting in a prominent appearance of the eyes often mistaken for proptosis. True proptosis, or increased ocular protrusion, occurs when the sutures of the cranial base are affected by synostosis and the orbits become too shallow for the globe. Particularly severe proptosis can occur in Pfeiffer syndrome type 3 (see the discussion on Pfeiffer syndrome in Chapter 7) [12].

The nasal bridge may be low, as typically seen in Apert syndrome. In CFNS, the nasal bridge and ridge are wide, often with a wide or bifid nasal tip. The nasal contour may be rounded and described as beaked in Crouzon syndrome, whereas deviation of the nasal septum is particularly common in Saethre-Chotzen syndrome. Fusion of the sutures on the calvarial base affects midfacial growth causing maxillary retrusion, which, in turn, results in relative mandibular prognathism. The latter finding becomes more evident as facial features mature in late childhood (see Chapter 19).

Evaluation of the oral region includes mouth shape, for example the inverted W-shape of the upper lip in young patients with Apert syndrome described as trapezoidal. Cleft lip, either isolated or in combination with cleft palate, can rarely be seen in females with CFNS [7]. A bifid uvula or cleft of the soft palate is frequently seen in Apert syndrome and should not be confused with the invariably present bilateral palatine ridges. While palatal clefting is less common in other craniosynostosis syndromes, a high or narrow palate is typical in syndromic craniosynostoses. Bite abnormalities including relative mandibular prognathism are frequent in older individuals (see Chapter 19).

The external ear position is evaluated and considered to be low-set if the insertion of the superior attachment of the pinna lies below an imaginary line between both inner canthi. The longest distance from the upper helical edge to the edge of the ear lobe, measured without touching the ear, is the ear length. Measurements can be compared with age-matched norms [5, 6]. The same imaginary line measuring ear length can be used to assess angulation of the ear, and standard values are available, as is a more detailed description of these measurements [6]. Individuals with Saethre-Chotzen syndrome often have small, rounded external ears with prominent antihelical crura. The external ear canals can be narrow in Crouzon, Pfeiffer, Apert, and occasionally Saethre-Chotzen syndrome.

Body proportions are assessed by inspection of the trunk and extremities. Some skeletal dysplasias present with craniosynostosis and dwarfism, such as thanatophoric dysplasia with cloverleaf skull, or Antley-Bixler syndrome with bowed femurs. Long fingers and arm span can be seen in Loeys-Dietz syndrome, a connective

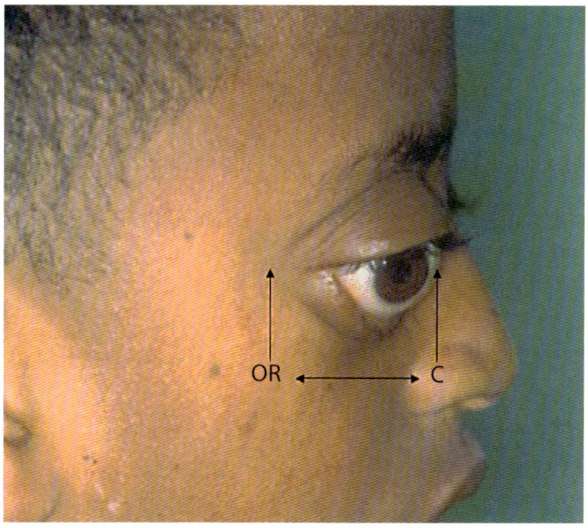

Fig. 6. Severe proptosis in a patient with Pfeiffer syndrome. C, cornea; OR, lateral orbital rim. Distance between OR and the maximal protrusion of the globe (C) is measured in millimeters to assess proptosis. Image courtesy of H. Collmann.

tissue disorder encompassing craniosynostosis, distinctive facial findings including hypertelorism and downslanting palpebral fissures, joint laxity, and arterial aneurysm (for discussion of these and other rare craniosynostosis syndromes, see Chapter 11). Attention should be paid to the clavicles and breasts, as females with CFNS can have hypoplastic clavicles, or unilateral breast hypoplasia. The latter is easily recognized in postpubertal women [7]. Genital anomalies are relatively rare in the well recognized craniosynostosis syndromes, with cryptorchidism occurring in about 10% of males with Apert syndrome.

Axillary pterygia, webbing notable upon abduction of the arm, sometimes occurs in females with CFNS. Limited abduction and internal rotation of the shoulder can result from glenohumeral joint dysplasia in Apert syndrome. Elbow ankylosis may limit range of motion in Apert and Pfeiffer syndromes type 2 and 3, and rarely in Pfeiffer syndrome type 1. Limited supination due to radioulnar fusion can occur in Apert, Crouzon, and Pfeiffer syndromes. Radial aplasia in combination with craniosynostosis is characteristic of Baller-Gerold syndrome (see Chapter 11).

Examination of the hands and feet often provides valuable information because patients with many of the common craniosynostosis syndromes have distinctive findings. Patients with Apert syndrome invariably have severe syndactyly affecting the hands and feet. Osseous or cutaneous syndactyly ranges from partial to complete fusion of the 2nd, 3rd, and 4th finger (type 1), with additional binding of the 5th finger (type 2), to fusion of all 5 digits (type 3) [13]. In most cases, the thumb is not involved in the fusion, giving rise to the descriptive term 'mitten hand'. Feet typically show syndactyly affecting all toes, with a broad and medially deviated distal phalanx of the hallux less involved in the fusion than the toes 2 through 5. The most characteristic finding in Pfeiffer syndrome is broad and medially deviated thumbs and 1st toes (fig. 7) [14]. Patients with Crouzon syndrome usually do not demonstrate abnormalities of the hands and feet. Brachydactyly associated with subtle radiographic changes, such as thimble-shaped middle phalanges, is often present in Muenke syndrome. In Saethre-Chotzen syndrome, partial cutaneous syndactyly between the 2nd and 3rd or 3rd and 4th fingers is frequent (fig. 7). This is appreciated most easily on the palmar view with fingers slightly spread. Often the 5th finger is curved, showing clinodactyly, and there may be a single palmar flexion crease. The 1st toe may be broad and in a valgus position, and partial cutaneous syndactyly between the 2nd and 3rd toes may be seen in Saethre-Chotzen syndrome. In CFNS, hands and feet may be short and wide, and mild cutaneous syndactyly can occur. Longitudinal ridging or grooving of the nails is characteristic for CFNS. The skin should be inspected for distinctive findings such as the thickened, darkened appearance of acanthosis nigricans, which develops during infancy in the Crouzon with acanthosis nigricans syndrome, or the furrowing on scalp and forehead in Beare-Stevenson cutis gyratum syndrome (for details see Chapter 11). During the evaluation for the more common dysmorphic findings, the examiner may note other rare abnormalities. Detailed documentation of unusual findings can be helpful, and photos are particularly valuable. Throughout the evaluation, the examiner will gain a general impression of the patient's cognitive development.

Evaluation of Specific Organ Systems and Their Function: Central Nervous System and Neurodevelopment

Synostosis of 2 or more sutures often causes increased intracranial pressure, and when fundoscopy reveals papilledema, urgent neurosurgical intervention is indicated. Because increased intracranial pressure develops in the majority of patients with multisutural synostosis and carries a risk of serious complications, vigilant follow-up is required [15]. Central nervous system

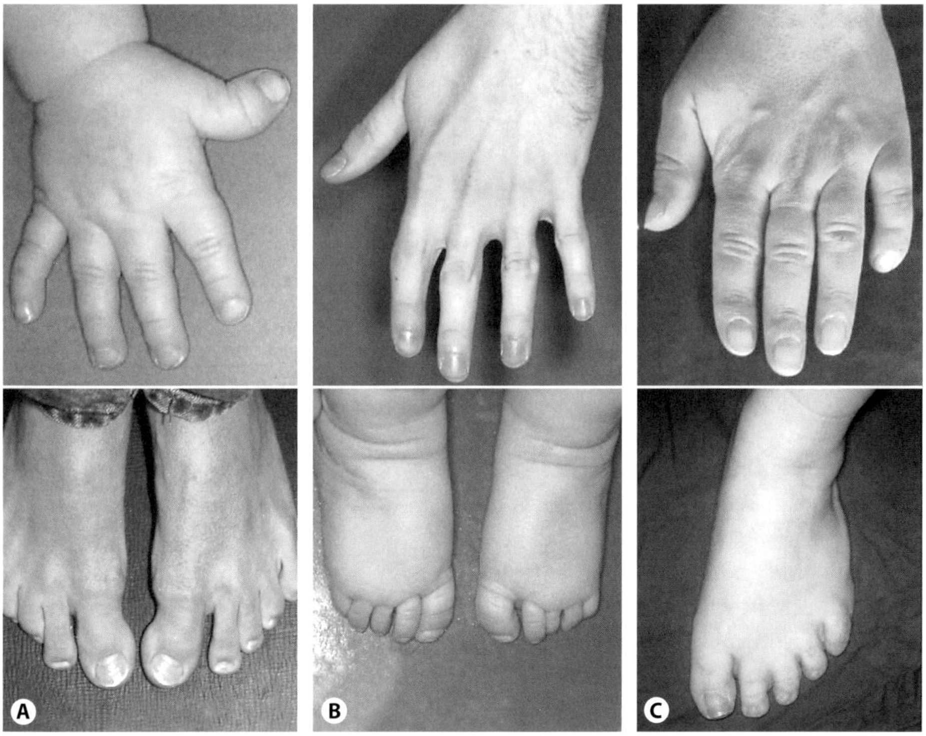

Fig. 7. Hand and foot findings in patients with Pfeiffer syndrome (**A**); Saethre-Chotzen syndrome (**B**); Muenke syndrome (**C**). Images courtesy of H. Collmann.

malformations, including agenesis of the corpus callosum and ventriculomegaly, are seen with increased frequency in Apert and Pfeiffer syndromes type 2 and 3. Increased intracranial pressure is more common in *FGFR2*-related synostoses [16]. A brain imaging study is recommended to identify congenital structural anomalies in individuals with Apert and Pfeiffer syndromes type 2 and 3, and in other patients with significant neurologic or developmental abnormalities.

Cognitive development ranges from normal, in most individuals with isolated synostosis, to severely delayed, as is typical for individuals with chromosome abnormalities. The expected range of abilities varies greatly for the different craniosynostosis syndromes due to single gene mutations. Many individuals with Apert syndrome are mentally retarded, with the mean IQ reported in different studies as 62 (range, 10–114) or 74 (range, 52–89), respectively [17, 18]. In contrast, individuals with Crouzon and Pfeiffer syndrome type 1 typically have normal intellectual development. Developmental delay is usually severe in patients with Pfeiffer syndromes type 2 or 3 [12]. Mild learning disabilities may be present in Muenke syndrome. Most individuals with Saethre-Chotzen syndrome have normal intellectual abilities; however, some have learning difficulties. Individuals with Saethre-Chotzen syndrome and severe developmental delay or mental retardation are more likely to have a microdeletion encompassing the complete *TWIST* gene [19, 20]. Thus, a brief screening test for developmental abnormalities should be considered for all patients with newly diagnosed craniosynostosis. Developmental specialists can perform more detailed evaluations as needed, and therapies should be provided as necessary. As in all developmentally delayed children, a hearing evaluation and an ophthalmologic examination may identify contributing treatable factors. If developmental problems are anticipated based on the syndrome diagnosis, early intervention can be initiated before significant delay is manifested.

Evaluation of Specific Organ Systems and Their Function: Ophthalmologic Considerations

The structural and functional integrity of the eyes can be affected in numerous ways in the craniosynostosis syndromes. As noted above, papilledema, an indicator for increased intracranial pressure, needs to be addressed urgently as it can result in optic atrophy. The optic nerve may be irreversibly damaged without concurring symptoms of intracranial hypertension, such as headache and vomiting. Thus, repeated fundoscopy is indicated in high-risk patients, such as *FGFR2*-related or pansynostosis. Synostosis may result in shallow orbits, which, in turn, leads to proptosis of the globes. If severe proptosis prevents complete closure of the eyelids, the cornea will develop exposure keratitis and ulcers, causing scarring and visual impairment. Lubricating medication is indicated if the palpebral fissure remains open more than 2 mm during sleep. Tarsorrhaphies or craniofacial surgical reconstruction may be necessary to correct severe proptosis. Less urgent problems include tear duct stenosis and ptosis, which are seen commonly in Saethre-Chotzen syndrome, and eye positional abnormalities, most often hypertelorism and downslanting palpebral fissures. The abnormal orbital anatomy and position often cause mechanical disturbances of the extraocular muscles resulting in strabismus, and untreated infantile strabismus can result in amblyopia. Reconstructive craniofacial surgery can change the orbital anatomy significantly, in turn affecting globe position and muscular function. Therefore, if possible, strabismus repair should be performed after craniofacial reconstruction. Long-term ophthalmologic follow-up is part of the team approach for patients with complex craniosynostosis, and surgical intervention should be coordinated, as craniofacial surgery impacts ocular structure and function.

Evaluation of Specific Organ Systems and Their Function: Otolaryngologic Considerations

Midfacial hypoplasia and retrusion with choanal stenosis occurs in syndromic craniosynstoses and can result in upper airway obstruction with its sequelae of feeding difficulties in infancy, failure-to-thrive, sleep apnea, and ultimately cor pulmonale [21]. Individuals with Apert and Pfeiffer syndromes type 2 and 3 are at increased risk for tracheal cartilaginous sleeve, an airway malformation in which distinct tracheal rings cannot be identified [22]. In place of normal cartilaginous arches, a continuous segment of cartilage extends from below the subglottis to the carina or the mainstem bronchi. This airway abnormality may be diagnosed by bronchoscopy, and in severe cases, the prognosis is poor despite tracheostomy.

The narrow nasopharyngeal space in patients with bicoronal synostosis impairs tympanic ventilation, and, in turn, leads to chronic otitis media. Conductive hearing loss due to acute and chronic otitis is common in individuals with Apert, Pfeiffer, Crouzon, and Saethre-Chotzen syndromes, and to a lesser degree in Muenke syndrome. The need for pressure equalization tubes can be anticipated in these patients. Low to mid-frequency sensorineural hearing loss is often noted in Muenke syndrome, and may be of consequence in environments with ambient noise, such as the classroom. Regular audiologic evaluations are important, and special accommodations such as sound field amplification and preferential seating in the classroom can improve speech perception in individuals with hearing loss.

Evaluation of Specific Organ Systems and Their Function: Growth and Feeding

Abnormal growth is relatively common in young patients with syndromic craniosynostosis and can be directly related to feeding difficulties. Feeding difficulties may be due to a cleft palate, seen in 43% of individuals with Apert syndrome [23], or due to upper airway problems, such as choanal stenosis. All infants with feeding problems should be evaluated for cleft palate and choanal stenosis or atresia, but midfacial hypoplasia with resulting narrow upper airway and abnormal tongue placement may be sufficient to impair breathing and feeding. Neurological abnormalities can cause feeding difficulties, and the head circumference should be measured and documented regularly in all infants. A sudden increase may raise concern for hydrocephalus and increased intracranial pressure. In addition to the abnormal skull shape directly related to the craniosynostosis, macrocephaly may be seen in Apert and Muenke syndromes. Microcephaly due to pansynostosis is occasionally the presenting finding in Crouzon syndrome, particularly when synostosis develops postnatally. Microcephaly occurs in isolated pansynostosis or Saethre-Chotzen syndrome. Linear growth may be slightly below average in Apert syndrome and decelerates with ages, typically resulting in height at the low end of the normal range [24]. Relative short stature is occasionally seen in Saethre-Chotzen syndrome. Height growth should be assessed regularly throughout childhood and adolescence, and a significant change in the growth velocity may require further investigation, including renewed concern for increased intracranial pressure.

Evaluation of Specific Organ Systems and Their Function: Internal Organs

Structural abnormalities of internal organs are frequently present in patients with underlying chromosome abnormalities, and specific abnormalities may be associated with certain structural differences (see Chapter 13 for a discussion regarding specific chromosome abnormalities). In addition, craniosynostosis syndromes can involve internal organs. For example, Apert and Pfeiffer syndromes type 2 and 3 can be associated with cardiac malformations and genitourinary tract malformations. About 10% of individuals with Apert syndrome have structural cardiac anomalies, including ventricular septal defect and pulmonic stenosis. Similarly, in about 10% of individuals with Apert syndrome, structural genitourinary anomalies are present. These anomalies include hydronephrosis, polycystic kidneys, bicornuate uterus, vaginal atresia, and cryptorchidism. An echocardiogram and an ultrasound of the kidneys and urinary tract should be performed in patients with Apert syndrome, Pfeiffer syndromes type 2 and 3, and in patients with chromosome abnormalities.

Evaluation of Specific Organ Systems and Their Function: Musculoskeletal Considerations

Additional skeletal abnormalities are not uncommon in craniosynostosis syndromes and include vertebral fusions in Apert, Pfeiffer, Crouzon, and Saethre-Chotzen syndromes, radiohumeral synostosis in Pfeiffer syndrome and shoulder girdle abnormalities with short humeri in Apert syndrome. Severe hand abnormalities can occur, such as the syndactyly seen in Apert syndrome. Patients with Apert syndrome should be evaluated by an experienced hand surgeon within the first 6 months of life, and syndactyly release typically will be performed in stages [25]. Other skeletal findings, such as carpal fusion, can only be identified on radiographs. Although many skeletal differences do not result in functional consequences and do not require surgical intervention, evaluation by an orthopedist should be considered.

Differential Diagnosis and Laboratory Testing

Based on the medical history and physical examination, craniosynostosis may appear to be an isolated finding or one component of a syndromic constellation. Both isolated and syndromic craniosynostosis may have an identifiable genetic cause. Isolated craniosynostosis of the sagittal suture is the most common form, typically without an identifiable genetic cause. Similarly, metopic synostosis without associated abnormalities rarely has an identifiable genetic cause. Unilateral coronal synostosis is most often an isolated finding but can be seen in Muenke or Saethre-Chotzen syndrome. Bicoronal synostosis suggests a genetic etiology, but the specific cause may not always be detectable with the currently available diagnostic studies. Wilkie et al. discourage genetic testing for sporadic non-syndromic sagittal and metopic synostosis since the diagnostic yield is low [26]. In contrast, individuals with bicoronal and unicoronal synostosis should have testing for the *FGFR3* mutation causing Muenke syndrome [26, 27], followed by *TWIST* sequencing for a mutation diagnostic of Saethre-Chotzen syndrome as indicated [28]. Pansynostosis, fusion of multiple cranial sutures, presenting with microcephaly rarely occurs in isolation and should prompt further evaluation of the brain structure. Lack of brain growth with secondary absence of stretching forces on the sutures may allow for synostosis to occur, and a brain malformation may remain asymptomatic in a young infant. Identification of a congenital brain abnormality changes the approach to differential diagnosis and genetic testing, with a focus on the primary abnormality rather than its secondary manifestations.

When additional abnormalities are noted in a patient with craniosynostosis, these suggest a syndromic condition. Identification of characteristic malformations, such as the severe syndactyly typical for Apert syndrome, or hypertelorism with a bifid nose and longitudinal ridging of nails typical for a female with CFNS, can lead to a clinical diagnosis. A clinical diagnosis may be confirmed with molecular gene studies [29–35], (see Chapter 15), and laboratories offering the specific tests can be identified through the gene tests directory [36]. Once the pathogenic mutation is documented in the proband, family members can be tested for this particular change. Such testing can be helpful if there is variable phenotypic expression and family members would like to know if their children are at risk for craniosynostosis. For example, a father of a female with CFNS carrying an *EFNB1* mutation will pass this mutation on to all daughters, and the daughters are expected to show clinical findings. In individuals with dysmorphic findings in addition to craniosynostosis, certain features suggest which gene is most likely to harbor a pathogenic mutation (table 1). In a patient with multiple anomalies not suggestive of a recognizable craniosynostosis syndrome, these additional findings deserve close attention. Identification of an unusual finding may allow for a database [37–40] and literature search and can ultimately result in the diagnosis of a rare syndrome: for example, bowing of the femora in Antley-Bixler syndrome (see Chapter 11). When no clinical diagnosis can be established in an individual with dysmorphia and developmental delay or mental retardation, a chromosome analysis should be performed. Craniosynostosis can result from small deletions, for example loss of 1 copy of the *TWIST* gene [20], loss of a commonly-deleted region of chromosome 22 [41], or gain of chromosomal material, such as duplication or triplication of the *MSX2* gene [42]. In addition to a high-resolution chromosome analysis that can identify translocations [43], an array-based comparative genomic hybridization (aCGH) study will provide more detailed information. The aCGH covers regions previously studied using fluorescent in situ hybridization (FISH), and FISH now generally serves as a confirmatory assay. A chromosome analysis and aCGH may be considered in all individuals with trigonocephaly. Interpretation of aCGH results may require parental studies, and available information changes continuously as this technology is used more widely. Patients lacking a definitive diagnosis should be reevaluated every few years because the understanding of medical genetics improves rapidly. Information about the genetic mechanism benefits not only the patient, but can be relevant for family members. In this context, it is important to note that a singleton case in a family can have a genetic origin. Even those family members in whom genetic testing documents the absence of recurrence risk may benefit from this knowledge. Thus, identification of an underlying genetic cause is worthwhile, even when it does not impact the treatment plan.

Multidisciplinary Treatment Approach

Surgical craniosynostosis repair is often performed by a plastic surgeon in collaboration with a neurosurgeon. Medical care of individuals with craniosynostosis is not limited to issues directly related to the synostosis, such as skull shape and facial appearance, but takes into consideration secondary effects, such as elevated intracranial pressure and strabismus. Shallow or abnormally positioned orbits, as well as midfacial retrusion, result from fusion of sutures on the cranial base. Growth and maturation of facial structures during adolescence need to be monitored because facial abnormalities can become more notable. Patients may perceive facial findings differently from medical professionals, family members, or peers, and self-esteem can be significantly impacted. Thus, while a single surgical procedure may suffice to repair uncomplicated synostosis, long-term follow up through a team approach may be necessary to address the complex medical needs encountered in many patients (see Chapter 18). The identification of a mutation or other genetic cause confirms a molecular diagnosis, and medical problems associated with any particular disorder are reviewed individually. To address all medical needs of patients, craniofacial teams should be composed of plastic surgeons, neurosurgeons, ophthalmologists, geneticists, orthodontists, speech therapists, audiologists, social workers, and other professionals.

References

1 Kane AA, Mitchell LE, Craven KP, Marsh JL: Observations on a recent increase in plagiocephaly without synostosis. Pediatrics 1996;97:877–885.
2 Rogers GF, Oh AK, Mulliken JB: The role of congenital muscular torticollis in the development of deformational plagiocephaly. Plast Reconstr Surg 2009;123: 643–652.
3 Mulliken JB, Vander Woude DL, Hansen M, LaBrie RA, Scott RM: Analysis of posterior plagiocephaly: deformational versus synostotic. Plast Reconstr Surg 1999;103:371–380.
4 van Vlimmeren LA, van der Graaf Y, Boere-Boonekamp MM, L'Hoir MP, Helders PJ, Engelbert RH: Effect of pediatric physical therapy on deformational plagiocephaly in children with positional preference: a randomized controlled trial. Arch Pediatr Adolesc Med 2008; 162:712–718.
5 Jones KL: Smith's Recognizable Patterns of Human Malformation, 6th ed. Philadelphia, Elsevier Inc., 2006.
6 Hall JG, Allanson JE, Gripp KW, Slavotinek AM: Handbook of Physical Measurements, 2nd ed. New York, Oxford University Press, 2007.
7 Saavedra D, Richieri-Costa A, Guion-Almeida ML, Cohen MM Jr: Craniofrontonasal syndrome: a study of 41 patients. Am J Med Genet 1996;61:147–151.

8 Wieland I, Jakubiczka S, Muschke P, Cohen M, Thiele H, et al: Mutations of the ephrin-B1 gene cause craniofrontonasal syndrome. Am J Hum Genet 2004; 74:1209–1215.
9 Moloney DM, Slaney SF, Oldridge M, Wall SA, Sahlin P, et al: Exclusive paternal origin of new mutations in Apert syndrome. Nat Genet 1996;13:48–53.
10 Honein MA, Rasmussen SA: Further evidence for an association between maternal smoking and craniosynostosis. Teratology 2000;62:145–146.
11 Cohen MM Jr, Kreiborg S: A clinical study of the craniofacial features in Apert syndrome. Int J Oral Maxillofac Surg 1996;25:45–53.
12 Gripp KW, Stolle CA, McDonald-McGinn DM, Markowitz RI, Bartlett SP, et al: Phenotype of the fibroblast growth factor receptor 2 Ser351Cys mutation: Pfeiffer syndrome type III. Am J Med Genet 1998;78:356–360.
13 Cohen MM Jr, Kreiborg S: Hands and feet in the Apert syndrome. Am J Med Genet 1995;57:82–96.
14 Cohen MM Jr, Kreiborg S: Growth pattern in the Apert syndrome. Am J Med Genet 1993;47:617–623.
15 Greene AK, Mulliken JB, Proctor MR, Meara JG, Rogers GF: Phenotypically unusual combined craniosynostoses: presentation and management. Plast Reconstr Surg 2008;122:853–862.
16 Marucci DD, Dunaway DJ, Jones BM, Hayward RD: Raised intracranial pressure in Apert syndrome. Plast Reconstr Surg 2008;122:1162–1170.
17 Cohen MM Jr: Apert syndrome; in Cohen MM Jr, MacLean RE (eds): Craniosynostosis: Diagnosis, Evaluation and Management, 2nd ed. New York, Oxford University Press, 2000, pp 316–353.
18 Yacubian-Fernandes A, Palhares A, Giglio A, Gabarra RC, Zanini S, et al: Apert syndrome: factors involved in the cognitive development. Arq Neuropsiquiatr 2005;63:963–968.
19 Johnson D, Horsley SW, Moloney DM, Oldridge M, Twigg SR, et al: A comprehensive screen for *TWIST* mutations in patients with craniosynostosis identifies a new microdeletion syndrome of chromosome band 7p21.1. Am J Hum Genet 1998;63:1282–1293.
20 Gripp KW, Kasparcova V, McDonald-McGinn DM, Bhatt S, Bartlett SP, et al: A diagnostic approach to identifying submicroscopic 7p21 deletions in Saethre-Chotzen syndrome: fluorescence in situ hybridization and dosage-sensitive Southern blot analysis. Genet Med 2001; 3:102–108.
21 Cohen MM Jr, Kreiborg S: Upper and lower airway compromise in the Apert syndrome. Am J Med Genet 1992;44:90–93.
22 Hockstein NG, McDonald-McGinn D, Zackai E, Bartlett S, Huff DS, Jacobs IN: Tracheal anomalies in Pfeiffer syndrome. Arch Otolaryngol Head Neck Surg 2004;130:1298–1302.
23 Slaney SF, Oldridge M, Hurst JA, Moriss-Kay GM, Hall CM, et al: Differential effects of *FGFR2* mutations on a syndactyly and cleft palate in Apert syndrome. Am J Hum Genet 1996;58:923–932.
24 Cohen MM Jr: Pfeiffer syndrome update, clinical subtypes, and guidelines for differential diagnosis. Am J Med Genet 1993;45:300–307.
25 Guero S, Vassia L, Reneir D, Glorion C: Surgical management of the hand in Apert syndrome. Handchir Mikrochir Plast Chir 2004;36:179–185.
26 Wilkie AOM, Bochukova EG, Hansen RMS, Taylor IB, Rannan-Eliya SV, et al: Clinical dividends from the molecular genetic diagnosis of craniosynostosis. Am J Med Genet A 2006;140A:2631–2639.
27 Gripp KW, McDonald-McGinn DM, Gaudenz K, Whitaker LA, Bartlett SP, et al: Identification of a genetic cause for isolated unilateral coronal synostosis: a unique mutation in the fibroblast growth factor receptor 3. J Pediatr 1998;132: 714–716.
28 Kress W, Schropp C, Lieb G, Petersen B, Büsse-Ratzka M, et al: Saethre-Chotzen syndrome caused by *TWIST1* gene mutations: functional differentiation from Muenke coronal synostosis syndrome. Eur J Hum Genet 2006;14:39–48.
29 Reardon W, Winter RM, Rutland P, Pulleyn LJ, Jones BM, Malcolm S: Mutations in the fibroblast growth factor receptor 2 gene cause Crouzon syndrome. Nat Genet 1994;8:98–103.
30 Muenke M, Schell U, Hehr A, Robin NH, Losken HW, et al: A common mutation in the fibroblast growth factor receptor 1 gene in Pfeiffer syndrome. Nat Genet 1994;8:269–274.
31 Wilkie AOM, Slaney SF, Oldridge M, Poole MD, Ashworth GJ, et al: Apert syndrome results from localized mutations of *FGFR2* and is allelic with Crouzon syndrome. Nat Genet 1995;9:165–172.
32 Schell U, Hehr A, Feldman GJ, Robin NH, Zackai EZ, et al: Mutations in *FGFR1* and *FGFR2* cause familial and sporadic Pfeiffer syndrome. Hum Mol Genet 1995;4:323–328.
33 Muenke M, Gripp KW, McDonald-McGinn DM, Gaudenz K, Whitaker LA, et al: A unique point mutation in the fibroblast growth factor receptor 3 gene *(FGFR3)* defines a new craniosynostosis syndrome. Am J Hum Genet 1997;60: 555–564.
34 el Ghouzzi V, Le Merrer M, Perrin-Schmitt F, Lajeunie E, Benit P, et al: Mutations of the *TWIST* gene in the Saethre-Chotzen syndrome. Nat Genet 1997;15:42–46.
35 Kan SH, Elanko N, Johnson D, Cornejo-Roldan L, Cook J, et al: Genomic screening of fibroblast growth-factor receptor 2 reveals a wide spectrum of mutations in patients with syndromic craniosynostosis. Am J Hum Genet 2002;70:472–486.
36 Genetests: NCBI, Seattle (WA), University of Washington. Available from: http://www.ncbi.nlm.nih.gov/sites/GeneTests/?db = GeneTests. Accessed February 12, 2010.
37 OMIM: Online Mendelian Inheritance in Man. NCBI, Baltimore (MD), Johns Hopkins University. Available from: http://www.ncbi.nlm.nih.gov/omim/. Accessed February 12, 2010.
38 London Medical Databases, 2006: Winter-Baraitser Dysmorphology Database (WBDD). Available from: http://www.lmdatabases.com/about_lmd.html#lddb. Accessed February 12, 2010.
39 POSSUMweb. Victoria (Australia): Murdoch Childrens Research Institute. Available from: http://www.possum.net.au/. Accessed February 12, 2010.
40 Gorlin RJ, Cohen MM Jr, Hennekam RCM: Syndromes of the Head and Neck, 4th ed. New York, Oxford University Press, 2001.

41 McDonald-McGinn DM, Gripp KW, Kirschner RE, Maisenbacher MK, Hustead V, et al: Craniosynostosis: another feature of the 22q11.2 deletion syndrome. Am J Med Genet A 2005;136A: 358–362.

42 Bernardini L, Castori M, Capalbo A, Mokini V, Mingarelli R, et al: Syndromic craniosynostosis due to complex chromosome 5 rearrangement and *MSX2* gene triplication. Am J Med Genet A 2007;143A:2937–2943.

43 Reid CS, McMorrow LE, McDonald-McGinn DM, Grace KJ, Ramos FJ, et al: Saethre-Chotzen syndrome with familial translocation at chromosome 7p22. Am J Med Genet 1993;47:637–639.

Karen W. Gripp, M.D.
Division of Clinical Genetics
Alfred I. duPont Hospital for Children
Wilmington, DE, 19803 (USA)
Tel. +1 302 651 5916, Fax +1 302 651 5033, E-Mail kgripp@nemours.org

Muenke M, Kress W, Collmann H, Solomon BD (eds): Craniosynostoses: Molecular Genetics, Principles of Diagnosis, and Treatment.
Monogr Hum Genet. Basel, Karger, 2011, vol 19, pp 216–231

Imaging Studies and Neurosurgical Treatment

H. Collmann[a] · T. Schweitzer[a] · H. Böhm[b]

[a]Section of Pediatric Neurosurgery, Neurosurgical Department, [b]Department of Maxillofacial Surgery, University of Würzburg, Würzburg, Germany

Abstract

The diagnosis of craniosynostosis is predominantly a matter of careful clinical examination. Imaging aids are used to verify the clinical diagnosis, but, more importantly, to detect the involvement of additional sutures, signs of intracranial hypertension, secondary sequelae of craniosynostosis, and associated anomalies. Treatment is aimed at preserving or restoring function as well as correcting disfiguring distortions. The formerly prevalent craniectomy techniques have now partly been replaced by plastic surgical techniques. Long-term postoperative surveillance is mandatory since recurrent deformity and/or elevated intracranial pressure may occur in a significant proportion of patients, particularly in progressive multisutural synostosis commonly seen in patients with syndromic craniosynostosis.

Technical Aids of Examination

Following comprehensive clinical evaluation, various supplementary studies are usually necessary in order to answer some basic questions. The following problems must be addressed: Has the fused suture been correctly identified by clinical exam? Are additional sutures involved? Is there elevated intracranial pressure? Are concurrent malformations of the brain, i.e. ectopic cerebellar tonsils, hydrocephalus, ventriculomegaly, or brain dysplasia present? Are there cranial pathologies that could potentially interfere with surgery?

To answer these questions various radiological techniques as well as pressure monitoring may be considered. Specifically, these techniques include ultrasonography, plain radiographs, computed tomography (CT), and magnetic resonance (MR) imaging.

Ultrasound is now considered an advanced technique that may partly substitute for CT in early infancy in order to avoid radiation exposure. The necessary bone window may be provided by the open fontanelle, or alternatively, by any other skull defect. During the first 6 months of life, ultrasound examination can readily differentiate between open and fused cranial sutures. In our institution, ultrasound is the primary radiological method used to confirm open sutures in suspected positional plagiocephaly or closed sutures in craniosynostosis [1].

Plain radiographs are used to detect sutural fusion in clinically less obvious cases and more importantly, to look for additionally affected sutures and for signs of intracranial hypertension. In fact, serial radiographs have demonstrated the basically dynamic nature of craniosynostosis. Progressive

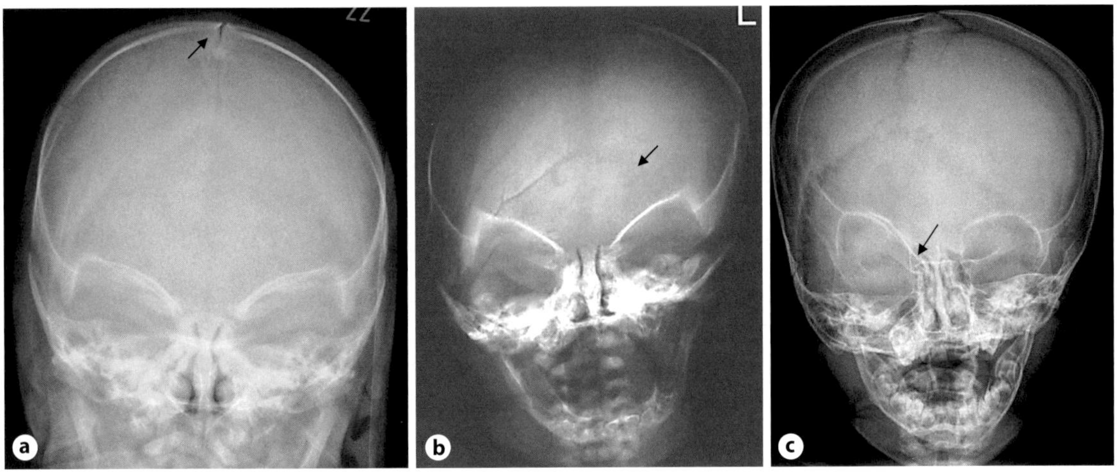

Fig. 1. a–c Plain radiographs of (**a**) sagittal suture synostosis simulating an open suture (arrow); (**b**) right-sided lambdoid synostosis: note the barely visible normal suture on the left side (arrow); (**c**) right-sided unilateral coronal synostosis: note the deformed right orbit and the elevated lesser sphenoid wing (arrow).

multisutural fusion is a common feature of the *FGFR2*-related syndromes, although the rate of progression may vary considerably. In our own study group, pansynostosis had occurred in 75% of Crouzon patients by the end of the 4th year, while in Apert patients the corresponding value was 40%. Progressive synostosis has also been reported in some cases of scaphocephaly, which is consistent with observations in our department. Plain radiographs also provide information about the molding of the inner cranial surface as well as abnormal vascular channels traversing the bone, e.g. dilated emissary veins. This information may be of particular importance for surgical planning. However, plain X-rays should not be performed routinely. For instance, in typical cases of scaphocephaly, trigonocephaly, anterior plagiocephaly, and brachycephaly, there is no need for radiographs just to confirm the affected suture, as this can be readily inferred from the abnormal head shape. Usually, there is no need for repeat plain X-rays during the first year of life, since additional information of any significance is rarely obtained by repeat X-rays within a few months period. Due to the radiation dose involved and the quality of the image, digital exposure technique is mandatory. With advancing age, repeated radiographs may sometimes reveal progressive multisutural fusion, thereby demonstrating that craniosynostosis is basically a growth failure, i.e. a dynamic process.

Some pitfalls may be encountered during evaluation of the sutures. In infancy, lateral radiographs quite often do not clearly depict the patent coronal suture, because the margins of the thin bone extensively overlap and interdigitate. This appearance should not be confused with sutural fusion. Conversely, a sharply delineated suture, as is often noticeable in scaphocephaly, indicates incipient osseous fusion rather than an open suture (fig. 1a, b). In doubtful cases of facial asymmetry the typical deformity of the ipsilateral orbit ('harlequin eye') and the elevated lesser sphenoid wing clearly indicate unilateral coronal synostosis (fig. 1c).

Increased molding of the endocranial vault surface may either represent copper beaten skull ('Wolkenschädel') due to increased intracranial

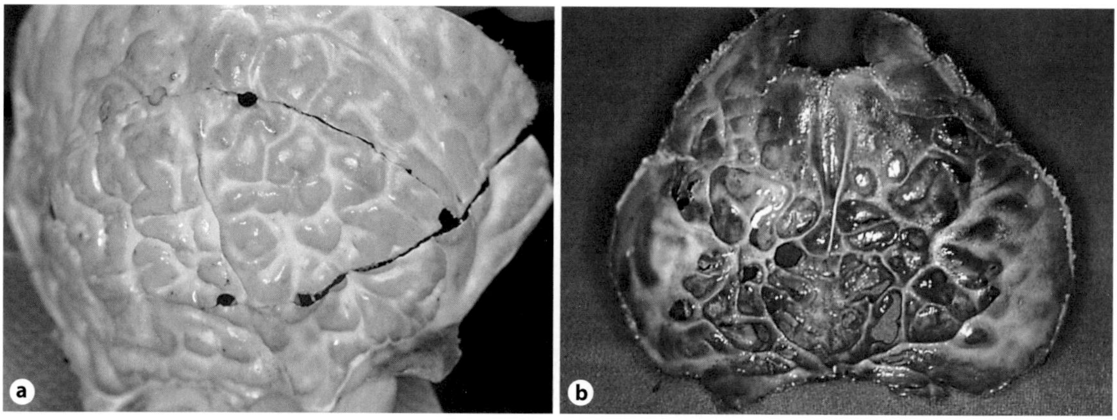

Fig. 2. Surgical specimen of copper beaten skull (**a**) and honeycomb pattern (**b**).

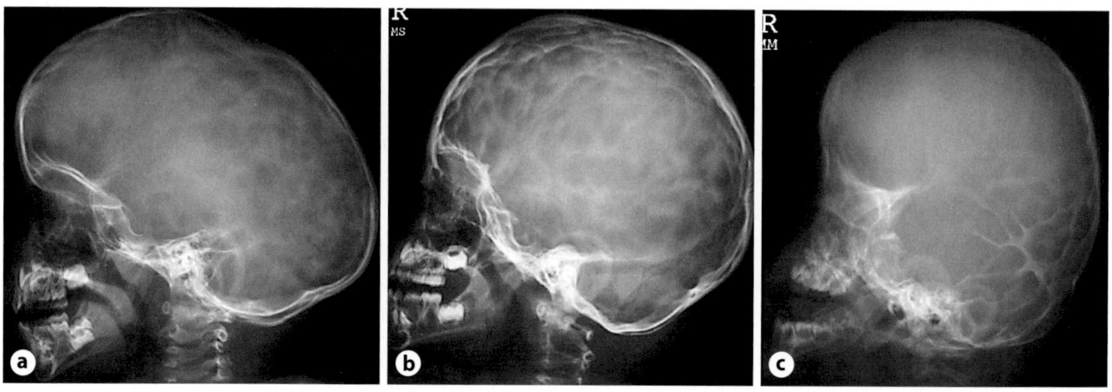

Fig. 3. Radiographs of normal digital markings (**a**); copper beaten skull (**b**); localized honeycomb pattern (**c**).

pressure, or the so-called 'honeycomb pattern' ('Lücken-Leistenschädel'), which corresponds to primary bone dysplasia (figs. 2, 3). Copper beaten skull is a negative imprinting of the gyral pattern on the cortical surface. It usually develops only after the first year of life, whereas the irregular honeycomb pattern is already present at birth or appears during the first months of life. Moreover, it usually disappears spontaneously within 2 or 3 years. The true nature of the honeycomb pattern has not yet been elucidated. In a few samples investigated at our institution, histology showed a high proportion of immature woven bone. Copper beaten pattern should be separated from normal digital printings, which is a common pattern during childhood. As the border between normal and pathological imprintings is ill-defined, the diagnostic value is reasonably high only in severe cases. Sensitivity is low, since molding of the endocranial surface is a time-consuming process of at least several months.

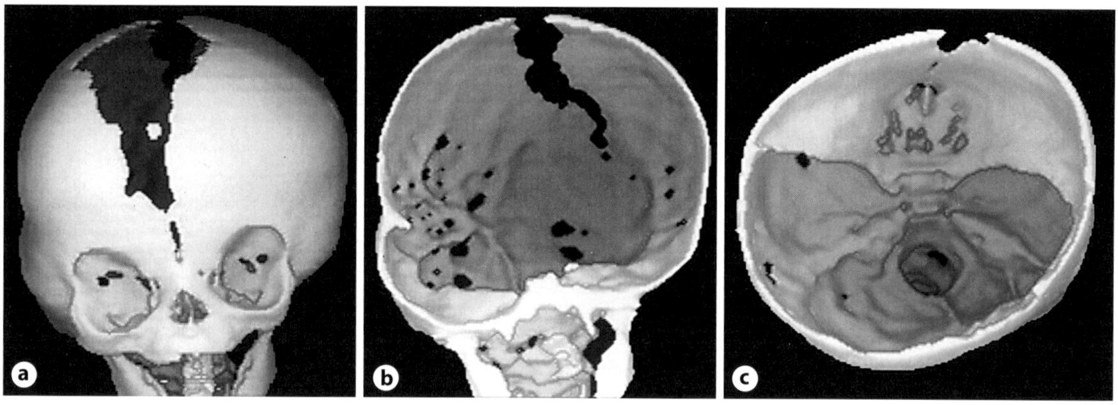

Fig. 4. a–c Three-dimensional computed tomography of an infant with Apert syndrome, demonstrating plagiocephaly, midline calvarial defect, and right-sided occipital honeycomb pattern.

CT allows for a more intricate insight into the structure of the cranial bones and, therefore, can differentiate more precisely between open and fused sutures, particularly in high definition and thin slices. In addition, abnormal emmissary venous channels are readily identified, which may be important for surgical planning [2]. Three-dimensionally reformatted images not only provide impressive views of the outer and inner surfaces of the deformed skull (fig. 4), but also enable quantitative analysis of cranial shape and volume [3]. In selected cases this technique allows creation of a scale plastic model for planning complex cranio-maxillofacial surgery (see Chapter 19). For routine use, however, the technique does not add significant information to what can be inferred from clinical examination and plain radiographs. Principally, the reformatted pictures are not conclusive as to the sutural state since they can be manipulated by the applied computer algorithm. Thus, in each individual case, the benefit of a CT scan use should be carefully weighed against the potential risk associated with radiation exposure, which is much higher than that of plain radiographs. In fact, recent studies suggest that each CT scan performed in early infancy causes a significant increase in cancer risk in later life [4].

MR imaging has become the gold standard for imaging of intracranial structures, although the need for sedation or even anesthesia for infants and young children should be kept in mind. In craniosynostosis, the most common pathologies identified on MR images include: enlargement of cerebrospinal fluid spaces; herniation of the cerebellar tonsils; abnormalities of the corpus callosum and other types of cerebral malformations; in some cases abnormal venous drainage of the brain and empty sella (fig. 5a–f).

Progressive hydrocephalus develops in 20–30% of patients diagnosed with Pfeiffer or Crouzon syndrome, and in a few percent of patients with Apert syndrome [5]. Progressive hydrocephalus may also occur in several of the less common craniosynostosis syndromes such as Crouzon syndrome with acanthosis nigricans [6]. In most cases, compromised cerebrospinal fluid (CSF) spaces in the posterior fossa and herniation of the cerebellar tonsils have been noted, which suggest impaired CSF outflow from the 4th ventricle (fig. 5a). However, a venous outflow problem leading to CSF malabsorption has also been postulated as a causative mechanism [5]. True hydrocephalus should be separated from non-progressive distortion ventriculomegaly, which is a common

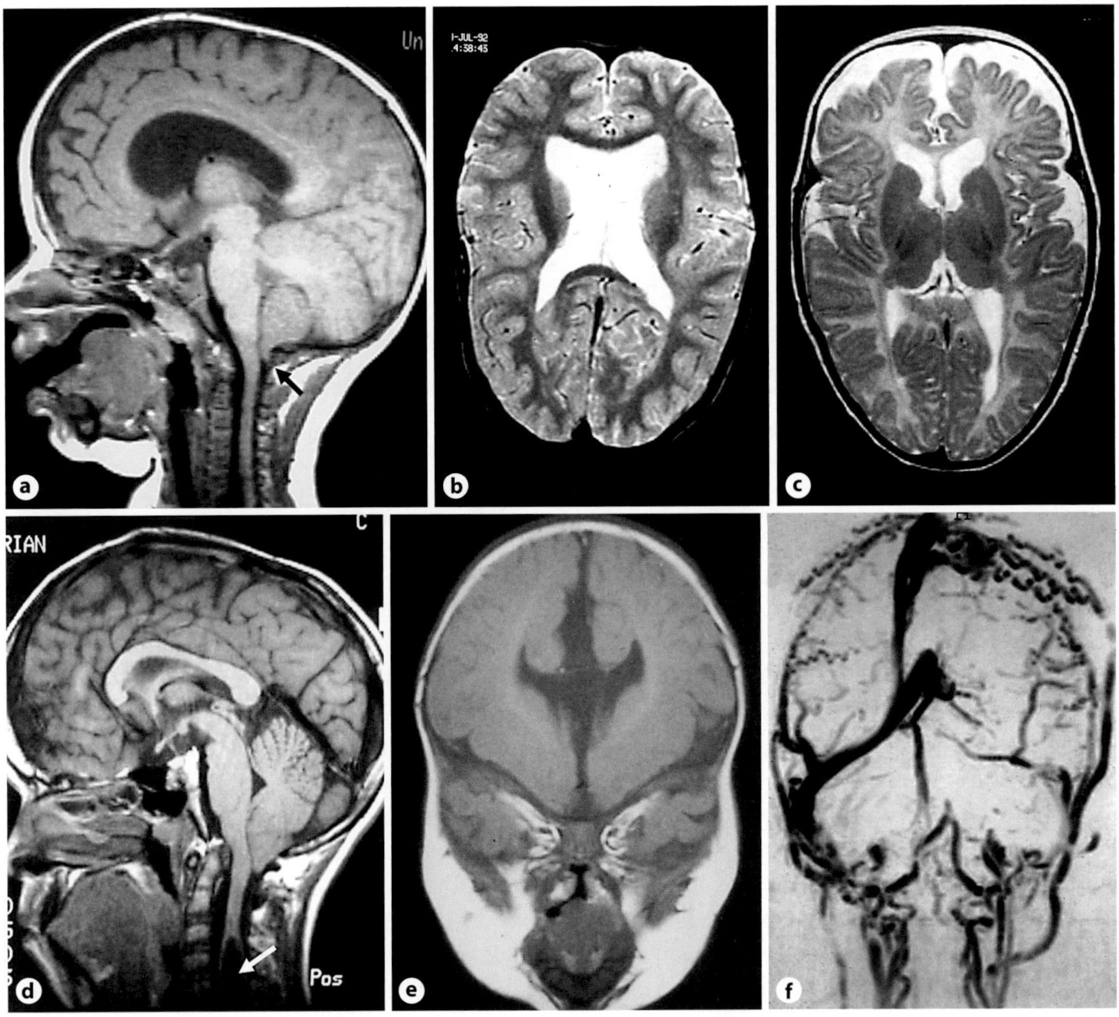

Fig. 5. Magnetic resonance imaging of hydrocephalus and Chiari I malformation (arrow) in a Crouzon patient (**a**); ventriculomegaly in Apert syndrome (**b**); dilated frontal subarachnoid space in simple scaphocephaly (**c**); ectopic cerebellar tonsils and hydrosyringomyelia (arrow) in isolated pansynostosis (**d**); agenesis of the corpus callosum in Apert syndrome (**e**); obstruction of the left transverse and sigmoid sinus leading to extensive curling venous collateral channels of the scalp (MR angiography) (**f**).

phenomenon in Apert syndrome and obviously part of a primary cerebral maldevelopment (fig. 5b). This type of ventriculomegaly has also been observed in Crouzon syndrome [6]. In this scenario, diagnosis of true hydrocephalus is not as straightforward as usual, since the rigid synostotic skull may prevent gross ventricular dilatation, while intracranial hypertension may also be attributable to craniostenosis. Clinicians must keep in mind that MR images do not generally allow reliable conclusions about intracranial pressure. Yet some signs on MR are apt to raise suspicion, such as compromised basal cisterns and subarachnoid spaces over the cerebral convexity, dilated optic nerve sheaths and extension of the suprasellar cistern into the sella turcica ('empty sella').

Enlargement of the subarachnoid space is a frequent finding in isolated monosutural synostosis, particularly in scaphocephaly (fig. 5c). Its clinical significance is a matter of ongoing debate: while some authors believe that there is a CSF absorption deficit [5], others hold the view that the CSF space dilates only passively to accommodate for local compensatory skull expansion caused by an intrinsically disparate bone growth [6].

Herniation of the cerebellar tonsils into the foramen magnum (Chiari I malformation) also occurs most often in patients with Crouzon or Pfeiffer syndrome, while it is fairly rare in Apert syndrome. Chiari I malformation in this context has been attributed to early synostosis of the lambdoid suture and, hence, deficient expansion of the posterior fossa [7]. In fact, the lambdoid suture usually closes during infancy in Crouzon and Pfeiffer syndromes, but only after the second year of life in most patients with Apert syndrome. If both cerebellar tonsils herniate into the upper spinal canal, hydrocephalus may be a consequence, as described above. In addition, CSF flow between the cranial and spinal subarachnoid spaces may be obstructed leading to hydrosyringomyelia and spinal cord dysfunction (fig. 5d). In these cases, hydrosyringomyelia may involve the majority of the cord, but may spare the upper cervical portions. Hence, on MR imaging, the entire cervical cord must be visualized in order to identify a syrinx. For timely identification of a Chiari I malformation or hydrocephalus, routine MR imaging is strongly recommended in all cases of congenital or infantile lambdoid suture fusion, i.e. isolated lambdoid synostosis, combined sagittal and lambdoid synostosis (so-called 'Mercedes-Benz syndrome'), Crouzon, Pfeiffer, Apert, *FGFR3*-related Crouzon (with acanthosis nigricans) and some other rare syndromes [6].

Finally, MR imaging is the most accurate available technique to visualize abnormalities of the cerebral anatomy, e.g. dysplasia or agenesis of the corpus callosum or the septum pellucidum in Apert syndrome (fig. 5e). In some cases of persistent intracranial hypertension, MR angiography may disclose constricted or even obstructed venous channels as the true underlying pathology (fig. 5f) [5, 8].

Elevated intracranial pressure due to brain constriction in a poorly expanding cranial cavity has been called craniostenosis in a strict sense [9]. It is the most important functional risk of craniosynostosis and, hence, the focus of diagnostic interest. While its potential impact on optic nerve function is beyond doubt, conclusive data describing the effect on brain function are still lacking. Consequently, the degree of intracranial hypertension that should prompt surgical intervention remains poorly defined. The diagnosis of intracranial hypertension in this context is not straightforward, since classical symptoms like headaches and vomiting are usually absent. The single demonstrative clinical sign of intracranial hypertension in craniosynostosis is papilledema, the presence of which therefore has to be routinely assessed. While repeated ophthalmoscopy, for instance in 3-month intervals, can detect impending damage to the optic nerve in time, this technique has low sensitivity for the detection of intracranial hypertension. The same holds true for the so-called 'copper beaten skull' on radiographs, which is conclusive only in its most severe form. As mentioned previously, CT scans or MR images are generally not applicable for proving or excluding elevated intracranial pressure.

Intracranial pressure monitoring – currently by means of an intracerebral probe – is considered the gold standard of diagnostic evaluation, but, of course, has the drawback of requiring a surgical procedure (fig. 6) [10]. Furthermore, in the growing skull, the results obtained are valid for a limited time only. Therefore, this method is restricted to cases that remain doubtful after non-invasive investigations have been performed. In some patients, the less accurate short-term recording of

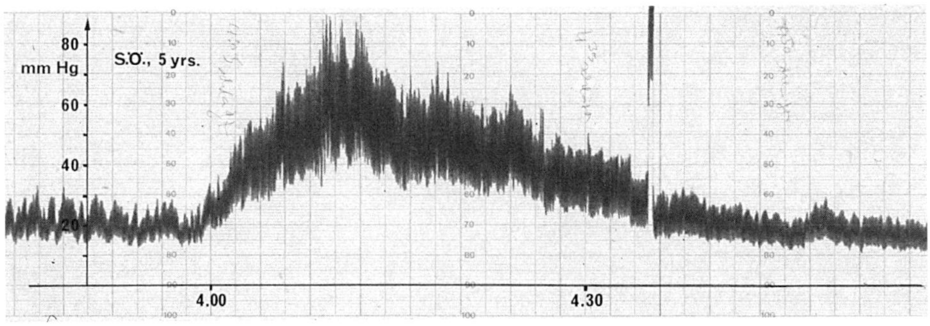

Fig. 6. Intracranial pressure monitoring showing abnormal pressure wave in Pfeiffer syndrome with recurrent craniostenosis.

CSF pressure via a lumbar puncture may yield conclusive values to warrant surgery.

Principles of Treatment

The indication for surgery for craniosynostosis is never based on the diagnosis per se, but exclusively on functional impact and/or psychosocial well-being. Treatment is aimed at optimizing both facets, preserving or restoring function as well as correcting disfiguring deformities. Surgical considerations must address all 3 portions of the cranial skeleton, each of which may be affected by the growth failure: the neurocranium, the orbits, and the midface.

In its ideal form, surgery should restore normal sutural function and skull growth. From the preceding chapters, it is obvious that such a goal cannot be achieved by the currently available techniques. Nevertheless, for many decades surgery consisted of small linear craniectomies in an implicit attempt to recreate some sort of functional suture. The morphological results were not satisfying, particularly in cases of forehead deformity. In a misguided attempt to prevent recurrent synostosis, surgeons then wrapped the bone margins with foils made of foreign material, thereby ignoring the fact that re-ossification originates from the underlying dura rather than from the margins of the cut bone plates [11]. Linear craniectomies were somewhat effective in form as well as function. From a modern-day perspective these techniques worked by partially and transiently restoring the compliance of the cerebral envelope, thus allowing the distorted brain to reshape the bone according to its own normal shape, until after a few weeks the vault solidified again through re-ossification. The surgical principle utilizing this process may be referred to as passive reshapement. Its effectiveness depends on an easily distensible dural envelope, and therefore this technique is largely limited to early infancy and to scaphocephaly in particular. In this deformity, the lateral portions of the dura can readily expand, while expansion in a longitudinal direction is limited by the falx and the tentorium. In contrast to the former small strip craniectomies, large-scale craniectomies are currently preferred (fig. 7a), as this latter approach has proven to be more effective. Once again, this type of craniectomy is confined to early infancy, since after the first 6 to 8 months of life the re-ossification potential rapidly declines, leaving the risk of a persistent bone defect. In older infants, this risk may be reduced by cutting the removed bone into pieces, which are then repositioned, termed the morcellation technique.

Since the late 1970s, more radical plastic-surgical techniques have been developed, allowing

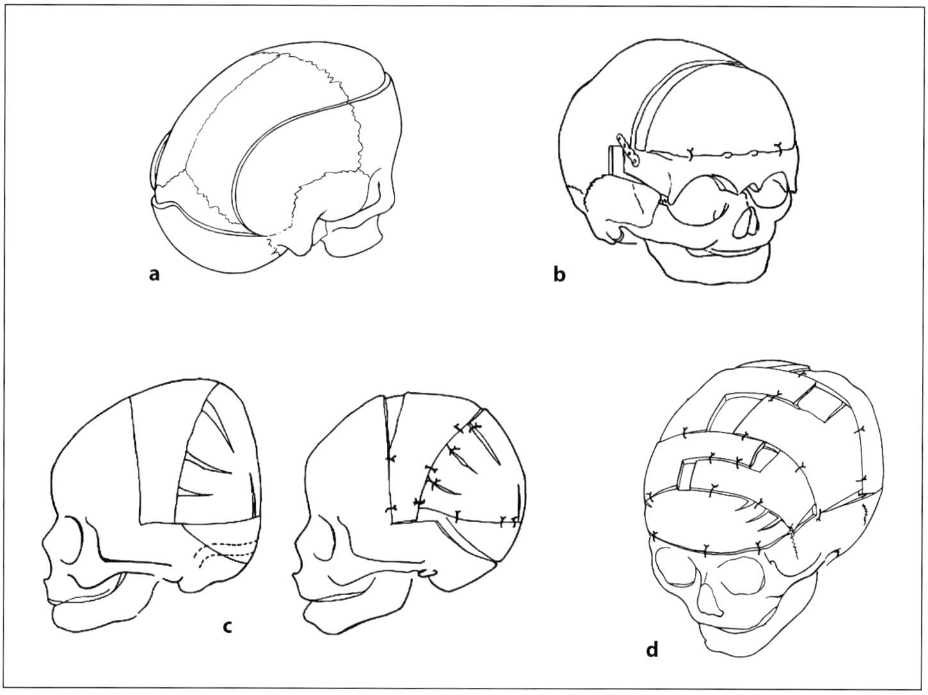

Fig. 7. Basic surgical techniques for craniosynostosis. **a** Craniectomy in scaphocephaly; **b** fronto-orbital advancement; **c** occipital advancement; **d** total vault reconstruction. (Reprinted from [12] with permission by Elsevier).

for an immediate and stable change of the cranial shape: active reshapement. In essence, these techniques consist of the removal of appropriate bone flaps, which are then recontoured and placed in a new position, according to the desired cranial shape and volume. Active remodelling is particularly effective in deformities involving the forehead and the frontal base or the occiput. Moreover, the technique is largely independent of the patient's age. The following various methods can be distinguished (table 1) [12].

Fronto-orbital advancement (figs. 7b, 8). In essence, the procedure consists of removing the frontal bone including the surpraorbital rims, which is then recontoured, repositioned as desired and fixed with miniplates or simply with sutures.

Occipital advancement (fig. 7c). In an analogous manner, an occipital growth deficit may be corrected by reshaping a large occipital bone flap, which is then repositioned in a tilted fashion in order to expand the occipital cranial space.

Calvarial reconstruction (figs. 7d, 9). With this technique, almost the whole calvarial bone is cut into appropriate segments, which are then reassembled in a manner allowing for correction of deformities and cranial expansion. In selected cases the procedure may be combined with forehead advancement.

There are other techniques incorporating the midface into the procedure: *midface advancement*, *monobloc fronto-facial* advancement and *orbital transposition*. These techniques will be addressed in Chapter 19.

For all the aforementioned techniques, a standard surgical approach is used, consisting of a bicoronal skin incision, which for cosmetic

Table 1. Timing and technique for surgical correction of various synostotic deformities. Timing according to the practice of the Würzburg craniofacial center

Synostotic deformity	Timing	Technique
Scaphocephaly	<6 months 6–12 months >12 months	craniectomy morcellation calvarial reconstruction
Trigonocephaly	>9 months	fronto-orbital advancement
Brachycephaly	>9 months	fronto-orbital advancement
Anterior plagiocephaly	>9 months	fronto-orbital advancement
Posterior plagiocephaly	>9 months	occipital advancement
Oxycephaly	not applicable	forehead advancement with calvarial reconstruction

reasons is usually performed in a curvilinear or a zig-zag fashion. Extensive hair clipping or shaving has turned out to be dispensable. Stable re-fixation of bone flaps is achieved by means of miniplates, wire loops, or even by simple sutures. Metallic plates have to be removed and are now largely substituted for by resorbable plates. Following osteosynthesis solid bone healing is accomplished within 3 weeks in infancy, and within approximately 6 weeks in later childhood.

Timing of surgery is critical for the management of craniosynostosis. Timing depends on several conflicting age-related factors, the effect of which remains to some degree unpredictable. For instance, the bone is more pliable and easier to mold in infancy than in later childhood. Large dural areas denuded from bone reliably re-ossify only during the first 6 to 8 months of life, while even minor bone defects of less than 3 cm diameter may remain open if created after the second year of life. It has also been suggested that early surgery prevents harmful effects on brain development [13], although there is little evidence substantiating this view [14]. On the other hand, recurrent deformity or cranial volume deficit is more likely to occur if surgery is performed at an early age since intrinsic osseous growth failure can hardly be corrected by mechanical means [12, 15, 16]. However, the significance of this age-related effect has not been clearly elucidated. As a consequence, optimal timing of elective surgery is a matter of discussion. While several centers prefer to perform any type of surgery in early infancy [17, 18], the Würzburg craniofacial team, like others [15], prefers to defer active plastic surgical procedures until the end of the first year, as in their opinion this policy can reduce recurrences. Optimal timing as discussed above is of secondary importance in any situation involving surgical urgency, e.g. overt intracranial hypertension or severe proptosis putting the cornea at risk. At present, the craniofacial team in Würzburg prefers to perform elective craniectomy during the first 6 months of life, while plastic reconstructive techniques are preferably deferred until an age of 9 to 18 months.

Surgical Risks

Any individual treatment protocol for correction of craniosynostosis must include a careful risk-benefit analysis. Serious problems may arise even during induction of anesthesia, since intubation in patients with Crouzon or Apert syndrome may

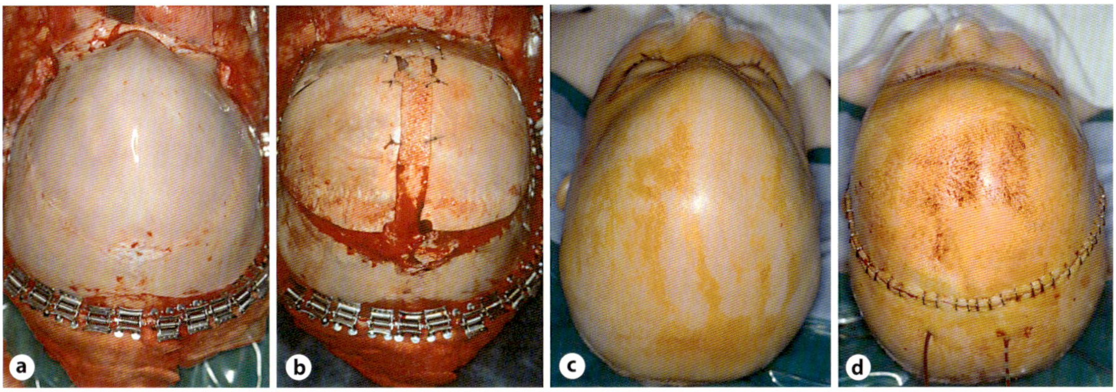

Fig. 8. Fronto-orbital advancement for trigonocephaly. Operative site (**a**, **b**) and outer aspect (**c**, **d**) prior to and after correction.

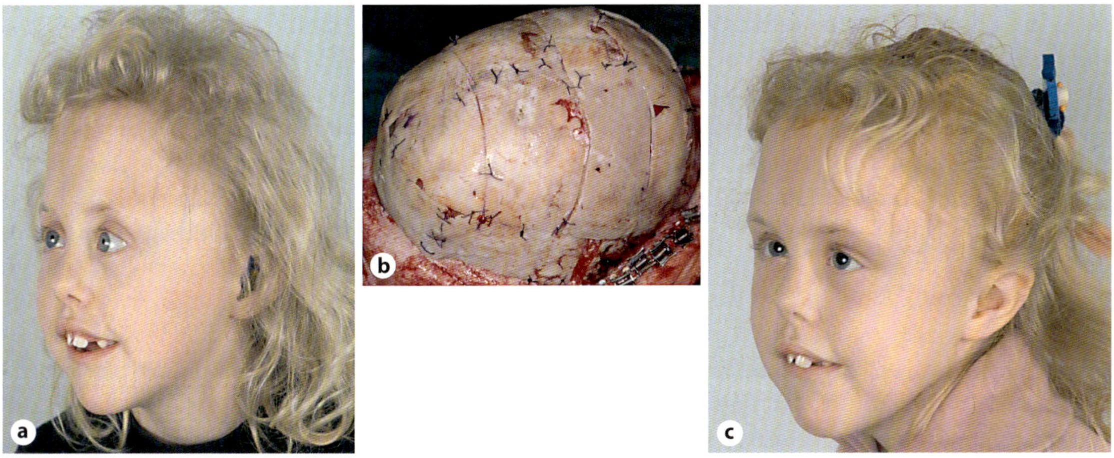

Fig. 9. Total vault reconstruction, re-operation for recurrent turricephaly. **a** Before operation; **b** intraoperative view; **c** 2 weeks after surgery.

be surprisingly difficult due to midface hypoplasia. Surgical risks include a mortality of roughly 0.3%, the predominant reason being intraoperative blood loss and re-bleeding [12]. Significant blood loss may result from inadvertent opening of a dural sinus, but is primarily an unavoidable consequence of the large-scale surgical field and the well vascularized bone and dural surface. Blood transfusion is usually necessary. The risk of re-bleeding is mainly confined to the first 12 postoperative hours and should be carefully monitored in the intensive care unit. In contrast, the risk of a significant brain injury or even injury to the optic nerve, often the most pressing concern to the patient's family, is remarkably low. Deep wound infections affecting some 2–5% of cases occur almost exclusively after reconstructive surgery, and may prolong the hospital stay considerably. Minor wound problems are more common. They are often attributable to skin tension after cranial expansion procedures, particularly over bulky plates used for osteosynthesis. Contrary to what may be expected, devascularisation of the bone flaps leaving almost no living cells hardly ever results in significant postoperative osteolysis. As mentioned above, persistent bone defects are to be expected after wide craniectomy performed beyond the age of 8 months, and when reconstructive techniques leave bony gaps of 3 cm or more in patients older than 2 years. The artificial epidural dead space usually left after plastic surgical augmentation of the vault is not a matter of major concern, as it is almost invariably filled up within a few weeks, first by expansion of the dura and the subarachnoid space, thereafter by the expanding brain. Keeping surgical risks at a minimum requires careful preoperative evaluation, meticulous surgical technique by a well-trained team of pediatric neurosurgeons, maxillofacial or plastic surgeons and pediatric anesthetists, and careful postoperative observation in a pediatric intensive care unit.

Postoperative Surveillance and Strategies

Documentation of surgical results is important not only to validate the applied treatment method but also for scientific reasons. Results may be more readily quantified with regard to function than to morphology. Preoperative papilledema should resolve at least partially within 2 to 4 weeks, but may need several months to disappear completely. If there is doubt, invasive pressure monitoring is warranted. One should keep in mind that intracranial hypertension may persist in cases of obstructive hydrocephalus [6] or impaired venous drainage of the brain [8]. Improvement of the cranial shape should be documented at least by photographs, optimally by means of 3-dimensional stereophotogrammetry. While some morphological parameters, e.g. horizontal cephalic index, are readily quantified by cephalometry, others are not, e.g. parietal width and height.

There are no data suggesting that surgery is able to correct intrinsic osseous growth failure. Consequently, even after adequate surgical correction, various degrees of recurrent deformity and/or elevated intracranial pressure may arise (table 2). In general, these problems seem to be more pronounced in patients treated at an early age and in those affected with syndromic craniosynostosis [12, 15, 16]. Recurrent intracranial hypertension seems to be related mainly to early progressive multisutural fusion, which is a predominant feature of the most common syndromes (Crouzon, Pfeiffer, and Saethre-Chotzen), with the exception being patients with Muenke syndrome (table 2). In isolated monosutural craniosynostosis, progressive involvement of other sutures is rare and mainly confined to scaphocephaly.

Long-term postoperative surveillance is highly recommended until brain bulk growth is completed by approximately 12 years of age. Routine check-ups should be tailored to the individual risk profile and may include ophthalmoscopy at 6-month intervals in patients with scaphocephaly and perhaps other types of single-suture craniosynostosis, but at 3-month intervals in any plurisutural synostosis including Crouzon, Pfeiffer, Apert, and Saethre-Chotzen syndromes. In these authors' practices, the oldest patient developing recurrent papilledema de novo was a patient with Apert syndrome who was almost 8 years old. Routine eye evaluations are supplemented by repeated radiographs at 1, 2, 4, 8, and 12 years of age.

Surgery for recurrence usually carries a higher risk due to wide-spread scarring and residual bone defects. Moreover, multiple recurrences of deformity may occur if re-operation has been performed before school age. These issues should be taken into account if re-operation is considered.

Co-existing pathologies like hydrocephalus and hindbrain herniation also deserve continued surveillance. In some cases, hydrocephalus may become apparent only after the brain has been

Table 2. Re-operations for recurrent deformity and/or intracranial hypertension. Data from the craniofacial center of Würzburg

Synostosis type	No. of surgical patients	No. of patients requiring re-operation (%)	No. of patients with elevated ICP at re-operation (%)
Scaphocephaly	384	21 (5)	14 (4)
Trigonocephaly	140	1 (1)	0
Brachycephaly	30	4 (13)	1 (3)
Anterior plagiocephaly	78	7 (9)	0
Posterior plagiocephaly	6	0	0
Oxycephaly	21	1 (5)	1 (5)
Crouzon	64	29 (45)	27 (42)
Pfeiffer	15	9 (60)	9 (60)
Apert	53	12 (23)	10 (19)
Saethre-Chotzen	48	18 (38)	8 (17)
Muenke	38	2 (5)	0
Craniofrontonasal	7	0	0

ICP, intracranial pressure.

released from its confined space. For treatment, surgical expansion of the posterior fossa has been advocated [7], but was not successful in a few of our own patients, who eventually needed conventional CSF shunting into the peritoneal cavity. Chiari malformation not only causes hydrocephalus but may also cause symptoms from brainstem compression or from an extending hydrosyringomyelia (fig. 5b). As these sequelae occur at an unpredictable age, long-term surveillance is mandatory. Treatment is aimed at restoring a normal craniospinal CSF flow. This goal may sometimes be achieved by surgical expansion of the posterior fossa [7], but more often by conventional surgical technique, namely enlargement of the foramen magnum and, if necessary, expansion duroplasty and partial resection of the cerebellar tonsils.

As mentioned above, due to the growth failure in the skull base, upper airway obstruction and, within this context, chronic middle ear effusions may be persistent problems needing appropriate attention and treatment.

Management of Specific Types of Craniosynostosis

Scaphocephaly

There are good reasons for leaving cases of non-disfiguring deformity untreated and to follow a 'wait-and-see' policy, as only few patients will develop intracranial hypertension requiring surgery [19, 20]. Elective surgery consists of a wide vertex craniectomy, performed in most centers at an age of less than 6 months (fig. 7a). This timing ensures satisfactory correction of the deformity as well as sufficient re-ossification within 2 to 3 months. In later infancy, the decreased potential of re-ossification may be compensated for by repositioning pieces of the removed bone on the exposed dura, thereby creating a morcellation technique [21]. By the second year at the latest, the technique of total cranial vault reconstruction (fig. 7d) is applied in most centers [17].

While the conventional techniques require a bicoronal skin incision for surgical exposure, more recently the vertex craniectomy has been modified: the endoscopically guided technique takes advantage of 2 small skin incisions at the vertex, which are even less visible later [22]. Roughly 5% of patients with non-syndromic scaphocephaly require re-operation for recurrent deformity [23] and/or overt intracranial hypertension, the latter often attributable to progressive multisutural fusion (table 2) [12, 24, 25]. These cases should clearly be separated from other types of progressive craniosynostosis, e.g. Crouzon syndrome and hypophosphatasia, which initially may appear similar to simple scaphocephaly in the present authors' experiences. Finally, there are no data suggesting that early surgery reliably prevents the need for a second operation because of elevated intracranial pressure.

Trigonocephaly

According to the current state of knowledge, surgery is mainly performed for psychosocial reasons, as the risk of intracranial hypertension is low. Therefore, the mildest form of trigonocephaly, merely consisting of a metopic ridge, may be left untreated, although shaving the ridge has been advocated by some authors. Typical trigonocephaly is treated by surgical reshapement of the forehead, which includes the supraorbital rims but leaves the hypotelorism untreated (fig. 7b, 8) [26]. As experience shows, the latter will be less conspicuous following surgery. The commonly present epicanthal folds usually disappear spontaneously with increasing age. In the long run, some degree of recurrent deformity will usually appear, but rarely requires major re-operation. Minor depressions at the lateral forehead may be corrected with an on-lay plastic in adolescence.

Brachycephaly

In essence, surgery consists of an advancement of the forehead and the supraorbital rims, termed fronto-orbital advancement. In some cases, the typically increased forehead width may be reduced at the same time. It is more difficult to alleviate the turricephalic aspect, since more than a 2-cm reduction of cranial height can rarely be achieved. In selected cases additional space can be gained by means of an occipital advancement procedure (fig. 7c). Recurrent deformity will prompt re-operation in some cases (fig. 9, table 2), but elevated intracranial pressure does not appear to be a significant problem, consistent with data from other centers [15].

Anterior Plagiocephaly

Because of the complex distortion of the forehead and the periorbital region, treatment of this deformity carries the greatest challenge for the surgeon in terms of cosmesis. The basic principle of surgical technique is the same as in brachycephaly. As surgery leaves the facial asymmetry untouched, perfect correction will rarely be achieved. During follow-up, approximately 10% of patients consider re-operation because of conspicuous deformity.

Posterior Plagiocephaly

Once again, the difference between synostotic deformity and positional molding has to be stressed, since the latter condition rarely if ever requires surgical treatment. Correction of posterior plagiocephaly due to unilateral lambdoid synostosis is challenging as the deformity includes a striking contralateral parietal bulging. During surgery, particular attention must be paid to the great venous sinuses, as significant injury may cause disastrous bleeding.

Oxycephaly

In this condition, surgery is mainly aimed at treating intracranial hypertension, as grossly disfiguring deformity is usually absent [27]. Typical concerns regarding optimal surgical timing are therefore beyond consideration. As in most patients the supraorbital rims are slightly retruded, calvarial reconstruction may be combined with fronto-orbital advancement in order to sufficiently expand the intracranial space. In contrast to the syndromic forms, isolated pansynostosis appears to carry no major risk of recurrent intracranial hypertension (table 2). Additionally, attention should be paid to ectopic cerebellar tonsils (fig. 5d) [7].

Crouzon and Pfeiffer Syndromes

In the *FGFR2*-related syndromes, preoperative considerations differ considerably from those in isolated synostosis for a number of reasons. First, in these entities, intracranial hypertension is often a leading problem and may require urgent surgery even in early infancy. Second, the re-operation rate for recurrent intracranial hypertension is much higher (table 2). Finally, cosmetic results are often less pleasing than in isolated forms, particularly in patients with severe proptosis or clover-leaf deformity. In any individual treatment protocol these nuances have to be taken into account. For instance, in clover-leaf deformity with elevated intracranial pressure, a large-scale posterior craniectomy may be the first step. This allows deferring the forehead advancement to a later age, thereby reducing the risk of re-operation on the forehead. Conversely, severe proptosis putting the cornea at risk may require early forehead advancement or even a combined advancement of the forehead and the midface (see Chapter 19). Herniation of the cerebellar tonsils and shunt-dependent hydrocephalus are other common problems, affecting roughly 20% of patients with Crouzon syndrome and up to 60% of patients with Pfeiffer syndrome [6]. Re-operation, most often for recurrent intracranial hypertension, is a frequent necessity in both syndromes (table 2) [12]. Compromised upper airways and chronic middle ear problems, both resulting from midface hypoplasia, may persist until late adolescence, when surgery on the midface is most feasible (see Chapter 19).

Apert Syndrome

Even more than in the previously discussed syndromes, surgery is directed towards functional problems, since the most conspicuous facial features can hardly be corrected to a sufficient degree. Upper airway obstruction may be the most striking feature in the neonatal period, and can be a challenging problem for the medical team. Craniosynostosis treatment usually starts with fronto-orbital advancement. Even with adequate cranial expansion, intracranial hypertension reappears in approximately 20% of patients [12]. While non-progressive ventriculomegaly is present in the majority of patients, shunt-dependent hydrocephalus may still occur and should certainly be suspected in the presence of a concurrent Chiari I malformation [7].

On a side note, the specific problem of severe syndactyly should be addressed as early as possible, by 6 months of age at the latest. Surgical reconstruction of the hands is usually performed in several steps, mainly during the first 2 years of life [28].

Saethre-Chotzen Syndrome

As most patients present with forehead deformity, they are primarily treated with fronto-orbital advancement. Recurrent intracranial hypertension has been noted in roughly 20% of our patients [29], while even higher rates have recently been reported by other surgical centers [16]. Hydrocephalus or Chiari malformation has never been observed in our own series of more than 70 individuals.

Muenke Syndrome

In contrast to the former syndromes, there is no major concern for elevated intracranial pressure. Thus, surgery aims mainly at correcting the disfiguring deformity. In the present authors' experiences, the fairly common turricephalic aspect can be corrected only to a limited extent, especially as after surgery it tends to re-appear to a significant degree. Recurrent deformity has been appreciated as a significant problem occurring much more frequently than in non-syndromic coronal synostosis [30]. Nevertheless, re-operation has to be carefully considered with due regard to the individual benefit and the limits and risks of repeated surgery. Comprehensive medical care also includes the specific problems of sensorineural hearing deficit and mental retardation.

Craniofrontonasal Syndrome
In this particular entity, surgical considerations have to address the severe hypertelorism in addition to brachy- or plagiocephaly, while intracranial hypertension obviously represents no significant problem. Several techniques of orbital frame shifting have been developed, which will be discussed in Chapter 19.

In summary, treatment of craniosynostosis requires a well-coordinated, multidisciplinary team of specialists familiar with the spectrum of phenotypes, associated abnormalities, surgical techniques and risks, potential late complications and sequelae, which assumes comprehensive care for patients in the most economic manner possible. This team includes the paediatrician, geneticist, pediatric neurologist, neurosurgeon, plastic or maxillofacial surgeon, radiologist, ophthalmologist, ENT surgeon, audiologist, orthodontist, clinical psychologist, and clinical photographer.

References

1 Regelsberger J, Delling G, Tsokos M, Helmke K, Kammler G, et al: High-frequency ultrasound confirmation of positional plagiocephaly. J Neurosurg 2006;105(suppl 5):413–417.
2 Jeevan DS, Anlsow P, Jayamohan J: Abnormal venous drainage in syndromic craniosynostosis and the role of CT venography. Childs Nerv Syst 2008;24: 1413–1420.
3 Posnick JC, Lin KY, Jhawar BJ, Armstrong D: Apert syndrome: quantitative assessment by CT scan of presenting deformity and surgical results after first-stage reconstruction. Plast Reconstr Surg 1994;93:489–497.
4 Hall EJ, Brenner DJ: Cancer risks from diagnostic radiology. Br J Radiol 2008; 81:362–378.
5 Cinalli G, Sainte-Rose C, Kollar EM, Zerah M, Brunelle F, et al: Hydrocephalus and craniosynostosis. J Neurosurg 1998;88:209–214.
6 Collmann H, Sörensen N, Krauss J: Hydrocephalus in craniosynostosis: a review. Childs Nerv Syst 2005;21:902–912.
7 Cinalli G, Spennato P, Sainte-Rose C, Arnaud E, Aliberti F, et al: Chiari malformation in craniosynostosis. Childs Nerv Syst 2005;21:889–910.
8 Hayward R: Venous hypertension and craniosynostosis. Childs Nerv Syst 2005; 21:880–888.
9 Schüller A: Craniostenosis. Radiology 1929;13:377–382.
10 Renier D, Sainte-Rose C, Marchac D, Hirsch JF: Intracranial pressure in craniostenosis. J Neurosurg 1982;57:370–377.
11 Shillito J Jr, Matson DD: Craniosynostosis: a review of 519 surgical patients. Pediatrics 1968;41:829–853.
12 Collmann H, Sörensen N, Krauß J: Craniosynostosis – treatment, results and complications; in Choux M, diRocco C, Hockley AM, Walker ML (eds): Pediatric Neurosurgery. London, Churchill Livingstone, 1999, pp 291–322.
13 Arnaud E, Renier D, Marchac D: Prognosis for mental function in scaphocephaly. J Neurosurg 1995;83:476–479.
14 Kapp-Simon KA, Speltz ML, Cunningham ML, Patel PK, Tomita T: Neurodevelopment of children with single suture craniosynostosis: a review. Childs Nerv Syst 2007;23:269–281.
15 Wall SA, Goldin JH, Hockley AD, Wake MJ, Poole MD, Briggs M: Frontoorbital reoperation in craniosynostosis. Br J Plast Surg 1994;47:180–184.
16 Woods RH, Ul-Haq E, Wilkie AO, Jayamohan J, Richards PG, et al: Reoperation for intracranial hypertension in *TWIST1*-confirmed Saethre-Chotzen syndrome: a 15-year review. Plast Reconstr Surg 2009;123:1801–1810.
17 Renier D, Lajeunie E, Arnaud, E, Marchac D: Management of craniosynostoses. Childs Nerv Syst 2000;16:645–658.
18 Öcal E, Sun PP, Persing JA: Craniosynostosis; in Albright AL, Pollack IF, Adelson PD (eds): Principles and Practice of Pediatric Neurosurgery, ed 2. New York, Thieme, 2008, pp 264–288.
19 Boltshauser E, Ludwig S, Dietrich F, Landolt MA: Sagittal craniosynostosis: cognitive development, behaviour, and quality of life in unoperated children. Neuropediatrics 2003;34:293–300.
20 Florisson JM, van Veelen ML, Bannink N, van Adrichem LN, van der Meulen JJ, et al: Papilledema in isolated single-suture craniosynostosis: prevalence and predictive factors. J Craniofac Surg 2010; 21:20–24.
21 Arnaud E, Marchac D, Renier D: Le traitement des craniosténoses: indications et techniques. Neurochirurgie 2006;52: 264–291.
22 Jimenez DF, Barone CM, McGee MC, Cartwright CC, Baker CL: Endoscopy-assisted wide-vertex craniectomy, 'barrel-stave' osteotomies and postoperative helmet molding therapy in the management of sagittal suture craniosynostosis. J Neurosurg 2004;100(5 Suppl Pediatrics):407–417.
23 Fearon JA, McLaughlin EB, Kolar JC: Sagittal craniosynostosis: surgical outcomes and long-term growth. Plast Reconstr Surg 2006;117:532–541.
24 Reddy K, Hoffman H, Armstrong D: Delayed and progressive multiple suture craniosynostosis. Neurosurgery 1990;26: 442–448.

25 Arnaud E, Capon-Degardin N, Michienzi J, DiRocco F, Renier D: Scaphocephaly part II: secondary coronal synostosis after scaphocephalic surgical correction. J Craniofac Surg 2009;20 (suppl 2):1843–1850.
26 Collmann H, Sörensen N, Krauss J: Consensus trigonocephaly. Childs Nerv Syst 1996;12:664–668.
27 Renier D, Cinalli G, Lajeunie E, Arnaud E, Marchac D: Oxycéphalie, une craniosténose sévère. A propos d'une serie de 129 cas. Arch Pédiatr 1997;4:722–729.
28 Guero S, Vassia L, Renier D, Glorion C: Surgical treatment of the hand in Apert syndrome. Handchir Mikrochir Plast Chir 2004;36:179–185.
29 Kress W, Schropp C, Lieb G, Petersen B, Büsse-Ratzka M, et al: Saethre-Chotzen syndrome caused by *TWIST 1* gene mutations: functional differentiation from Muenke coronal synostosis syndrome. Eur J Hum Genet 2006;14:39–48.
30 Honnebier MB, Cabiling DS, Hetlinger M, McDonald-McGinn DM, Zackai EH, Bartlett SP: The natural history of patients treated for FGFR3-associated (Muenke-type) craniosynostosis. Plast Reconstr Surg 2008;121:919–931.

Hartmut Collmann
Section of Pediatric Neurosurgery, Neurosurgical Department
University of Würzburg, Josef-Schneider-Str. 11
97080 Würzburg (Germany)
Tel. +49 931 201 24809, Fax +49 931 25540, E-Mail collmann.h@nch.uni-wuerzburg.de

Muenke M, Kress W, Collmann H, Solomon BD (eds): Craniosynostoses: Molecular Genetics, Principles of Diagnosis, and Treatment.
Monogr Hum Genet. Basel, Karger, 2011, vol 19, pp 232–243

Maxillofacial Examination and Treatment

H. Böhm[a] · T. Schweitzer[b] · A. Kübler[a]

[a]Department of Maxillofacial Surgery, [b]Department of Paediatric Neurosurgery, University of Würzburg, Würzburg, Germany

Abstract
Syndromic craniosynostosis is often associated with malformations of the midface. Growth failure of the skull base results in midface and maxillary hypoplasia, which in turn causes proptosis, upper airway obstruction, dental malocclusion, as well as other functional impairments. For treatment, various standard maxillofacial surgical procedures have been developed, including Le-Fort-III distraction, fronto-orbito-maxillary advancement, monobloc frontofacial advancement, and orbital transposition. These operations require an experienced surgeon in a specialized centre in order to optimize outcome and to reduce the risk of complications. As craniofacial malformations are related to growth, surgical correction should preferably be performed in adolescence unless the degree of the symptoms demands an earlier intervention.

Development of the Midface

The face of a young child is not simply a smaller version of the adult face. During postnatal development, the facial proportions as well as the relationship to the neurocranium change considerably (fig. 1). While the morphology of facial growth has been well described, the mechanisms of growth regulation remain largely unknown [1].

Physiologically, a newborn exhibits a relatively underdeveloped viscerocranium. At the age of 2 years, the viscerocranium has only reached one-quarter and at the age of 8 years about one-half of its final adult size. In comparison, neurocranial growth is nearly completed by 8 years of age. With the eruption of the first teeth, a considerable growth spurt of the whole viscerocranium takes place. With ongoing growth, the viscerocranium develops anteriorly and caudally [2, 3].

The key for understanding the typical growth failure in craniosynostosis is knowledge regarding the growth of the anterior base of the skull. During the 5th to 6th week of embryological development (Carnegie 13), a mesenchymal aggregation in the area of the axial mesoderm of the head transforms into a blastema at the base of the skull. During the 6th week (Carnegie 17), this blastema matures to become the cartilaginous chondrocranium, representing a primary growth centre. From that point on, growth depends on chondroblast activity, which is almost exclusively regulated by as yet largely undefined endogenous factors. In the 7th to 8th week (Carnegie 18, 19, 20), the cartilaginous structure progressively transforms into bone through the process of endochondral ossification (fig. 2). During this stage, defective ossification of the skull base results in the typical malformation of craniosynostosis. Abnormal chondroblast

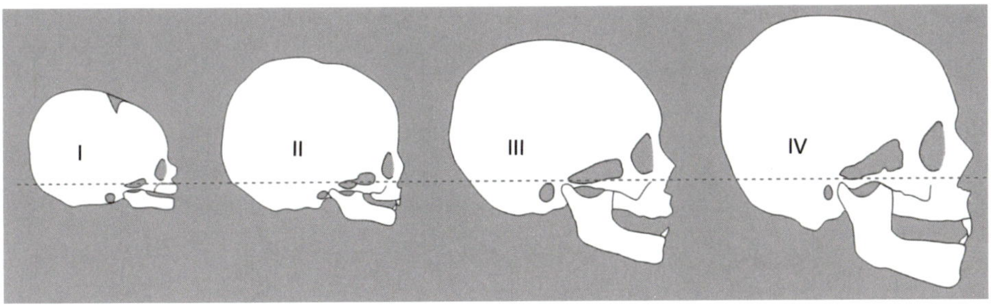

Fig. 1. Skull at different ages showing the changing relationship between the neurocranium and viscerocranium at birth (I), 1 year (II), 6 years (III), and 20 years of age (IV). (Modified and shown with permission from [46]).

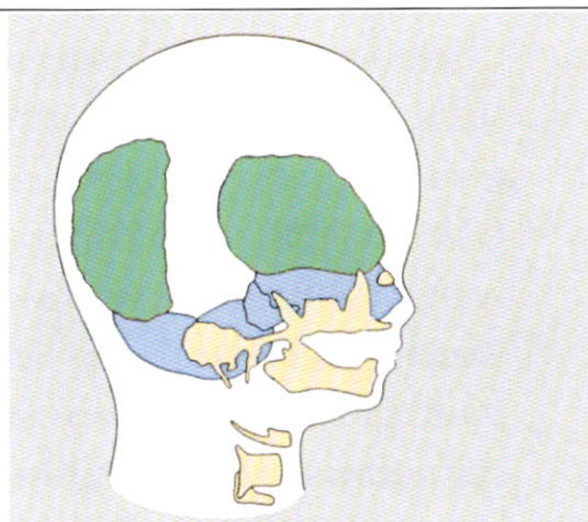

Fig. 2. Embryonic development of the cartilaginous skull base and the cranial vault, 8th–9th week of gestation. (Modified and shown with permission from [47].

activity is thought to lead to a diminished increase in volume of the cartilaginous skull base. As a consequence, the normal growth of the attached midface in the vertical, sagittal, and transverse dimensions is reduced. In summary, the typical facial deformities seen in craniosynostosis originate at the cranial base.

Abnormalities of the Viscerocranium in Craniosynostosis

Most craniofacial syndromes are associated with growth failure of both the neurocranium and the viscerocranium. Growth failure may affect the orbits and the midface in different manners.

Exophthalmus due to shallow orbits is the most striking feature. The skull base forms the upper border of the orbit, while the midface represents the lower border. Both structures have an important influence on the geometry of the orbit [4]. In 1971, Tessier stated that flattening the eye socket by 10 mm would result in a 6-ml loss of volume [5]. Depending on the affected sutures, the degree of exophthalmos may vary. In oxycephaly and brachycephaly, only the orbital roof is involved, while concurrent midface hypoplasia results in shallowness of the whole eye socket. Incomplete closure of the eyelids may give rise to exposure keratitis and corneal ulceration.

Hypertelorism and asymmetric orbital anatomy are related to impaired ocular motility, which

Table 1. Main aesthetic and functional sequelae of premature craniosynostosis in the viscerocranium

Main sequelae of premature craniosynostosis in the viscerocranium	
Shallow orbits:	proptosis, exposure keratitis
Hypertelorism:	strabismus, impaired binocular vision
Midface hypoplasia:	upper airway compromise, impaired ventilation of the middle ear
Deformity of maxilla and/or mandible:	malocclusion, dental crowding
Asymmetry and scoliosis of the face	

frequently causes strabismus and impedes the development of binocular vision [6].

Abnormal growth of the midface also affects the maxilla in all 3 dimensions and impairs the normal rotational growth of the upper jaw [7]. This may result in a flat midface with a small nose, an open bite (i.e. malocclusion with absent contact of the frontal teeth) and retrusion of the maxilla (retrognathia) leading to an aspect of mandibular protrusion (pseudoprogenia). Additionally, facial scoliosis may occur. Intraorally, the hypoplastic and narrow maxilla causes malocclusion and dental crowding. Dental crowding is found in the mandibula as well. The teeth of the lower jaw, in trying to compensate for pseudoprogenia, are pushed backwards. As a consequence, the affected individual suffers from difficulties in chewing and biting. Taken together, these problems may lead to failure to thrive and also may result in caries due to difficult dental hygiene.

Many patients present with a high-arched and narrow palate. In patients with Apert syndrome, a median furrow caused by lateral submucous swellings is almost invariably present, and should not be confused with a cleft palate. The latter abnormality is nevertheless a common feature of Apert syndrome: at our institution, significant clefts involving the velum and sometimes the posterior part of the hard palate were noted in 36% of 66 patients with Apert syndrome. Minor clefts or a bifid uvula may occur in up to 75% of patients with Apert syndrome [8]. This abnormality has also been observed in a few patients with Pfeiffer syndrome and Saethre-Chotzen syndrome [9, 10].

Depending on the degree of midface hypoplasia, a narrow nasal meatus, stenotic choanae and a narrow epipharyngeal space may be present. Consequently, a considerable number of patients suffer from upper airway compromise [11, 12], which in addition may lead to failure to thrive, poor growth, and ultimately to life-threatening cor pulmonale. The individual risk resulting from respiratory distress can be measured using standardized monitoring techniques such as polysomnography. This technique provides a basis for treatment decisions and for surveillance (see Chapter 17). Less severe midface hypoplasia leaving respiratory function intact may still impair the ventilation of the middle ear by the Eustachian tube, thereby causing recurrent middle ear effusions and infections.

Most functional and aesthetic sequelae of viscerocranial growth failure in craniosynostosis can be improved or even corrected by surgical treatment (table 1). Basically, surgery is not able to return deviant growth to normal. Therefore, as long as growth of the midface is not completed, one must consider in each patient whether (1) surgery is the only way to improve function; (2) the benefit of surgery reasonably outweighs the risks; (3) recurrent deformity requiring a second operation is anticipated; (4) the planned operation interferes with other prospective surgery. These considerations clearly influence both the selection of the specific treatment modality as well as timing of interventions.

Apart from physical examination and common imaging techniques (see Chapter 18), there are some specific diagnostic aids in maxillofacial surgery which are particularly helpful for planning surgery and postoperative surveillance:

A lateral cephalogram allows accurate measurement of the deformities in a standardized manner (fig. 3), while plaster jaw casts are useful for the planning of both orthodontic treatment and maxillofacial surgery (fig. 4). A 3-dimensional model of the entire skull may aid in the planning of complex surgical procedures (fig. 5).

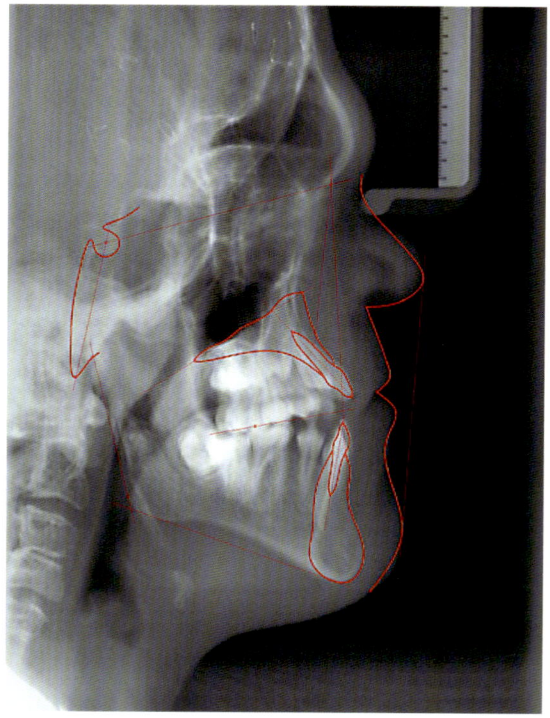

Fig. 3. Lateral cephalogram showing tracing of the frontal teeth, jaws, and central skull base for analysis of spatial relationships.

Principles of Maxillofacial Treatment in Patients with Craniosynostosis

A wide variety of surgical techniques exists for the correction of facial malformations in patients with craniosynostosis. The principles of the most common techniques will be described here. Most of these procedures require lengthy training, excellent surgical skills, and extensive and specific experience. In addition, the pediatric anaesthetist needs to have particular expertise with regards to difficult intubation in patients with midface hypoplasia, significant intraoperative blood loss, and potential early postoperative complications. Therefore, the surgical treatment of patients with craniosynostosis is usually confined to specialized centres that are able to provide a well-trained team of maxillofacial surgeons, neurosurgeons, anaesthesiologists, paediatricians, ENT surgeons, and orthodontists.

Tracheostomy

In life-threatening upper airway obstruction, e.g., in the case of frank cor pulmonale, a tracheostomy may be warranted as a minor, immediately effective procedure. However, in view of a reported mortality rate of 2–8.5% [13], a permanent tracheostomy should be avoided if possible. In addition, an early tracheostomy leads to delayed speech development, requiring prolonged speech therapy. Instead, nasopharyngeal tubes or CPAP (continuous positive airway pressure) masks will satisfactorily improve respiration in most cases. A permanent tracheostomy should be considered only if these measures fail [14], but a midface advancement may be an option as well [15].

Midface Advancement

Le-Fort-III Distraction. Severe hypoplasia of the midface can be corrected by means of a Le-Fort-III osteotomy, which essentially consists of detaching the maxilla including the infraorbital rim, the nasal skeleton, and the zygoma, from the cranial base. The procedure is indicated not only in cases of severe upper airway compromise but

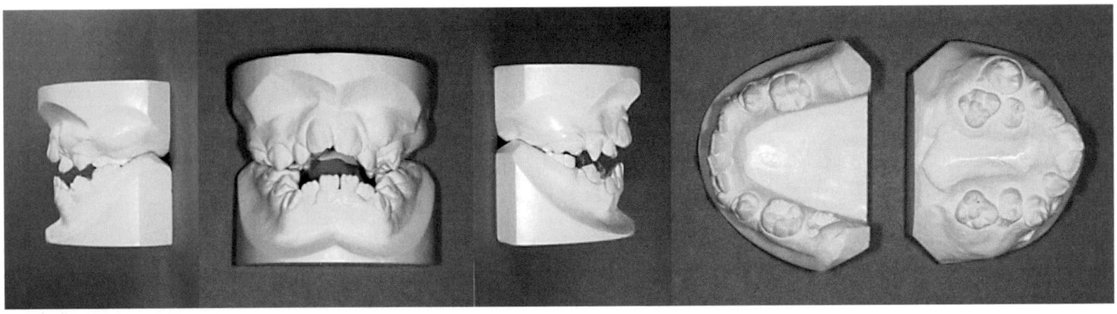

Fig. 4. Plaster cast of a patient with Apert syndrome. Note the absent occlusion of frontal teeth (open bite), small maxilla with dental crowding, and narrow palate.

also in patients with severe proptosis putting the cornea at risk, or simply for aesthetic (i.e., psychosocial) reasons. It is important to note that the procedure allows only for correction of maxillary retrognathia, while the reduced height and width of the maxilla are left untreated.

Midface advancement is currently performed by applying the technique of distraction osteogenesis (fig. 5) [16]. Surgical exposure of the midface is achieved via a bicoronal scalp incision, which may be supplemented by intraoral, infraorbital, and transconjunctival incisions as necessary. After elevating the frontal scalp flap, the nasal bone, the upper parts of the maxilla, and the zygomatic arches are exposed, after which Tenon's capsule is carefully separated from the orbital walls. Using oscillating saws and chisels, the viscerocranium is then completely separated from the cranial base. Additional approaches through the oral cavity and through the infraorbital region may be used to gain access to the orbital floor and to the pterygomaxillary joint. In order to facilitate this difficult type of surgery, the use of intraoperative computer aided navigation has been established [17].

Following detachment of the midface, wires or rigid bars are fixed to the bone laterally from the nasal aperture or at the maxillary teeth, and guided through the skin or between the lips. After wound closure, a headframe is fixed to the parietal bones and distractors are attached to the frame. These devices allow well-controlled traction at the midface using the wires or bars (fig. 5). Proper positioning of the distractors is crucial, as it defines the vector of midface movement [18]. After a period of 7 to 10 days, the newly generated, unmineralized callus at the osteotomy line is gradually distended at a rate of about 1 mm per day by activating the distractors. In this way, the midface is moved forward without interrupting continuity of immature bone. An overcorrection of about 30% of the desired advancement is recommended, since mild recurrence is likely to occur after distraction has been terminated. Following an inpatient hospitalization of 3 to 4 weeks, the distraction process may be continued by the patient and family on an outpatient basis. After completing the distraction, a 12-week period of retention is necessary, in which the position of the midface is maintained in order to allow mineralization of the callus tissue. Thus, about 18 to 20 weeks after surgery, the headframe and the distraction device can be removed under local anesthesia.

Since its introduction in craniofacial surgery, the distraction osteogenesis technique has been modified several times, e.g. by using individually prefabricated devices which permit an accurate and well defined movement of the midface [19], or by internal distraction devices [20, 21], or by combinations of external and internal distracters

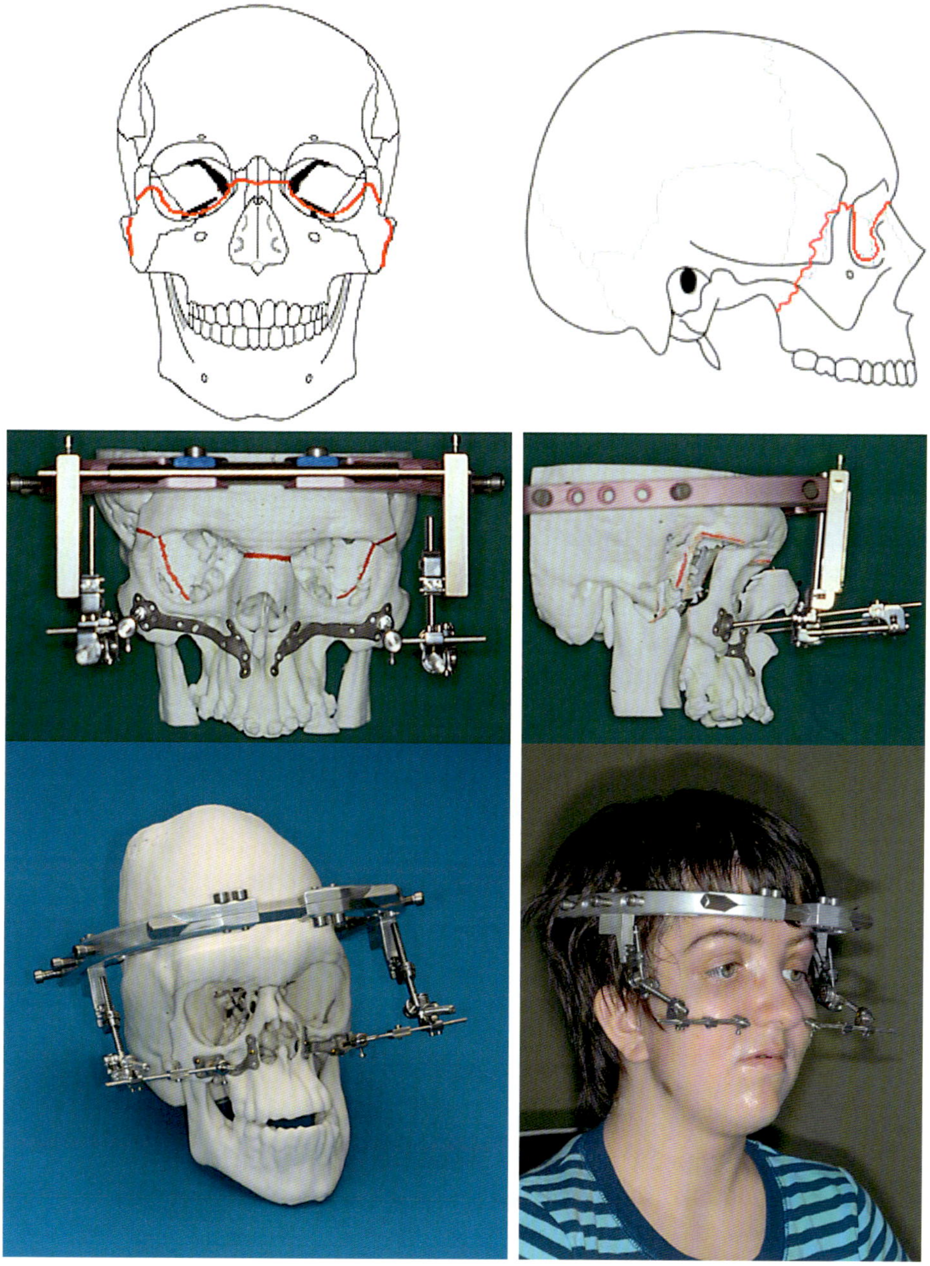

Fig. 5. Le-Fort-III-distraction osteogenesis, showing osteotomy lines and position of the distractors.

[22]. In the present author's experience, external distraction allows for improved control of the distraction vector and assures better functional and aesthetic results.

The previously customary single-step midface advancement with rigid fixation is now considered obsolete because of a high risk of poor bony healing and subsequent pseudarthrosis. At present this technique is only rarely applied. It may still be justified in cases where only minor advancement is necessary.

As the movement of the midface in conjunction with the maxilla profoundly alters dental occlusion, close cooperation with an orthodontist is mandatory. Prior to surgery, the dental arches must be properly aligned. In many cases the maxilla has to be widened by orthodontic devices, a treatment that may require surgical support. In particular, the teeth of the maxilla and mandibula should fit together in a neutral occlusion in the planned postoperative position of the midface. The orthodontic pretreatment may last 12 to 18 months, and in most cases has to be continued after surgery for about 6 months.

While the Le-Fort-III distraction usually dramatically improves respiration [15], it often does not result in relatively normal dental occlusion despite orthodontic pretreatment. Due to the deficient rotational growth of the maxilla, an open bite usually persists; i.e., the opposing molar teeth contact each other before the incisors overlap. In this case, normal occlusion is achieved by combining the Le-Fort-III distraction with a Le-Fort-I distraction procedure, i.e., separating the lower from the upper maxilla. This enables the surgeon to move the teeth-carrying maxillary portion independently from the upper midface. Alternatively, a classical Le-Fort-I osteotomy may be performed after the midface distraction treatment has been completed. Depending on the individual anatomy and specifics of each patient, the classical osteotomy pattern may be modified accordingly.

Optimal timing of surgery on the midface is a matter of ongoing debate. In our centre, we prefer to defer the Le-Fort-III distraction to early adulthood, as it is only in this age that recurrent midface retrusion is not to be anticipated. Other centres emphasize the need for early functional improvement as well as concerns directly related to social issues, and, therefore, prefer an age of 8 to 12 years [14, 15]. However, as surgery can only compensate for the actual growth deficit, the persisting growth failure will usually result in recurrent deformity requiring a second midface advancement in young adulthood [23]. Re-operation is usually more difficult and carries a higher surgical risk due to scar formation and irregular bone regeneration in the distracted areas. Nonetheless, there is a generally accepted lower age limit, since below 3 years of age the cranial vault is not stable enough to resist the pressure exerted by the pins of the head frame.

In infancy a single-step Le-Fort-III osteotomy may be justified as an alternative option to a permanent tracheostomy in patients in whom there is severe upper airway obstruction refractory to less invasive treatment [14, 15].

Surgical risks of the Le-Fort-III osteotomy include extensive blood loss, deep wound infection due to opening of the paranasal sinuses, injury of the second trigeminal branch, and because of extensive intraorbital dissection in rare instances, damage to the optic nerve. Fatalities have also been reported [24]. Therefore, the indication for this procedure should be carefully scrutinized in any patient, and the operation should be performed in specialized centres.

Fronto-Orbito-Maxillary Advancement (Tessier). In patients in whom there is severe proptosis due to shallow orbits, even more complex surgical procedures may be necessary in order to prevent corneal damage and to avoid tarsorrhaphy, which in infants inevitably leads to amblyopia.

Fronto-orbito-maxillary advancement allows for correction of both the frontocranial and the midfacial malformations, thereby simultaneously improving function as well as aesthetics. The

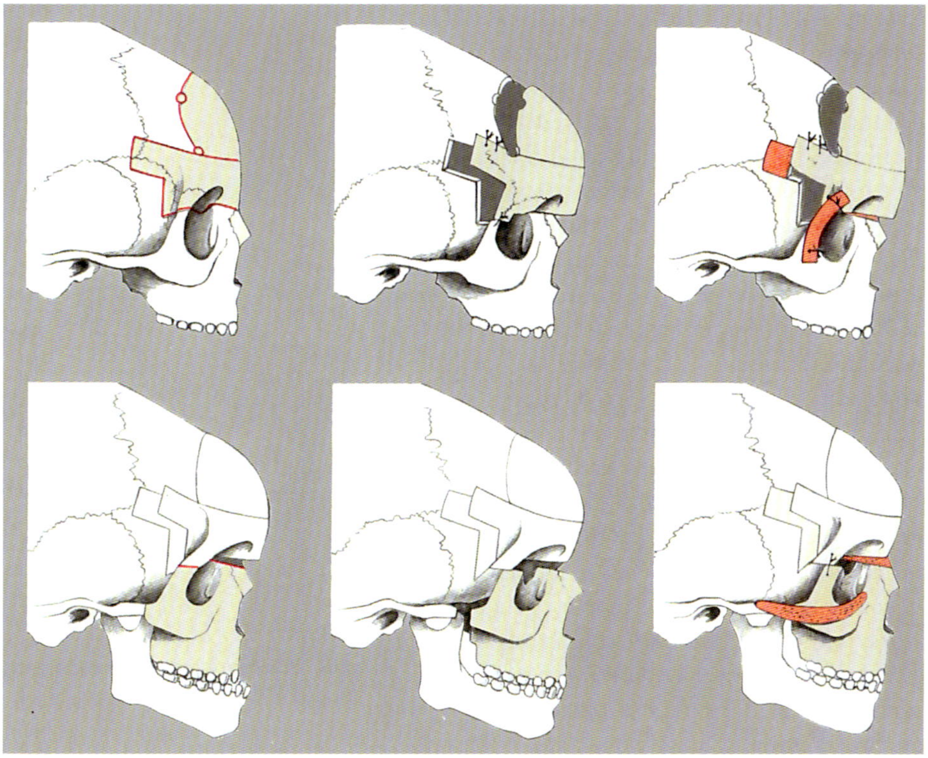

Fig. 6. Fronto-orbito-maxillary advancement. Note the coloured bone struts for stabilisation and bridging of bone gaps. (Reproduced with permission from [16]).

French plastic surgeon Paul Tessier was the first to combine fronto-orbital advancement and a Le-Fort-III osteotomy [5]. The principles of both procedures have been described previously. As shown in figure 6, bone grafts harvested from the iliac crest were necessary to fill the gaps resulting from the advancement of the osteotomized segments.

By moving forward a bifrontal bone flap and a fronto-orbital bandeau, the frontal growth deficit is compensated for and the orbital roof is expanded. The simultaneous advancement of the midface provides additional orbital space, thereby correcting exophthalmos. In addition, this procedure markedly improves the dental occlusion as well as the facial appearance [16].

In its initial version all 3 segments (frontal segment, fronto-orbital segment and midface) have been sectioned and repositioned in a single procedure. As the segments can be moved independently from each other according to the individual requirements of each, satisfactory aesthetic results are usually achievable. However, the technique involves a high rate of complications as it breaks down the natural barrier between the neurocranium and the nasal airways. Inadvertent dural tears may readily occur and can lead to CSF fistulas and ascending infections. Fatalities due to meningitis have been reported [25]. The risks are considerably reduced if fronto-orbital advancement and Le-Fort-III osteotomy are performed separately as a staged procedure.

Monobloc Fronto-Facial Advancement (Ortiz-Monasterio). This technique represents the logical progression of the fronto-orbito-maxillary advancement (fig. 7). It allows a satisfactory correction of the periorbital region in the case of severe proptosis, and at the same time allows for effective treatment of midface retrusion provided there is normal dental occlusion [25, 26]. Optimal timing is estimated to be between 5 and 10 years of age [16, 25, 26], but infants have also been subjected to this technique. In this procedure, a bifrontal bone flap is first elevated via a bicoronal incision. The anterior skull base is sectioned transversally and a circular osteotomy is made in the orbit. After dividing the zygoma, the maxilla is separated from the pterygoid and the nasal septum is transsected. Then the osseous monobloc, consisting of the midface and the complete orbital framework, is mobilised and shifted to an advanced position. In order to secure the advancement, 2 bone grafts, harvested from the parietal region, are put as spacers into the lateral bony gaps of the orbits. Another graft is placed between the nose and the crista galli in the midline. Titanium miniplates aid in stabilising the monobloc (fig. 7) [16].

The procedure carries considerable surgical risks. Several fatalities have been reported [25, 27]. A wide opening of the paranasal sinuses without the chance of re-creating an effective barrier to the neurocranium is associated with a high risk of ascending infection.

If the technique is modified as the distraction osteogenesis procedure, the perioperative risk decreases markedly [28, 29], but severe complications such as optic nerve injury have nonetheless been reported [30]. If distraction is performed with internal devices, the technique can be applied to small children and even infants for the treatment of severe upper airway obstruction and/or exophthalmos [31].

Another modification used in a few centres capitalizes on the distensibility of the open sutures at the cranial bases, thereby avoiding risky transsection of the paranasal sinuses [von Gernet, München, personal communication]. Despite these possible modifications, this procedure should only be considered if there is a clear indication, after careful planning, and with the availability of a skilled surgical team and ancillary staff.

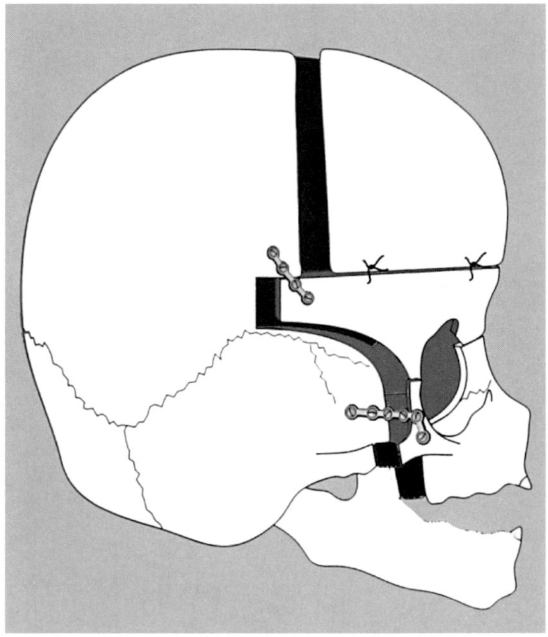

Fig. 7. Monobloc frontofacial advancement. (Reproduced with permission from [48]).

Correction of Ocular Hypertelorism

Ocular hypertelorism indicates the occurrence of an increased intraorbital distance. Assessing hypertelorism by using several soft-tissue landmarks has been suggested as a way to screen for the presence of hypertelorism [32]. However, it is important to keep in mind that a flat nasal bridge, epicanthal folds, exotropia, widely spaced eyebrows, narrow palpebral fissures, and dystopia can create the false impression of hypertelorism. Bony structures allow an accurate measurement [33]. Therefore, ocular hypertelorism may be defined as bony interorbital distance (BIOD) greater than

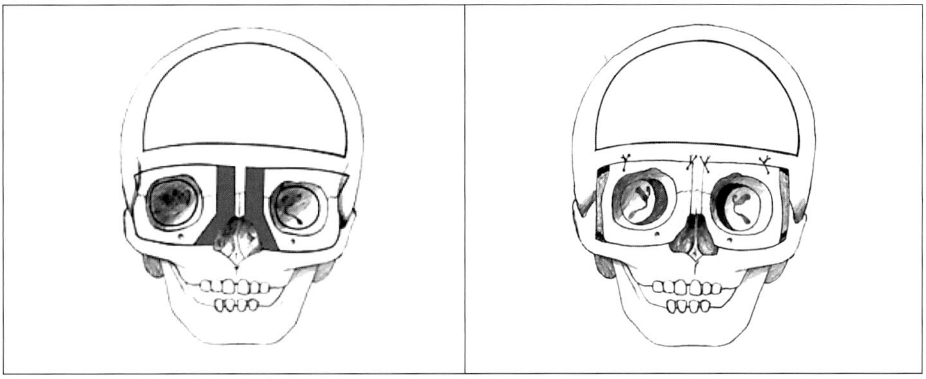

Fig. 8. Orbitotomy for surgical correction of hypertelorism. (Reproduced with permission from [16]).

Table 2. Mean bony interorbital distance (BIOD) [45]

Age	BIOD, mm	Age	BIOD, mm	Age	BIOD, mm
2	15, 3	8	19, 3	14	21, 9
4	17, 1	10	20, 3	16	22, 3
6	18, 4	12	21, 0	18	22, 6

2 standard deviations above the normal mean age- and race-related value (table 2).

Mild hypertelorism with a BIOD of 30–34 mm in adults is classified as degree 1/first degree. Degree 2/second degree indicates a BIOD >34–40 mm, and degree 3/third degree a BIOD >40 mm [34]. Munro and Das suggested 4 different types of hypertelorism on the basis of BIOD and orbital shape [35].

A degree 1/first degree hypertelorism is barely noticeable, and usually needs no correction. Degrees 2 and 3 hypertelorism are considered to warrant surgical treatment for psychosocial reasons.

Orbitotomy for the Correction of Hypertelorism. In 1960, Tessier and Guiot developed a procedure that they called the 'functional orbit' [36]. Since then, this technique has been modified several times [37]. As an example, the functional orbit method with 'frontal crown' is described here (fig. 8) [16].

First, via a bicoronal incision, the bony forehead is exposed and Tenon's capsule is separated from the orbital walls. Next, a bifrontal bone flap is lifted, leaving in place a frontal bar of about 1 cm width just above the supraorbital rim – the 'frontal crown'. The hypertrophic medial bone is removed and the frame of the eye socket is osteotomised. The orbital roof is cut via the intracranial approach while the medial and lateral walls as well as the orbital floor are cut using an extracranial approach. At this point, the mobilised orbital frames are approximated to each other. Either resorbable sutures or plates, or metallic miniplates or wires are used for rigid fixation [38, 39]. The osseous procedure usually has to be supplemented by soft tissue correction in order to reduce the abnormal intercanthal distance (see Chapter 17).

Some authors have suggested a correction at the age of 3 to 5 years in order to assure stereoscopic vision [40, 41]. However, at this age the tooth germs of the second (adult) dentition are in a very high position, and thus are prone to injury during operation. Therefore the intervention should be deferred until an age of 6 to 8 years. At this age, surgery is less difficult, and the danger for damage to the dentition is less. Moreover, functional and aesthetic improvement is more predictable. However, adolescents and adults are no longer able to retrieve stereoscopic vision after surgery. As with other procedures, 3-dimensional imaging allows for preoperative planning [42]. Surgical risks include postoperative strabismus and even loss of vision from optic nerve damage.

It is worth mentioning that this kind of osteotomy does not appear to significantly influence the growth and development of the face [26, 43, 44]. However, improved self-esteem and reduced psychosocial distress through an improved appearance is beyond doubt [16].

References

1 Enlow DH: Growth and the problem of the local control mechanism. Am J Anat 1973;136:403–405.
2 Björk A: The face in profile. Svensk Tandläk Tidskr 1947;40, (suppl 55).
3 Goose DH, Appleton J: Human Dentofacial Growth. Oxford, Pergamon Press, 1982.
4 Tessier P: Craniofacial surgery in syndromic craniosynostosis, in Cohen MM (ed): Craniosynostosis: Diagnosis, Evaluation and Management. New York, Raven, 1986, pp 321–411.
5 Tessier P: Relationship of craniostenosis to craniofacial dysostosis, and to faciostenosis. Plast Reconstr Surg 1971;48: 224–237.
6 Morax S: Ocularmotor disorders in craniofacial malformations, in Caronni EP (ed): Cranifacial Surgery, 1st ed. Boston, Little Brown, 1985, pp 97–107.
7 Langford RJ, Sgouros S, Natarajan K, Nishikawa H, Dover MS, Hockley AD: Maxillary volume growth in craniosynostosis. Plast Reconstr Surg 2003;111: 1598–1604.
8 Kreiborg S, Cohen MM Jr: The oral manifestations of Apert syndrome. J Craniofac Genet Dev Biol 1992;12:41–48.
9 Stoler JM, Rogers GF, Mulliken JB: The frequency of palatal anomalies in Saethre-Chotzen syndrome. Cleft Palate Craniofac J 2009;46:280–284.
10 Stoler JM, Rosen H, Desai U, Mulliken JB, Meara JG, Rogers GF: Cleft palate in Pfeiffer syndrome. J Craniofac Surg 2009;20:1375–1377.
11 Moore MH: Upper airway obstruction in the syndromal craniosynostoses. Br J Plast Surg 1993;46:355–362.
12 Schafer ME: Upper airway obstruction and sleep disorders in children with craniofacial anomalies. Clin Plast Surg 1982;9:555–567.
13 Gianoli GJ, Miller RH, Guarisco JL: Tracheotomy in the first year of life. Ann Otol Rhinol Laryngol 1990;99:896–901.
14 Bannink N, Nout E, Wolvius EB, Hoeve HL, Joosten KF, Mathijssen IM: Obstructive sleep apnea in children with syndromic craniosynostosis: long-term respiratory outcome of midface advancement. Int J Oral Maxillofac Surg 2010;39:115–121.
15 Flores RL, Shetye PR, Zeitler D, Bernstein J, Wang E, et al: Airway changes following Le Fort III distraction osteogenesis for syndromic craniosynostosis: a clinical and cephalometric study. Plast Reconstr Surg 2009;124:590–601.
16 Zöller JE, Kübler AC, Lorber WD, Mühling JFH: Kraniofaziale Chirurgie. Stuttgart, Thieme, 2003.
17 Jeelani NU, Khan MA, Fitzgerald O'Connor EJ, Dunaway D, Hayward R: Frontofacial monobloc distraction using the StealthStation intraoperative navigation system: the ability to see where you are cutting. J Craniofac Surg 2009;20: 892–894.
18 Shetye PR, Giannoutsos E, Grayson BH, McCarthy JG: Le Fort III distraction: Part I. Controlling position and vectors of the midface segment. Plast Reconstr Surg 2009;124:871–878.
19 Klammert U, Böhm H, Schweitzer T, Würzler K, Gbureck U, et al: Multidirectional Le Fort III midfacial distraction using an individual prefabricated device. Craniomaxillofac Surg 2009;37: 210–215.
20 Pelo S, Gasparini G, Di Petrillo A, Tamburrini G, Di Rocco C: Distraction osteogenesis in the surgical treatment of craniostenosis: a comparison of internal and external craniofacial distractor devices. Childs Nerv Syst 2007;23:1447–1453.
21 Satoh K, Mitsukawa N, Tosa Y, Kadomatsu K: Le Fort III midfacial distraction using an internal distraction device for syndromic craniosynostosis: device selection, problems, indications, and a proposal for use of a parallel bar for device-setting. J Craniofac Surg 2006;17: 1050–1058.
22 Wall SA, Butler L, Byren J, Carls PF, Greenwood S, et al: Combined internal and external Le Fort III distraction osteogenesis–the 'elusive vector'. J Craniofac Surg 2009;20(suppl 2):1806–1808.
23 Meazzini MC, Mazzoleni F, Caronni E, Bozzetti A: Le Fort III advancement osteotomy in the growing child affected by Crouzon's and Apert's syndromes: presurgical and postsurgical growth. J Craniofac Surg 2005;16:369–377.
24 Nout E, Mathijssen IM, van der Meulen JJ, van Veelen ML, Koning AH, et al: Internal carotid dissection after Le Fort III distraction in Apert syndrome: A case report. J Craniomaxillofac Surg 2010 [Epub ahead of print].

25 Tessier P: Discussion. The monobloc frontofacial advancement: do the pluses outweigh the minuses? Plast Reconstr Surg 1993;91:988–989.
26 Ortiz-Monasterio F, Fuente del Campo AF, Carillo A: Advancement of the orbits and the midface in one piece, combined with frontal repositioning, for the correction of Crouzon's deformities. Plast Reconstr Surg 1978;6:507–516.
27 Wolfe SA, Morrison G, Page LK, Berkowitz S: The monobloc frontofacial advancement: do the pluses outweigh the minuses? Plast Reconstr Surg 1993; 91:977–987.
28 Cruz AA, Akaishi PM, Arnaud E, Marchac D, Renier D: Exorbitism correction of faciocraniosynostoses by monobloc frontofacial advancement with distraction osteogenesis. J Craniofac Surg 2007; 18:355–360.
29 Meling TR, Høgevold HE, Due-Tønnessen BJ, Skjelbred P: Comparison of perioperative morbidity after LeFort III and monobloc distraction osteogenesis. Br J Oral Maxillofac Surg 2010 [Epub ahead of print].
30 Alonso N, Goldenberg D, Fonseca AS, Kanashiro E, Matsushita H, et al: Blindness as a complication of monobloc frontofacial advancement with distraction. J Craniofac Surg 2008;19:1170–1173.
31 Arnaud E, Marchac D, Renier D: Reduction of morbidity of the frontofacial monobloc advancement in children by the use of internal distraction. Plast Reconstr Surg 2007;120:1009–1026.
32 Cohen MM Jr, Richieri-Costa A, Guion-Almeida ML, Saavedra D: Hypertelorism: interorbital growth, measurements, and pathogenetic considerations. Int J Oral Maxillofac Surg 1995;24:387–395.
33 Currarino G, Silverma FN: Orbital hypotelorism, arhinencephaly, and trigonocephaly. Radiology 1960;74:206–217.
34 Tessier P: Orbital hypertelorism. I. Sucessive surgical attempts. Material and methods. Causes and mechanisms. Scand J Plast Reconstr Surg 1972;7:135–155.
35 Munro IR, Das SK: Improving results in orbital hypertelorism correction. Ann Plast Surg 1979;2:499–507.
36 Tessier P: Notes on the history of craniofacial surgery; in Jackson IT, Munro IR, Slayer KE, Whitaker LA (eds): Atlas of Craniomaxillofacial Surgery, 1st ed. St. Louis, Mosby, 1982, pp VII-XII.
37 Habal M: Surgical correction of orbital hypertelorism: a surgical evolution through time. J Craniofac Surg 2009;20: 715–717.
38 Mühling J, Collmann H, Reuther J, Sörensen N: Functional and anatomic aspects of the orbitotomy in craniofacial surgery. Neurosurg Rev 1989;12:21–23.
39 Tessier P: Experiences in the treatment of orbital hypertelorism. Plast Reconstr Surg 1974;53:1–18.
40 Edgerton MT, Jane JA: Vertical orbital dystopia – surgical correction. Plast Reconstr Surg 1980;67:121–138.
41 Epstein F, Wood-Smith D, Converse JM, Benjamin MV, Becker MH, Ransohoff J: Radical one-stage correction of craniofacial anomalies. J Neurosurg 1975;42: 522–529.
42 Moreira Gonzalez A, Elahi M, Barakat K, Yavuzer R, Brinkmann B, Jackson IT: Hypertelorism: the importance of three-dimensional imaging and trends in the surgical correction by facial bipartition. Plast Reconstr Surg 2005;115:1537–1546.
43 Caronni EP: Facial bipartition in hypertelorism. Cleft Palate J 1986;(suppl 23):19–26.
44 McCarthy JG: A study of gustatory and olfactory function in patients with craniofacial anomalies. Plast Reconstr Surg 1979;64:52–58.
45 Costaras M, Pruzansky S, Broadbent BH Jr: Bony interorbital distance (BIOD), head size, and level of the cribriform plate relative to orbital height: I. Normal standards for age and sex. J Craniofac Genet Dev Biol 1982;2:5–18.
46 Miethke RR: Schädelentwicklung; in Diedrich P (ed): Kieferorthopädie I: Orofaziale Entwicklung und Diagnostik. München, Urban & Fischer, 2000, p 31.
47 Joos U, Kleinhenz J: Klinisch relevante Syndrome im Kopfbereich; in Horch HH (ed): Mund-Kiefer-Gesichtschirurgie. München, Urban & Fischer, 2007, p 400.
48 Zöller JE, Mühling J: Kraniofaziale Fehlbildungen. Teil I: Prämature Schädelnahtsynostosen; in Horch HH (ed): Mund-Kiefer-Gesichtschirurgie. München, Urban & Fischer, 2007, p 433.

Hartmut Böhm
Department of Maxillofacial Surgery, University of Würzburg
Pleicherwall 2
97070 Würzburg (Germany)
Tel. +49 931 201 72940, Fax +49 931 201 72941, E-Mail boehm_h@klinik.uni-wuerzburg.de

Author Index

Arnheim, N. 58

Beenken, A. 45
Benson, M.D. 13
Böhm, H. 216, 232

Calabrese, P. 58
Cohen Jr., M.M. IX, 67
Collmann, H. VIII, 1, 98, 165, 216
Connerney, J.J. 28

Fanganiello, R.D. 152
Feret, H. 143

Gripp, K.W. 199

Hehr, U. 177

Jehee, F.S. 152

Kress, W. VIII, 1, 98, 165
Kübler, A. 232

McDonald-McGinn, D.M. 143
Mohammadi, M. 45
Müller, U. 8
Muenke, M. VIII, 1, 89, 119, 165

Nah, H.-D. 143

Opperman, L.A. 13

Passos-Bueno, M.R. 152

Raam, M.S. 119

Schmid, M. VII
Schramm, T. 184
Schweitzer, T. 165, 216, 232
Solomon, B.D. VIII, 1, 89, 165
Spicer, D.B. 28

Wieland, I. 107

Zackai, E.H. 143

Subject Index

Bold numbers refer to figures and tables.

Abnormal head shape 199, 200
Acrocallosal syndrome (ACLS) 143, 148
Active reshapement 223
Age-dependence 58
Anterior plagiocephaly **92**, 169, 178, **200**, 201, **224**, **227**, 228
Antley-Bixler syndrome 123
Apert syndrome 3, **3**, 34, 35, 38, 47, 50, 58ff, **64**, 67ff, **179**, **189**, **192**, 195, **205**, 206ff, **219**, **220**, **227**, 229, 243, **236**
  adult cranial volume **69**
  birth length/weight **69**
  cartilage sleeve abnormalities 72, **74**
  central nervous abnormalities 69
  craniofacial abnormalities 71
  cutaneous manifestations **78**, 79
  development 67
  discovery/history 3
  ear and aural findings 73
  gene mutations 47, 61, **80**
  growth 67
  hands/feet 74, **75**, **76**
  IQ 70
  lack of cartilaginous segmentation 74, **74**, **75**
  molecular genetics 80
  ophthalmologic abnormalities **71**, 72
  oral manifestations 72, **73**
  paternal age effect 63
  phenotype **68**, **71**, **73**
  prenatal diagnosis 79
  radiographic findings **68**, 72, **75**, **76**, **77**, **78**
  respiratory problems 72
  skeletal findings 76, **77**, **78**
  sperm mutation frequency 62, **64**
  surgery 229
  ventriculomegaly 69, **220**
  visceral anomalies 69
Array CGH 152, 180, 212
Autosomal
  dominant 8, 67, 81, 83, 89, 98, 150, 124, 129, 131, 135, 178
  recessive 124, 126, 129, 174

Baller-Gerold syndrome **124**, 126
Beare-Stevenson cutis gyrata syndrome **124**, 127
Bisutural synostosis 172, **173**
Bohring-Opitz syndrome **125**, 128
Bone morphogenetic protein (BMP) 39
Boston type craniosynostosis 8ff, 36, **205**
  causative mutation 10
  phenotypic spectrum 8, **9**
Boundary formation 17
Brachycephaly **92**, **99**, **124**, 170, **171**, 178, **179**, 186, **200**, 202, **224**, 228

C syndrome 128, **154**
Calvarial
  bone growth regulation 13ff
  reconstruction 223, **224**
  sutures 15, 134
Candidate genes 158
Carpenter syndrome **125**, 129, 180
Cartilaginous segmentation 74ff, **74**, **75**, 77, **84**
Cellular interference 107ff
  concept 115, **115**
Central nervous system 67, 69, 81, 84, 208
Chromosomal alterations 152ff, **154**
  candidate gene identification 158

deletions 157
submicroscopic rearrangements 159
Clinical approach 199ff
Clinical evaluation 178, 204ff
differential diagnosis 212
family history 204
growth 211
internal organs 211
musculoskeletal considerations 211
neurodevelopment 208
ophthalmologic considerations 210
otolaryngologic considerations 210
past medical history 204
physical examination 206
Clinical features **84**, 91, **93**, 107, **108**
Cloverleaf skull (Kleeblattschädel) 8, **9**, 83, **84**, **124**, 186, **190**, 204, **205**
Cognitive
development 100, 209
impairment 89, **93**
Computed tomography (CT) **92**, **171**, **172**, **173**, 216, **219**
Copper beaten skull (Wolkenschädel) **174**, 217, **218**
Coronal suture **11**, 14, **14**, **18**, 28ff, **30**, **31**, **154**, **185**, 186, **186**, **187**, **188**, **191**, **194**, 202
synostosis 37, 91, **92**, **93**, 98, **100**, 107, **109**, 154, 169, **170**, 172, **173**, 178, 201, **203**, **205**
Cranial bones **14**, **21**, **30**
Cranial vault 13, 14, **233**
anatomy 14
origin 14
Craniectomy 199, **223**, **224**
Craniofacial abnormalities 71, 82, 84, 99, 108
Craniofrontonasal syndrome (CFNS) 107ff, **179**, **205**, **227**, 230
cellular interference 115
clinical features 107ff, **108**, **109**
craniofacial symptoms 108
development 109
EFNB1 mutations 110ff, **112**, **113**, **114**
extracranial features 109
genetic mouse models 116
inheritance 109
molecular genetics 107
pathomechanism 114
sex-dependent manifestations 114
surgery 230
Craniosynostosis 1, 8, 13, 28, 45, 58, 67, 89, 98, 107, 119, 143, 152, 165, 177, 184, 199, 216, 232
Crouzon syndrome 3, 67, 81ff, **179**, **205**, **220**, **227**, 229
adult cranial volume **69**
aural findings 83
central nervous system 81
cervical anomalies 82
craniofacial abnormalities 82
discovery/history 3
FGFR2 mutations **80**
molecular genetics 83
ophthalmologic findings 82
oral findings 83
phenotype **81**
radiographic findings 82
respiratory problems 82
surgery 229
Crouzon syndrome with acanthosis nigricans **125**, 130

3D CT scan 146
2D ultrasound 184
3D ultrasound 184
De novo mutation 59, 90, 98, 104, 111, **112**, 123, 129, 134, 137, 145, 157, 182
Dura mater 15, 16, 30, **30**
Dwarfism syndromes 45ff

EFNB1 17, 37, 40, 107ff, **114**, **179**, 180, **205**
germline mutations 113
mutation spectrum 111, **112**
Environmental factors 153
Eph/ephrin signaling 17, **18**, **20**, 36, 110, **111**
Etiology 203
Extracranial malformation 101, 109, 178, **179**
Eye positions **206**

FGFR activation 45ff
FGFR1/2/3 20ff, 35ff, 45ff, 58ff
gain-of-function mutations 46
ligand-dependent 47, **48**, **51**
ligand-independent 46, **52**, 54
Fibroblast growth factor (FGF)/FGF receptor (FGFR) signaling 19ff, 34ff, 45ff
Fontanelle **124**, 166, **167**, **188**, 191, 202, 206
Fronto-orbital
advancement 223, **223**, **224**, **225**, 228, 239
recession 8, **9**, **205**
Fronto-orbito-maxillary advancement (Tessier) 238

Gain-of-function mutation 8, 35, 46ff, **48**, **51**, **52**, 54
Genetic
counseling 90, 181
paradox 110
Genetic testing 89, 177ff
clinical evaluation 178
genetic counseling 181
genetic workup 178, **179**
laboratories 181
result interpretation 181
Germline
mutations 58ff, 113
nucleotide substitutions 58ff
selection model 59, 60
GLI3 Disorders 143ff
genotype-phenotype correlation 148
mouse models 149
mutations 143ff, 148
pathogenesis 148
Greig cephalopolysyndactyly syndrome (GCPS) 144

Historical overview 1ff
treatment aspects 5
Honeycomb pattern (Lücken-Leistenschädel) 218, **218**, **219**
Hot spot model 59
Hydrocephalus 70, 82, 91, **191**, 219, **220**
Hypertelorism correction 240

IgIII domain 35, 80, 83
Imaging studies 202, 216ff
technical aids 216
Internal organs **205**, 211
Intracranial
hypertension 2, **99**, 102, 166, 173, 216, 221, **227**, 228, 229
pressure (ICP) 5, 16, 70, 98, 166, 208, 216, 221, **222**, **227**

Jackson-Weiss syndrome 131, **132**, **179**
Jacobsen syndrome (JBS) 132, **132**, 157

Lambdoid suture **11**, **14**, 72, 82, **154**, **185**, **187**, **189**
synostosis **154**, 171, 172, **172**, **173**, **201**, **203**, **217**, 221
Le-Fort-III distraction 235ff, **237**
Ligand-dependent mutation 47, **48**, **51**
Ligand-independent mutation 46, **52**, 54
Loeys-Dietz syndrome **133**, 136

Magnetic resonance imaging (MRI) **167**, **174**, 216ff, **220**
Male bias 58
Maxillofacial
examination 232
treatment 232, 235
Mechanism of craniosynostosis 37
Megalencephaly 67, **68**
Metopic suture 11, 28, 153, **154**, 159, 168, **186**, **187**, **188**, **196**
synostosis **100**, 143ff, **146**, **148**, **154**, 180, 159, 168, 172, **173**, 180, 203
Midface
advancement 235ff
development 232
Molecular genetic testing 177ff
Molecular genetics 80, 83, 86, 107ff
Monobloc frontofacial advancement 240, **240**
Monosomy 9p syndrome 157
Mouse models 37, 95, 105, 116, 149
MSX2 mutation 36, 40, 159, **205**
discovery 8ff
functional analysis 10
transgenic mice **11**
Muenke syndrome 4, 89ff, 102, 186, **189**, **191**, **193**, **205**, **209**, 229
clinical findings 91, **93**, **94**, **209**
discovery 4
gene mutation 90
genetic counseling 90
inheritance 90
management 93
molecular pathogenesis 93
phenotype **92**
surgery 229
Multidisciplinary treatment approach 213
Mutation
clusters 60, 62
frequency 58ff, **64**
hot spot model 59, 60

Neurodevelopment 100, 208
Neurosurgical treatment 216ff
Nonsyndromic (isolated) craniosynostosis 165ff, 184, 212
Nucleotide substitution mutations 58, 59
distribution in testis 61

Occipital advancement 223, **223**, **224**

Ophthalmologic
  abnormalities 72, 82
  considerations 210
Opitz trigonocephaly syndrome **125**, 128, **154**, **179**
Orbitotomy 241, **241**
Osteoblast
  commitment 13, 16
  differentiation 16, 19, 38, 39
  function 24
  proliferation 19, 38
Osteogenic
  fronts **30**, 32ff
  layer **15**
Osteoglophonic dysplasia **132**, 134
Otolaryngologic considerations 210
Oxycephaly 173, **174**, 186, **224**, **227**, 228

P450 Oxidoreductase (POR) deficiency 123
Pansynostosis 173, **179**, 203, **205**
Passive reshapement 222
Paternal
  age-dependence 58ff
  age effect 58
  origin 113
  skewing 58ff
Pedigree **9**
Performance 70
Pericranium **30**, 32
Pfeiffer syndrome 4, 50, 52, 67, 83ff, **179**, 186, **189**, **205**, **207**, **209**, **222**, **227**, 229
  central nervous system 84
  craniofacial features 84
  discovery 4
  hands/feet 85, **209**
  molecular genetics 86
  phenotype **84**
  subtypes 83, **85**
  surgery 229
  vertebral abnormalities 86
Phenotypic overlap 89, 98, 126, 136
Physical examination 206
Plagiocephaly **92**, 169, 171, **179**, 200, **200**, **201**, **219**, **224**, **227**, 228
Polysyndactyly 143ff
Posterior plagiocephaly 171, **200**, **201**, **224**, **227**, 228
Postoperative surveillance 226
Premature craniosynostosis sequelae **234**
Prenatal
  detection 182
  diagnosis 79, 182, 184ff
  ultrasound 184ff

Radiography **10**, **68**, 72, **75**, **76**, 77, 82, **84**, **132**, **133**, **146**, **174**, 216ff, **217**, **218**
Recurrence risk 182
Recurrent mutations 58
Re-operation **227**
Runx2 16, 22, 39

Saethre-Chotzen syndrome 3, **30**, 98ff, **154**, 158, **179**, **205**, **209**, **227**, 229
  craniofacial features 99
  discovery/history 3
  extracranial features 101
  mouse model 105
  neurodevelopmental findings 100
  phenotypic features 98, **99**, **100**, **101**, **209**
  surgery 229
  treatment 105
  TWIST mutations 102ff
Sagittal suture **11**, **14**, **30**, **154**, **167**, **189**, **191**
  synostosis 154, 172, **173**, 180, 203, **217**
Scaphocephaly 166ff, **167**, **179**, 180, **200**, **220**, **223**, **224**, 227, **227**
  subgroups 166, **167**
Shprintzen-Goldberg syndrome **133**, 136
Signal transduction pathways 28ff, 148
  integration 37ff
Skeletal abnormalities 76
Skull shapes **200**
Sonography 184ff
Sperm mutation frequency 63, **64**, 65
Spermatogonia 60, 62
Submicroscopic rearrangements 159
Surgical
  risks 224
  techniques 222, **223**, **224**
  timing **224**
Suture
  anatomy 29, **30**
  maintenance 24
  mesenchyme **15**, 29, 32
Syndactyly phenotypes 50
Syndromic craniosynostosis 2, 28ff, 34, 119, 153, 184, **205**, 232
  associated genes 34
  chromosomal alterations **154**ff

Technical aids 216
Telecanthus **206**
Testis 58ff
TGFβ signaling 24, 37
Tracheostomy 235
Transcriptional control 16
Transgenic mice 8, 30
Trigonocephaly 143ff, **144**, **147**, **154**, 168, **168**, 180, 186, **190**, **200**, 203, **224**, **225**, **227**, 228
Turribrachycephaly 8, **9**, **10**, **155**, **205**
Turricephaly 170
TWIST1 17, 18, 33, 36, 40, 41, 98, 102ff, 158, 180
  mutational spectrum 104

Ultrasound examination 184ff, 216
Uncommon craniosynostosis syndromes 119ff, **120**
Underlying etiology 203

Variable expressivity 89, 98, 107, 109
Ventriculomegaly 220
Viscerocranium 13, 28, 232, 233

X-linked 109